Super Healthy Kids
A Parent's Guide
to Maharishi Ayurveda

Kumuda Reddy, M.D.
Linda Egenes

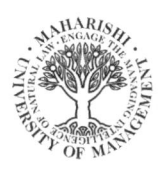

MAHARISHI UNIVERSITY OF MANAGEMENT PRESS
Fairfield, Iowa

Maharishi University of Management Press
Fairfield, Iowa 52557
www.mumpress.com

Cover and book design by Shepley Hansen. Cover photograph by Ken West. Illustrations by Kathryn Alders.

©2010 by Maharishi Vedic Education Development Corporation and Kumuda Reddy, M.D. ®Maharishi Ayurveda, Maharishi Ayur-Veda, Maharishi Vedic Medicine, Maharishi Vedic Approach to Health, Maharishi Vedic Health Center, Transcendental Meditation, Quiet Time, TM, Maharishi Transcendental Meditation, Maharishi Ayurveda Health Center, TM-Sidhi, Word of Wisdom, Maharishi Vedic, Maharishi Vedic Science, Vata, Pitta, Kapha, Maharishi Vedic Vibration Technology, MVVT, Maharishi Amrit Kalash, Amrit Kalash, Maharishi Rejuvenation, Maharishi Vedic Architecture, Fortune Creating, Maharishi Vastu, Maharishi Gandharva Veda, Maharishi Sthapatya Veda, Maharishi Jyotish, Maharishi Yagya, Maharishi Vedic Astrology, Maharishi Yoga, Maharishi, Maharishi University of Management, Maharishi International University, Maharishi Vedic University, Maharishi School of the Age of Enlightenment, Maharishi Peace Palace, Consciousness-Based, and Consciousness-Based education are registered or common law trademarks, licensed to Maharishi Vedic Education Development Corporation, a 501(c)(3) non-profit educational organization, and used under sublicense or with permission.

All rights reserved. No part of this book may be reproduced or transmitted in any form or by any means, electronic or mechanical, including photocopying, recording, or by any information storage and retrieval system, without permission in writing from the authors.

Library of Congress Control Number 2009943943
ISBN   978-0-923569-11-2

We gratefully acknowledge permission to use material from the following published sources. The charts and accompanying text on pages 40, 41, and 87 are adapted from *Scientific Research on the Maharishi Transcendental Meditation and TM-Sidhi Programs: A Brief Summary of 500 Studies* (Fairfield, IA: Maharishi University of Management Press), ©1996 by Maharishi University of Management, and from *Scientific Research on the Maharishi Technology of the Unified Field: The Transcendental Meditation and TM-Sidhi Program* (Fairfield, IA: Maharishi International University Press), ©1988 by Maharishi International University. The chart and accompanying text on page 156 is adapted with permission from *Summary of Research Findings* (Colorado Springs, CO: Maharishi Ayurveda Products International, Inc.), ©1996. The charts and accompanying text on pages 85, 86, and 210 are borrowed with permission from *Growing Up Enlightened* by Drs. Sanford and Randi Nidich.

Printed in the United States of America.

What Parents and Health-Care Professionals Are Saying about *Super Healthy Kids*

"This knowledge of Maharishi Ayurveda for your child's health is invaluable for preventing imbalances and promoting strength and happiness. Thanks to Reddy and Egenes for providing this for parents and health-care professionals."
—**Chris Clark, M.D.**, *author of* ***Contemporary Ayurveda: Medicine and Research in Maharishi Ayur-Veda***

Super Healthy Kids by Dr. Kumuda Reddy and Linda Egenes is a wonderful resource for parents who want to use a holistic approach in raising their children. In this era of media madness, overuse of medications, fast food, and stressful lifestyles, parents are searching for answers. I highly recommend this informative guide for using natural, preventive approaches such as proper balanced nutrition, lifestyle changes, and herbal remedies."
—**Swatantra K. Mitta, M.D.**, *practicing pediatrician for over 25 years*

"This book should be a principal reference book for all mothers and mothers-to-be who want to nurture and care for their children using the best natural preventive methods available, as laid out in Maharishi Ayurveda for maintenance of health and a disease-free life."
—**Mousumi Dey, M.D.**, *former consultant for the World Health Organization (WHO)*

Super Healthy Kids is easy to read and gives parents a solid foundation in the Ayurvedic way to help children stay healthy. As a mother and a practitioner of Maharishi Ayurveda, I recommend that every household have a copy."
—**Sankari Wegman**, *Ayurvedic Expert at The Raj Maharishi Ayurveda Health Center*

"As a mother of three children ages 14, 12, and 10, I truly think this book is a gold mine of information for daily life and ensuring the health of our children. Ayurveda is the ancient science of life, and the remedies and suggestions are time-tested, natural, and efficient. With so many man-made medications with unknown long-term side effects, it is reassuring to have this book as an ally in the ongoing effort to keep our children healthy in mind and body."
—**Caterina Titus,** *President of Ruby Star Productions*

"Dr. Reddy and Ms. Egenes have written the definitive complementary medical book on pediatrics. They have a deep appreciation for ancient Vedic wisdom and offer potent Ayurvedic recommendations for such common problems as respiratory and ear infections, headaches, digestive problems, anxiety and ADHD. At a time when many parents are leery about overusing antibiotics and prescription drugs, Dr. Reddy makes a clear case for natural medicine. This book is a 'must have' for all creative, responsible parents."
—**John C. Peterson, M.D.,** *Board Certified in Family Practice, practicing family physician, practitioner of Maharishi Ayurveda health care since 1984, adjunct faculty at Indiana University School of Medicine, and medical director of a freestanding birthing center*

To Maharishi Mahesh Yogi,

who has given us the direct experience of pure consciousness,

the key to a disease-free society and lasting peace for

the whole world

The Vedic Approach to Health is the approach of Natural Law, which is inscribed in every grain of the human physiology and is easily accessible to anyone within the intelligence of his own body.

This has provided a direct path for prevention, restoration, and maintenance of balance in the natural relationship between intelligence and the physiology—between the body and its own inner intelligence. With this, the possibility has arisen for the individual to really enjoy balanced, healthy life in happiness—the goal of an affluent society.

—Maharishi Mahesh Yogi

NOTE FROM THE AUTHORS

The educational information included in this book is intended to help parents improve the health of their children and is not in any way intended as a substitute for standard medical care from a primary-care medical doctor or pediatrician. No part of this book is intended to diagnose or treat any disease or to replace standard medical care. While the self-care approaches outlined in this book have been safely used by hundreds of children and adults, as with any health approach, the results cannot be guaranteed. The authors, publisher, and Maharishi Ayurveda Products International are not responsible for any adverse effects that may result from the herbal and self-care approaches outlined in this book. Consult with your health-care professional before giving your child any herbal products, remedies, or procedures described in this book and before making any changes in your child's current medical treatment.

Maharishi Ayurveda offers valuable complementary recommendations to supplement the advice of the medical doctor but is not meant in any way to replace it. Even to use Maharishi Ayurveda properly, it is recommended that you consult a medical doctor or expert who is trained in Maharishi Ayurveda to receive a proper diagnosis and individualized treatment program.

Contents

Acknowledgements		13
Preface		15

Part 1 • A New View of Children's Health

1	Why Not Choose the Most Effective Health Care for Your Child?	19
2	Nature Knows Best	31
3	Treating Individual Differences	51
4	Why Kids Get Sick and How to Prevent It	67

Part 2 • Reconnecting with the Source

5	How to Eliminate Stress and Restore Immunity	79

Part 3 • Healthy Foods, Food Supplements, and Eating Habits

6	Six Keys to a Healthy Diet	91
7	Foods That Build Immunity and Foods That Destroy It	103
8	Foods for Different Ages	129
9	Ten Healthy Eating Habits for Powerful Digestion	141
10	Boosting Immunity and Creating Balance with Maharishi Ayurveda Herbal Food Supplements and Rasayanas	149

Part 4 • Behaviors That Create Health

11	Sleep and the Bedtime Routine	165
12	Ayurvedic Massage and the Wake-Up Routine	177
13	Improving Health with Ayurvedic Exercise	193
14	Emotions, Behavior, and a Nourishing Family Environment	207

CONTENTS

PART 5 • **Using the Near and Far Environment to Enhance Immunity**
15 Ten Ways to Protect Your Child
    from Environmental Risk Factors   227

PART 6 • **The *Maharishi Ayurveda* Approach to Common and Chronic Disease in Children**
16 Prevention and Treatment of Common Childhood Illnesses 245
17 Prevention and Treatment of Chronic Disease in Childhood 263

Part 7 • **A Vision of Your Child's Future with Maharishi Ayurveda**
18 Your Cosmic Child   281

Glossary   299
Quick Reference Guide   305
Appendix   313
Notes   319
Index   329

ACKNOWLEDGEMENTS

With great gratitude to our parents and families, all of whom have supported us in this endeavor in untold ways. We'd also like to thank the people who worked so hard to make this manuscript a book. Many thanks to Mary Zeilbeck for editing; Martha Bright and Fran Clark for proofreading; Carol de Giere, Maryanne Eagleson, and Marjan de Jong for research; Bonita Pedersen for food recipes; and Keith Wegman for diagrams, charts and layout. Special thanks to Craig Pearson, Harry Bright, and everyone at Consciousness-Based Books and the Maharishi University of Management Press who brought this book to completion.

—Kumuda Reddy, M.D., and Linda Egenes

PREFACE

The world is my family. That is what the Sanskrit words *Vasudhaiva kutumbukam* say in English, and that is exactly how I feel at this moment in my life. When I look in my mind's eye at the millions of children of all ages—along with their parents, teachers, and associates—I am filled with awe. There is such perfection and orderliness in nature, from the blade of grass beneath our feet to the soaring mountaintops to the starry galaxies. Just as there is perfection in nature, there is the same perfection within each child. Maharishi Ayurveda tells us that all children contain the seat of perfection within them, wherever they are and whatever they do in this life.

Yet the world that we live in is far from perfect. It has taken the enlightened wisdom of Maharishi Mahesh Yogi, who with infinite love and compassion has given us a vision of oneness for the whole universe, to remind us of our perfection. He has taught that we are an ocean of consciousness, even as we appear to be a wave. We are the underlying unity at the basis of the enormous diversity in nature.

We are nature itself, and thus we need natural health care to bring perfect health to the mind, body, emotions, intellect, behavior, and environment. Maharishi Ayurveda not only brings balance to these different areas of life, it offers practical techniques to develop our full human potential and higher states of consciousness. Development of consciousness is the central principle of Maharishi Ayurveda, and that is what sets it apart from other systems of health care.

It is by realizing who we really are—an infinite ocean of consciousness—that we can transcend the tiny barriers and boundaries which divide families and nations. As parents, we have the responsibility to nurture individuals who can transform this world. What a joy this world will be when we can look into each other's eyes and say happily, "You are indeed the extension of myself. I respect you in the same way that I respect myself."

I sincerely hope that this book will provide parents the vision and practical solutions not only to solve normal health concerns for their children, but to help them cultivate the perfect individuals and leaders that our world so desperately needs. Now is the time to begin.

—Kumuda Reddy, M.D.

PART 1
A New View of Children's Health

CHAPTER ONE

Why Not Choose the Most Effective Health Care for Your Child?

Of all the gifts you offer your child, nothing is as precious as good health. As a parent, you have the power to guide your child to a lifetime of healthy habits and healthy living.

While this is certainly an enormous responsibility, it doesn't have to be a burden. With the natural, simple principles outlined in this book, parents throughout the world are helping their children grow in health and happiness day by day.

Unlike Western medicine, which focuses on crisis intervention (and is very good at it), the natural health-care system presented in this book, called Maharishi Ayurveda®, will improve your child's health every day of the year. It will answer those important questions every parent asks: What can I do to keep my child as healthy as possible? What are the right foods for my child to eat? What if my child doesn't like the "standard" diet? How much exercise does my child need? What if my child is not "average" but is his own special case?

The fact is, every child is his own special case. In nearly thirty years as a practicing physician, I have never met two children who are exactly alike. Every child needs to be treated as an individual, by taking into account his or her own mental, physical, and emotional makeup. Maharishi Ayurveda recognizes that every child has different needs, and therefore may require different foods, daily routines, or exercise programs to stay healthy.

If this sounds complicated, don't worry. When you start using these natural health-care principles, your job will become easier. For it is my experience that when a child starts to follow his natural rhythms and eats the foods his system needs, he will immediately feel healthier and will spontaneously start making healthier choices.

My Own Story

Let me reassure you by telling my story.* When my twin daughters were born, I was a practicing physician in upstate New York. I had been born and raised in India, and my parents relied on many natural remedies from the traditional system of medicine in India (called Ayurveda) while I was growing up. However, my husband and I were trained as medical doctors and thus consulted medical doctors to treat our daughters.

After a complicated pregnancy, the twins were born ten weeks early and were underweight. Because their digestive systems were very weak, they had to remain in the hospital for six weeks. I was not able to breastfeed them and they couldn't tolerate many of the baby formulas that the hospital tried.

The girls' immunity was also very weak, and even after they left the hospital, they were constantly sick. They were not able to eat much and their weight remained low. It was a great challenge for me to follow the pediatrician's recommendations. Antibiotics were repeatedly prescribed for my tiny girls. They even had to take prophylactic antibiotics to prevent ear infections.

The antibiotics produced many unwanted side effects: low appetite, further weakening of the digestive system, and diarrhea. The girls were generally unhealthy, unhappy, cranky, and poor sleepers. This meant three years of sleepless nights for me.

Exhausted and fed up with the negative side effects of the prescribed treatments, I decided, "Enough is enough." I turned to my own roots, to the health-care system of my ancestors. In the late 1980s, I was fortunate to learn about Maharishi Ayurveda, which was available in the West at that time and was so much more comprehensive and complete than the Western medical approach I had been using. It appealed to me, and I started using it immediately.

---

* Throughout the book, "I" or "me" refers to Dr. Kumuda Reddy speaking from her experience as a mother and physician.

In just a short time, my daughters' health turned around 180 degrees. The simple, natural treatments of Maharishi Ayurveda simultaneously built up their immune systems while repairing problem areas. Once their immune systems were restored, they seldom came down with colds or ear infections.

Now that they are grown, they recognize that they can prevent health problems with the natural treatments of Maharishi Ayurveda and rarely have to consult a doctor. If they start to feel ill, they know how to quickly restore balance to their bodies. They see clearly that when they take herbal compounds instead of antibiotics, they don't suffer negative side effects. Instead they feel stronger, healthier, and more energetic. They are extremely healthy and happy, and excel in many different sports.

Since that time, I have taken the training to become a physician trained in Maharishi Ayurveda. This has been an amazing and gratifying experience, especially when I treat children. Let me tell you the stories of two of my young patients.

Marta

Marta[†] was eight years old when her mother brought her to see me. She was chronically ill, unhappy, and exhausted, with large dark circles under her eyes.

Her mother explained that Marta had allergies, seasonal asthma, and a facial tic (involuntary muscle spasm). I also saw that her head constantly jerked around, her eyes blinked incessantly, and her legs and arms spasmed unexpectedly.

Marta's movements annoyed her classmates, which made her self-conscious and caused the movements to increase. She had very few friends. A neurologist had prescribed conventional medications, but these drugs had not helped reduce the movements and had actually created additional side effects, such as constipation, headaches, fatigue, and loss of appetite. In addition, Marta suffered from a severe sleep disorder, which her mother thought could be due to the medication or the allergies. Marta's mother had already made the decision to stop the medications before consulting me. She also said that her daughter

---

† The names of the children and parents have been changed throughout the book to protect their privacy.

was frightened of anyone in a white coat who would prescribe or perform more blood tests and other diagnostic tests.

Right away I reassured Marta that she was going to be all right. I told her that her health would improve and that we would be using natural and gentle treatments that would not harm her. I tried to explain that we were partners in this game, that I would try to help her get better and that she could help me by taking her herbal preparations and following the instructions I gave her. I said that she would be making herself better. Marta seemed relieved but understandably skeptical.

I also told her which foods would help restore balance to her body, and taught her how to do a special herbal oil massage, called an *abhyanga*, to soothe and balance her nervous system. Maharishi Ayurveda herbal supplements were recommended to treat her allergies, asthma, digestive weakness, and constipation.

Within just a few weeks, her mother reported that these treatments had created a remarkable improvement in Marta. She was eating better, sleeping better, and was no longer awakened by asthma attacks in the night.

At that point, I started her on herbal preparations to improve her neurological disorders. Over the next few months, Marta steadily improved. The involuntary movements in her legs diminished by 90 percent. The uncontrollable bobbing of her head and neck was remarkably reduced. Soon it only happened occasionally, when she was under stress or tired or when exposed to a situation that made her feel very self-conscious.

In the process of restoring balance, Marta learned which foods, behaviors, and routines helped correct her imbalances. She learned what triggered health problems and how to prevent them. She learned how to take care of herself. Without realizing it, she started experiencing greater self-awareness, understanding her own physiology and how its biological inner intelligence functioned. She tuned in to her body in a very natural way without any struggle, without analyzing or rationalizing.

Six years later Marta is a young teenager. She looks beautiful and seems confident. Her asthma is completely gone. She has not had movements for many years, although she still has an occasional facial tic when under stress. Marta looks forward to living the life of her dreams.

Jonah

I'll never forget the first day that I met Jonah, an extremely thin eleven-year-old who looked like he might be nine or ten. He was tired and withdrawn. His mother was exasperated and told me that he had been diagnosed with irritable bowel syndrome (IBS). It was beyond her belief that a child could have an adult disease like that.

I first reassured her that IBS could be treated easily with Maharishi Ayurveda, especially in its early stages. While relating his medical history, his mother said that Jonah was always a fussy eater. He didn't like many foods, ate irregularly, and had the habit of drinking ice-cold sodas from an early age. His routine meal was a peanut butter sandwich. He hated any fruits, vegetables, lentils, or beans.

As a young child, Jonah was prone to constipation. Things gradually worsened after he turned nine, and he experienced gas and bloating and was under stress at school. He was also developing sleep problems. He loved sports, but he dropped out of the soccer team because he was not able to keep up with it. He played music in a band, but he felt that he was not enjoying anything. Jonah found school and homework to be tedious, and he was not able to perform at his optimal level. Lately he had started missing days at school, and he was also having bouts of diarrhea along with constipation. His mother thought that he was getting depressed.

With all these problems, he became even more of a picky eater, because he felt uncomfortable after eating just about everything. He had lost twenty pounds in the last six months. Conventional medical doctors had prescribed antidepressants, vitamins, and foods with roughage, but he could not tolerate any of them because they made his stomach hurt.

My first recommendation was a simple diet that included rice, pasta, and easy-to-digest vegetables such as asparagus, sweet potatoes, and cooked carrots. I also recommended herbal supplements to restore balance to his digestion and elimination. Other herbal formulas helped relieve the mental stress, insomnia, and fatigue.

Over the next few weeks, I kept a close eye on his diet, gradually adding foods that he could tolerate. Within a month his physiology started functioning normally. He began sleeping better, reported less stress, started eating regular meals, and was able to digest many foods without experiencing bloating or indigestion. Best of all, he said he was feeling happier inside.

At this point I strongly recommended that he learn the Transcendental Meditation® technique for stress reduction, which he did along with his mother. That proved to be a turning point in his life. Over the next few months he enjoyed a tremendous boost in energy and put on the weight that he had lost. Now after three years, he and his mother feel that IBS is far behind him.

What is Maharishi Ayurveda?

Before going any further, you probably want to know exactly what "Maharishi Ayurveda" means. *Veda* means "knowledge," and *Ayur* means "life." The word *Ayurveda* means "knowledge of life." Ayurveda is the oldest continuously used health-care system on earth. It is part of the Vedic tradition of knowledge that originated in India.

The word "Maharishi" refers to Maharishi Mahesh Yogi, the founder of the Transcendental Meditation technique. Starting in the 1980s, Maharishi has revived the Ayurvedic health-care system and has brought this valuable knowledge to the West. While much of the original knowledge of Ayurveda had been lost, Maharishi has revived its true basis—consciousness—and its integration with body, emotions, and the environment. This restored knowledge of Ayurveda is called Maharishi Ayurveda.

Maharishi Ayurveda is sometimes used interchangeably with the terms *Maharishi Vedic Approach to Health*℠ or *Maharishi Vedic Medicine*℠, but for simplicity's sake, we'll use *Maharishi Ayurveda* here.

In the next chapters, I'll explain in detail the natural, simple preventive measures and treatments that are offered by Maharishi Ayurveda. For now, I just want to point out some of the major differences between Maharishi Ayurveda and Western medical treatments.

When you and your child walk into the office of a physician who practices Maharishi Ayurveda, you can expect a completely different experience from your standard visit to the doctor. For one thing, a physician trained in Maharishi Ayurveda is never too busy to listen. In fact, listening to the patient is an important part of the diagnostic procedure.

WHY NOT CHOOSE THE MOST EFFECTIVE HEALTH CARE?

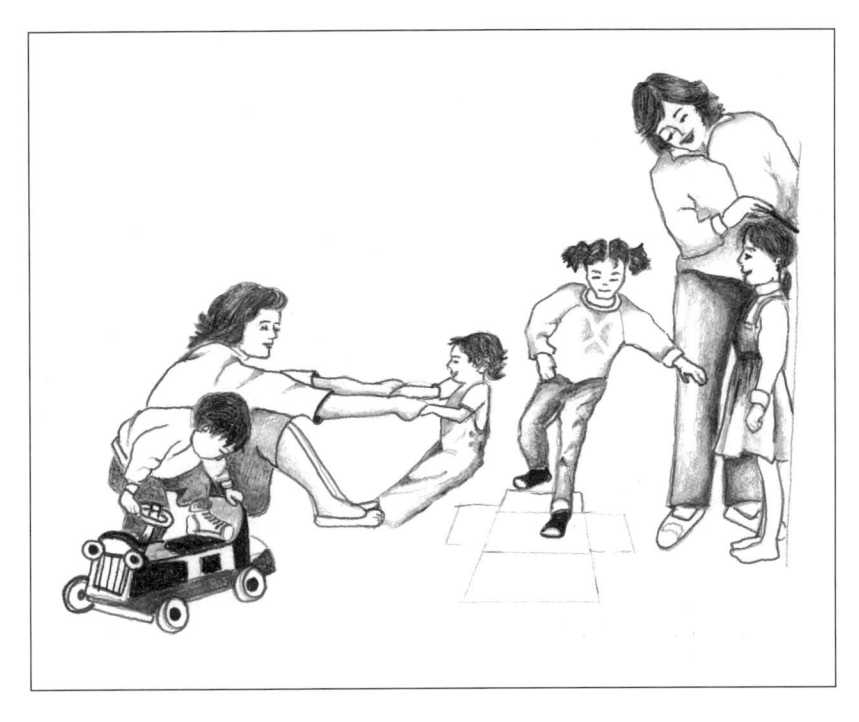

In Maharishi Ayurveda, the health expert trained in traditional Ayurvedic principles and practice (called a *Vaidya*), considers not just the headache or stomachache or insomnia, but looks deeply into the diet, lifestyle, and behavior of the child to see what might be causing the imbalance. In fact, during the diagnosis the mother fills out a questionnaire to describe in detail the child's likes and dislikes, dietary habits, daily routine, and emotional makeup as well as the standard medical history.

Rather than being confronted with frightening machines and clinical smells, the child is diagnosed using a simple, caring technique called pulse diagnosis. By placing three fingers on the child's radial pulse at the wrist, the physician trained in Maharishi Ayurveda is able to diagnose the child's psycho-physiological tendencies, body type, and the underlying cause of imbalances and symptoms. With this gentle and noninvasive technique, the physician gains insight into the underlying imbalances and specific causes of the health problems that the child is displaying. For this reason, the physician is able to give a completely

25

individualized treatment program, based on the child's pulse assessment.

The treatments are simple and natural, and children tend to like following them because they bring relief in a gentle, natural way. Let's say the child has trouble sleeping. After determining the cause, the physician trained in Maharishi Ayurveda may recommend simple changes to bring the entire system back into balance. These may include changes in the diet or the daily routine (such as eating the main meal at noon instead of at night, or eating more cooked foods instead of raw foods). Other pleasant treatment modalities such as aroma therapy, music therapy, or stress reduction techniques may be recommended to bring the body back into alignment with its own natural rhythms. Maharishi Ayurveda herbal formulas may also be recommended to correct the specific imbalance. If the cause is more emotional or mental in origin, treatments will take that into account.

You can see how effective it is to treat the health problem by adjusting the diet and daily routine. This is a more permanent and effective solution than simply prescribing a pill to mask the symptoms and letting the child continue to make the same mistakes in diet and daily routine that created ill health in the first place. Rather than creating negative side effects, these natural treatments of Maharishi Ayurveda boost immunity and actually create side *benefits*, or unexpected positive changes in overall mental, physical, and emotional health.

Maharishi Ayurveda is adept at preventing problems before they arise. It is such a sophisticated system of health care that it even takes the seasons and weather into account, including adjustments in diet and routine to prevent seasonal illnesses such as colds, flu, and sun sensitivity from cropping up. Seasonal checkups can keep the whole family at a level of health that you might not think possible.

The following chart more clearly outlines the differences between Maharishi Ayurveda and the modern medical approach.

Why Maharishi Ayurveda Is Healthier for Your Child	**Why Standard Western Medicine May Be Harmful**
1. *Relies on the body's own healing system to heal itself.* Maharishi Ayurveda aims to awaken the inner intelligence of nature, which has vast and enormous healing qualities. When the body is able to repair itself from within, the results are powerful and long lasting.	1. *Disrupts the body's natural rhythms and healing mechanisms.* Many Western treatments actually inhibit the immune system. Antihistamines, for instance, are used to treat allergies, but they actually suppress immunity.
2. *Treats the whole child, not just the illness.* Maharishi Ayurveda includes complete and profound treatments for improving your child's mental acuity and learning ability, mind-body coordination, immunity, and emotional balance. Every treatment restores balance to the whole child.	2. *Uses powerful drugs* to destroy the germ or virus causing the illness, and in the process often destroys balance in the child's physical, emotional, and mental health.
3. *Does not cause harmful side effects.* All of the treatments used are completely natural and noninvasive. Rather than creating negative side effects, every treatment boosts overall immunity and the mental and emotional well-being of your child.	3. *Creates new diseases.* Drugs and other medical treatments create many new iatrogenic diseases every year. Loss of appetite, low immunity, headache, and dizziness are just a few of the detrimental symptoms that children experience from routinely prescribed antibiotics and other drugs for common health symptoms such as colds. Side effects from drugs used to treat chronic illnesses such as asthma and diabetes are far more severe.
4. *Eliminates the root cause of the illness and restores balance.* Maharishi Ayurveda works at the fundamental level of	4. *Treats the symptoms without eliminating the cause.* Western medicine is famous for providing relief for

Why Maharishi Ayurveda Is Healthier for Your Child	Why Standard Western Medicine May Be Harmful
nature's intelligence itself. It identifies the source of the illness and from there treats the underlying imbalance. It corrects the source of the problem instead of just providing superficial relief for the symptoms.	symptoms but not actually addressing the underlying problem. This means that the problem continues to recur, especially when the toxic effects of prescribed drugs further weaken the body. This creates a vicious cycle, paving the way for further disease.
5. *Focuses on prevention of disease before it manifests.* Simple, noninvasive diagnostic techniques used in Maharishi Ayurveda aim to detect underlying imbalances and correct them before they manifest into physical symptoms, before they become full-blown diseases. If your child says he "just doesn't feel right," the underlying imbalance can be identified and treated with diet or herbal compounds before it manifests into an illness.	5. *Is crisis-oriented.* Most modern diagnostic tests cannot detect illness until it has already manifested. If you bring a child to see a doctor when he is "just not feeling right," your doctor can't help until it becomes flu, a cold, or a serious symptom of some sort.
6. *Health care is individualized.* The body type, diet, behavior, emotions, personality, likes, and dislikes of the child are considered in determining the cause and treatment of the problem. The deeper causes of illness are examined and considered, and thus the treatments may vary even if several children in your family are complaining of the same symptoms.	6. *Prescribes the same "magic-bullet" treatment for everyone.* Because treatment is focused on the invading germ or organism rather than the psychophysiology of the host, all treatments for a particular illness are virtually the same. The treatments don't take into account the vast differences in people, and the fact that the causes of the disease may be widely different from case to case.
7. *Cultivates self-sufficiency rather than dependency in the child.* Your child can	7. *Cultivates dependence on drugs, doctors, and machines.* The child is taught that

WHY NOT CHOOSE THE MOST EFFECTIVE HEALTH CARE?

Why Maharishi Ayurveda Is Healthier for Your Child	Why Standard Western Medicine May Be Harmful
learn how to prevent illness through diet, exercise, stress management, and simple procedures such as oil massage that are suited for his health needs. All of these can be done at home as part of the daily routine, to bring balance and health day by day. The child learns that his choices and habits can make a difference in how he feels now and throughout his life.	the doctor "heals" and "makes him well." Children are given the message that they can mistreat their bodies on a daily basis and the doctor "fixes" them.
8. *Is child-friendly, self-motivating, and unthreatening.* Children gravitate toward things that make them feel good. The treatments of Maharishi Ayurveda motivate children to stay healthy, because they immediately feel better with treatment and like how they feel.	8. *Treatments may be traumatic or frightening to children.* Many children who receive extensive medical treatments want to run away when they see a doctor or hospital.

In the coming chapters, you will learn more about this remarkable health-care system. Maharishi Ayurveda is for every child, whether he is generally healthy or suffers from a chronic illness. As a physician I have seen time and time again that the natural treatments of Maharishi Ayurveda are far more effective than standard medications in treating chronic illnesses such as asthma, chronic sinus and ear infections, weak appetite, hyperactivity, and chronic fatigue. This is because they treat the underlying imbalance, eliminating the disease at its source. These natural treatments are able to make deep, long-lasting improvements.

And for the healthy child, the simple but profound recommendations found in this book help prevent illness and boost immunity. Children who use Maharishi Ayurveda seldom fall prey to common childhood ailments such as colds, flu, and congestion. But even more than that, Maharishi Ayurveda opens a whole new world of possibilities for growth and fulfillment. As your child unfolds his or her full mental, physical, and emotional potential, you will be filled with wonder at the remarkable power latent in the human mind and body.

Along with other physicians throughout the world, I have seen children who were sick, depressed, and unable to be helped by the current system of medicine thrive when prescribed these natural treatments. I have seen disillusioned mothers, who came to me because frequent doctor visits resulted in a cycle of sickness for their children, become enthusiastic supporters of Maharishi Ayurveda. In this book, you will read the stories of these mothers and children. You can learn to apply these effective and natural recommendations for your own family and for generations to come, creating a world of enlightenment, peace, and harmony for your children to grow up in.

CHAPTER TWO
Nature Knows Best

The health care of American children is among the most expensive in the world. Americans spend a much higher portion of the country's gross domestic product on health care than any other country. The shocking news is that it is not the most effective, not by a long shot. In performance our health-care system ranked thirty-seventh of ninety-one countries according to a year 2000 World Health Organization report. Worse, Americans ranked twenty-fourth in life expectancy and infant mortality. In contrast, Japan, with the lowest infant mortality rate in the world, spends half as much on health care as the U.S.

Even more troubling, there has been a dramatic rise in chronic disease and in new emotional, psychological, and behavioral diseases among children in the U.S. It seems our health-care system, which was so effective in combating infectious disease in the last century, is not meeting the needs of today's children.

Children's Health Advances in the Twentieth Century

It's true that the health of American children increased dramatically in the last hundred years. This was mainly due to the decline in infectious diseases. The statistics tell the story: in 1920 the death rate was 987 per 100,000 children one to four years of age. By 1970 it had been reduced to forty-one per 100,000. This is a decline of 1,000 percent. Today the leading cause of death among children is no longer disease, but accidental injuries, of which half are caused by car crashes.

A number of factors are given credit for the decline in death rates, including immunizations, improved water safety standards, increased sanitation, better living conditions, stricter production standards for milk, and modern child labor laws. In more recent years, better care for premature and low-birth-weight infants has increased survival rates as well.

Development of penicillin and modern antibiotics are, of course, thought to be the major reasons that death rates have declined. Yet if you look into the matter more closely, the majority of that decline took place in the first half of the century, before antibiotics and other modern drugs became available.

Perhaps the most disappointing thing is that although infectious diseases such as smallpox and polio have been virtually wiped out, they have been replaced by other new diseases that do not often cause death but which greatly diminish a child's enjoyment and participation in life.

Some researchers even feel that there is a direct correlation between the eradication of infectious disease and the rise of chronic illness in children during the last century. An intriguing study involving 1,000 children, published in the *New England Journal of Medicine*, for instance, showed that children who had older siblings or attended day care as early as age six months, and therefore contracted more infectious disease early in life, had less than half the risk of asthma after age six.

According to the "hygiene hypothesis," the fact that the number of children with asthma has doubled in developing nations during the last twenty years may be due to the super-clean, germ-free environment that affluent city children grow up in. Farm children, who are exposed to germs and bacteria in animal droppings and dirt, and children in underdeveloped countries, do not experience these epidemic levels of allergies and asthma. The theory holds that our affluent society's war on germs, using detergents, antibiotics, and vaccines, has been too successful. We contract fewer infections from the bad germs that used to cause infectious disease; at the same time, we don't encounter the "good" bugs that can stimulate the immune system to function better. It is estimated that one in three children, and up to 50 percent of adults, have become hypersensitive to some aspect of their environment, making allergies an epidemic.

Thus some researchers feel that modern drugs and vaccines for squelching infectious disease not only led to the well-known problem of resistant viral and bacterial strains, but also may be contributing to the rise of chronic ailments. This curious phenomenon is summed up in a recent editorial in *The Economist*: "As the incidence of childhood infections has fallen, a number of chronic ailments, such as diabetes and asthma, have become more frequent. In parts of the world where childhood diseases are still common, these chronic ailments are rare. . . . All this suggests that in curing disease there are no easy fixes: every silver bullet leaves a cloudy trail. . . ."

In any case, whatever the causes, we are seeing a dramatic increase in chronic health problems among children. It is estimated that 30 percent of children in America today suffer from at least one chronic disease. While the majority of these are not life-threatening or debilitating diseases, up to 6.5 percent of school-age children have significant functional limitations. It is a sobering thought that millions of American children are weighed down by a long-standing, so far incurable physical condition. The number of children with asthma, for instance, is now estimated at 9 percent of the population, and disabling asthma increased by 232 percent since 1969, as reported in the National Health Interview Survey.

Most disturbing of all, there is a rise in new problems such as child abuse, suicide, and a host of behavioral, emotional, and psychological disorders associated with stress. These include attention deficit disorder, depression, autism, and behavioral disturbances. For instance, about 6 percent of school age children are currently diagnosed with Attention Deficit Hyperactivity Disorder (ADHD). Most of these health problems were not even mentioned in medical journals a few decades ago.

Why then, when we are spending so much money on our children's health, are our children so unhealthy?

One answer is that the health-care system no longer matches children's health-care needs. In the face of rising epidemics in obesity, allergies, asthma, and Type 2 diabetes—as well as the new threats of behavioral problems, learning disorders, child abuse, and neglect—medical experts are calling for a more integrated system of health care. There are many reasons to choose a holistic rather than a fragmented approach to medical care for your child. One of the main reasons is that the fragmented approach is not as effective. Let's look at other problems your child may face with the current system.

Today's Health Care Is Too Expensive

With changing employment patterns and economic challenges, even middle-income American families are finding themselves unable to afford the high cost of health care for their children. There are currently 8.1 million American children without health insurance. One study reported that of twenty-nine industrialized nations, the U.S., Turkey, and Mexico were the only three without universal health care—and less than half of the U.S. population is eligible for publicly supported health-care coverage under current federal legislation.

At the same time, the cost of prescription drugs and other medical treatment is soaring. A recent article in a newsweekly showed people "screaming for relief" from the exorbitantly high costs of drugs in the U.S.

Many expectant mothers in the U.S. do not have adequate prenatal care, resulting in high infant mortality rates. In 2004, the U.S. had a higher rate of infant mortality than 28 countries, including Singapore, Japan, Cuba, and Hungary. Compare that to 1960, when the U.S. had a higher rate than only eleven other countries. Researchers have found a leading reason for the high rate: preterm delivery. There was a 10 percent increase in preterm deliveries in the U.S. from 2000 to 2006, according to recent figures from the Centers for Disease Control and Prevention.

The high cost of health care is especially troubling in low-income families, given the high correlation between poverty and ill health among children. Mental retardation, learning disorders, emotional and behavioral problems, and vision and speech impairments are more prevalent among children living in poverty. Children in poverty have a higher death rate.

Nearly one in five children in America live in poverty today, according to the 2009 federal report "America's Children: Key National Indicators of Well-Being." For many other nations, the ratio is even higher.

Antibiotics Lower Immunity

It's a common family scene. A child of five develops a sniffle, and then a head cold and a slight fever. Being a responsible parent, the mother takes her child to the doctor before the illness gets out of hand. The doctor prescribes antibiotics, and the mother goes home satisfied that she has done the best for her child.

Common as this practice of prescribing antibiotics is, it is fraught with problems. Antibiotics can weaken the child's immunity, making him or her more susceptible to disease. Worse, antibiotics do not work on common cold viruses.

It has recently been recognized by the medical community that antibiotics have been overprescribed. Yet many doctors continue to prescribe antibiotics for colds and flu, even though antibiotics cannot treat viruses, which are the cause of most colds and flu. Antibiotics only treat bacteria.

There are two problems created by this tendency to overprescribe antibiotics. One is that bacteria have become increasingly resistant to commonly used antibiotics. There are new strains of tuberculosis, for instance, that current antibiotics can no longer kill. Bacterial resistance has progressed to such a point that many infections, which thirty years ago were easily controlled with antibiotics, are no longer easily treatable. As a result, drug makers have to come up with increasingly powerful antibiotics to overcome increasingly powerful strains of bacteria. Current antibiotics used to fight as many as four major diseases have already been rendered ineffective due to overuse and the growth of resistant strains.

Also, the more powerful the drug, the more damaging the side effects for the child. This is especially alarming, considering that antibiotics are known to weaken the immune system of adults, and children are more sensitive. Antibiotics have been shown to destroy the body's natural antibodies and white blood cells. Infections tend to increase when antibiotics are prescribed, perhaps because antibiotics destroy natural bacteria in the body, causing the harmful bacteria that have grown resistant to antibiotics to blossom.

I remember a saying from Maharishi Ayurveda: that life will always triumph over death. As long as we use a destructive approach to healing, in which we try to destroy harmful organisms with powerful drugs, those organisms will only grow stronger than our drugs.

What is needed instead is a life-strengthening approach. If we choose a health-care system that strengthens the immune system, then germs and other organisms will not be able to harm us.

Modern Drug Therapy Is Hazardous to the Health of Children

Another problem is that few drugs that are prescribed for children are actually tested for children, and most are not specifically licensed for children's use. Yet pediatricians still prescribe them, with an attitude of "try it and see."

This is especially disconcerting considering the serious side effects of many modern drugs. Here is a startling statistic: injury from drugs and other medical treatments in the U.S. dwarfs the annual automobile accident mortality count of 45,000 and accounts for more deaths than all other accidents combined.

Side effects can be much worse for children, due to their lower body weights and developing bodies and brains. Even more surprising, in 1998 the *Journal of the American Medical Association* (JAMA) published a study of hospital patients from 1966 to 1996, estimating that adverse drug reactions (which means the side effects from single drugs or their combinations) kill an estimated 100,000 people a year, with an additional 2 million seriously injured. And that statistic doesn't even include drug abuse or prescription errors.

Recently I read the headline, "Too much Tylenol can harm children." Accidental overdoses of Tylenol's active ingredient (acetaminophen) resulted in liver damage and even deaths of a number of children in the U.S., and thus caused the pharmaceutical company to change the labeling. As a physician and mother, this understated assessment of deadly harm dealt by an over-the-counter drug rings in my mind like a loud warning bell.

Our Current System Does Not Focus on Prevention

There is no better time to prevent disease than during childhood. Many research studies show that a wide range of adult illnesses can be prevented if good health habits are started in the critical early years. This is true even of hereditary diseases, such as hypertension, heart disease, and diabetes.

Childhood diseases, if not treated properly, tend to continue into adulthood. One-third of all disability—including some of the most debilitating and costly conditions for the entire U.S. population—began with childhood disorders. One longitudinal study conducted in England found that children who suffered from chronic illness in childhood tended to be even unhealthier at age twenty-three.

General ill health in childhood can also contribute to specific chronic diseases later on. A recent study conducted by Pennsylvania State University's Population Research Institute found that people with poor health in childhood were twice as likely to develop cancer or chronic lung disease by late middle age. Childhood illness was also linked to cardiovascular conditions, arthritis, and rheumatism as well. These findings were true regardless of the socioeconomic status of the patient.

Yet despite this obvious connection between childhood health and lifelong health as adults, in our current system *there is much, much less research on prevention for children than for adults*. And, as mentioned earlier, Western medicine has not been successful in preventing or treating chronic disease in either children or adults.

A recent three-year study conducted at Johns Hopkins University predicts that 157 million Americans will suffer from chronic disease by 2020, with a cost of $1.07 trillion in treatment. As the authors concluded, our country can't begin to reduce those costs without addressing the fundamental problem in our current health-care system: it doesn't encourage prevention.

Maharishi Ayurveda, on the other hand, is primarily focused on prevention. It teaches parents and children alike how to form the dietary and lifestyle habits now that will create health throughout life. And for a child who already has a chronic disease, Maharishi Ayurveda is effective in eliminating the underlying cause of the illness, so it does not continue into adulthood.

A New Paradigm for a New Millennium: An Integrated Approach

What is needed is a new paradigm, a more integrated system of health care that treats not just the disease but considers the child's mind, body, behavior, and emotions. What we need is a health-care system that focuses on life, on healthy living, on the elimination of disease at its source rather than the treatment of symptoms alone. We need a system that focuses on increasing the immunity of the child rather than attacking the germs inside the child with powerful drugs that have caustic side effects and deplete overall health, happiness, and well-being. Today, more than ever before, we need a health-care system that goes beyond medicine, enlivening the core of human consciousness itself.

As you read this book about Maharishi Ayurveda, you'll see how the healing power of nature can be employed to bring health and happiness to your child without huge expense or the crippling side effects of modern drugs.

Since I have learned of this integrated and complete health-care system, I cannot convey to you the relief I feel, knowing that here is a way to practice medicine that builds health and never destroys it. Here is a system of medicine that can truly end the mental, physical, and emotional suffering that a large percentage of the world's children face. I have hope that the children of today can grow in health, happiness, and fulfillment.

Let me give you an example from my practice.

Dylan: An Example of Curing A Chronic Disease Without Drugs

Dylan's mother brought him to me when he was barely five years old. He had asthma and was on three different inhalers and two oral preparations, which he needed around the clock. He was enrolled full-time in kindergarten and needed assistance from the school nurse to administer his medicine on schedule.

Despite all these efforts, Dylan did not feel enough relief from his symptoms. He was often fatigued, had a poor appetite, and picked at his food. His mother was told that he was hyperactive in class, constantly needing help, and was unable to focus on class projects.

Even at home his mother often found him hyperactive and cranky. She felt drained by her efforts to make him eat enough to stay healthy. Many times his asthma kept him awake at night. Overall, his behavior with his parents and siblings was challenging.

Besides his asthma, he suffered from constant colds and sinus problems, and was always the first to catch the flu bug if it was circulating at school or among family members. He had already been taken to the emergency room several times for asthma attacks.

Like any child in his situation, he was afraid of doctors, needles, and treatment protocols. Dylan's face reflected anxiety and insecurity, and it took some time for me to reassure him and build his confidence in the natural, noninvasive treatments of Maharishi Ayurveda. But young as he was, it was clear to me that he wanted to believe me because he just wanted to feel better.

I discovered that he was determined to play on the soccer team when he got older. "You help me with your treatment and I'll help you grow strong enough to join the soccer team," I said. And thus began a long-term, holistic recovery from a seemingly hopeless disease.

That day we started treatments from Maharishi Ayurveda without taking Dylan off his conventional asthma medications. During the next few months, as the symptoms subsided and Dylan gradually felt better, we slowly cut back his conventional medications until he was only using one asthma spray. This brings up an important point: It is not necessary for children to stop their prescribed medications in order to participate in the treatments of Maharishi Ayurveda. Maharishi Ayurveda is complementary to Western medicine, and can help remove some of the side effects caused by medications.

During this process of many visits, it was heartening to see Dylan walk happily into my office, as if he were coming to visit a family friend rather than a scary doctor. Dylan recognized right away that he felt healthier and happier. He was at ease with the treatments and willingly followed the diet and took the herbal preparations. Of course, he was just a young child and needed gentle reminders and direction from his mother not to indulge in the wrong foods.

Physiological and Psychological Improvement

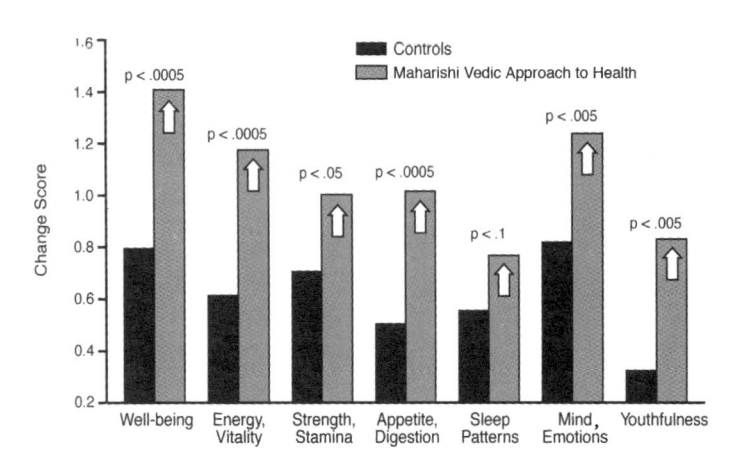

[Bar chart comparing Controls vs. Maharishi Vedic Approach to Health across: Well-being (p < .0005), Energy/Vitality (p < .0005), Strength/Stamina (p < .05), Appetite/Digestion (p < .0005), Sleep Patterns (p < .1), Mind/Emotions (p < .005), Youthfulness (p < .005). Y-axis: Change Score from 0.2 to 1.6.]

This study found that people who participated in a one-week Maharishi Rejuvenation[SM] program of the Maharishi Vedic Approach to Health improved significantly across a wide range of measures. Control subjects who received only intellectual knowledge of this program and its principles for the same amount of time did not show the same amount of improvement. These findings indicate that the Maharishi Rejuvenation program, which is recommended to be applied seasonally to remove accumulated physiological toxins of the season, promotes physiological and psychological balance.

Another study, published in a German medical journal, examined various physiological and psychological changes that occurred in subjects participating in a two-week Maharishi Rejuvenation program. Improvements included reduced cholesterol and urea, reduced bodily complaints and strains, reduced irritability and psychological inhibition, and greater stability and openness.

References: 1. R.H. Schneider, K.L. Cavanaugh, H.S. Kasture, S. Rothenberg, R. Averbach, D. Robinson, and R.K. Wallace, "Health Promotion with a Traditional System of Natural Health Care: Maharishi Ayur-Veda," *Journal of Social Behavior and Personality*, 5 (3) (1990), pp. 1–27.

2. R. Waldschutz, "Influence of Maharishi Ayur-Veda Purification Treatment on Physiological and Psychological Health," *Erfahrungsheilkunde-Acta Medica Empirica*, 11 (1988), pp. 720–729.

Decreased Health-Care Expenditures

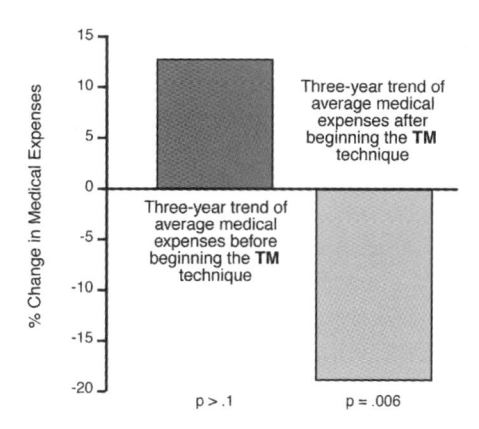

Three-year trend of average medical expenses after beginning the **TM** technique	(bar at ~+12%, p > .1)
Three-year trend of average medical expenses before beginning the **TM** technique	(bar at ~-18%, p = .006)

Y-axis: % Change in Medical Expenses (-20 to 15)

This chart shows three-year averages of medical expenses for physicians' services of participants before and after practice of the Transcendental Meditation program. In this study, government payments for physicians' services (approximately 20% of total medical expenses) were examined for 677 Quebec health plan enrollees who learned the Transcendental Meditation program. During the three years prior to beginning the Transcendental Meditation program, subjects' expenses (adjusted for inflation, age, and gender) did not change significantly. After learning the Transcendental Meditation program, subjects' adjusted expenses declined significantly, by 5-7% annually.

Reference: R.E. Herron, S.L. Hillis, J.V. Mandarino, D.W. Orme-Johnson, and K.G. Walton. "The Impact of the Transcendental Meditation Program on Government Payments to Physicians in Quebec," *American Journal of Health Promotion*, 10, (3) (1996), pp. 208-216.

During the next two or three years his concentration and self-esteem increased dramatically. He stopped catching the constant colds, sinus infections, and flu viruses that once plagued him. He is doing well at school now, and does not have the symptoms of hyperactivity. Today, he is a self-assured, gentle, relaxed eight-year-old. And he made the soccer team this year.

Dylan was cured by the simple, natural therapies that you have already read about in this book: proper diet, a healthy daily routine, and Maharishi Ayurveda herbal food supplements. These brought balance to his body, and cleared the blocks to his body's own healing intelligence to repair itself.

Why the Best Medicine Is Nature's Intelligence

When I say that there are simple and natural ways for your child to always feel happy, to become immune to disease, to enjoy perfect health throughout life, to mature into a productive, blissful adult who does not make mistakes and is a blessing to all whom he meets, you probably will think I am greatly exaggerating.

Yet this is surely the unspoken but deeply felt desire of every parent—for their children to be healthy and happy each day of their lives.

It is a completely natural desire. Why, then, shouldn't it be a possible one? When you look at nature, you see that all around there is perfection. The planets rotate around the sun, the moons rotate around the planets, the galaxies spin in the skies, and like a perfectly orchestrated symphony, they do not collide. Every day the sun rises and sets, every night the stars shine. It stretches the imagination just to think about the intelligence that orchestrates all the millions of details to make this happen every day.

What is even more incredible is that the perfection that you see all around you in nature is also inside your child.

Your child's body is an amazing creation. Each cell is packed with information to keep his or her body working properly. If you were to extract one DNA molecule from the nucleus of one human cell, and unwind the spiral, it would turn out to be a strand six feet in length. Multiply that times one trillion, the number of cells in an average human body, and you come up with a mind-boggling amount of information encoded in your child's DNA.

Your child's brain is equally astounding. It contains one hundred billion neurons (nerve cells). And the heart is far more efficient than any man-made machine. Over the course of a lifetime, your child's heart will pump 180 million quarts of blood through his or her body—enough liquid to fill the fuel tanks of fifty-six rockets. The heart does this without calling a conference of NASA scientists to replace any parts, without your child even knowing about it. Your child's heart, like the rest of his human body, constantly renews, repairs, and refurbishes itself without your child consciously doing anything.

The intelligence of the human body is nothing short of miraculous. And it is that intelligence of nature—which keeps your child's body functioning every day for a lifetime—that is at the basis of true health. Given the power of nature and the ability of the body to maintain and take care of itself, it seems like the most powerful medicine is nature itself.

As a physician trained in Maharishi Ayurveda, I know that it is not I, the doctor, who can make your child healthy. I know that it is the healing intelligence of nature inside your child—which can be awakened through all the therapies of Maharishi Ayurveda—that heals your child if he or she is sick. Let's look at how the intelligence of nature is part of the health equation.

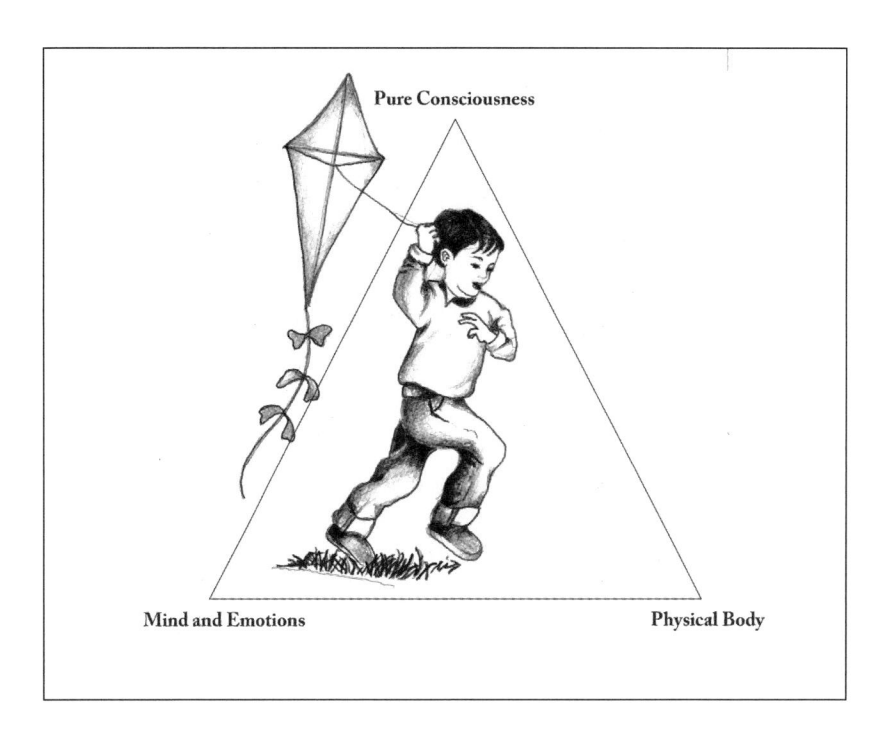

Health Equals a Balanced Body, Mind, and Consciousness

The word "health" is from the same root as "wholeness." If you had a choice, would you like your physician to take into account all aspects of your child's health—physical characteristics, mental tendencies, feelings, and behaviors—or just his physical symptoms? Any parent would surely want the most holistic approach.

In Maharishi Ayurveda, the whole person is considered to be much more than the human body. The body, in fact, is only one-third of the health equation.

Human life is made up of three basic parts:
1. Pure consciousness (nature's intelligence)
2. Mind and emotions
3. Physical body

You could also think of these as the spiritual, mental, and physical realms of life. It is interesting to note that until just recently, Western medicine only recognized the last one-third of this equation, the physical body. Because they could not be physically measured and quantified, the mind and emotions were disregarded as possible causes of disease. Today, of course, the role of the mind and emotions in health is widely recognized. The role of consciousness, or nature's intelligence, however, is still not acknowledged. Yet it is the key to good health.

The Role of Consciousness

In Maharishi Ayurveda, nature's inner intelligence, or consciousness, is considered to be more important in creating health than the body or even the mind. This fundamental level of consciousness, also called the Self, or *Atma*, in the Vedic tradition, is the source of intelligence, energy, and happiness. By enlivening consciousness, you nourish and bring balance to body, mind, and emotions.

It might help to think of consciousness in terms of an analogy. If you imagine an ocean, then consciousness is the silent, steady depth of the ocean. The mind and body are waves on the surface. If the ocean is stirred at the surface by a breeze, tiny waves form. If it is stirred at a deeper level by a strong wind, larger waves form. Yet the ocean is so deep that it always remains silent at its source, at the bottom of the ocean.

In the same way, nature's intelligence, or consciousness, is the silent, unseen source of the mind and the body. If there is balance at this fun-

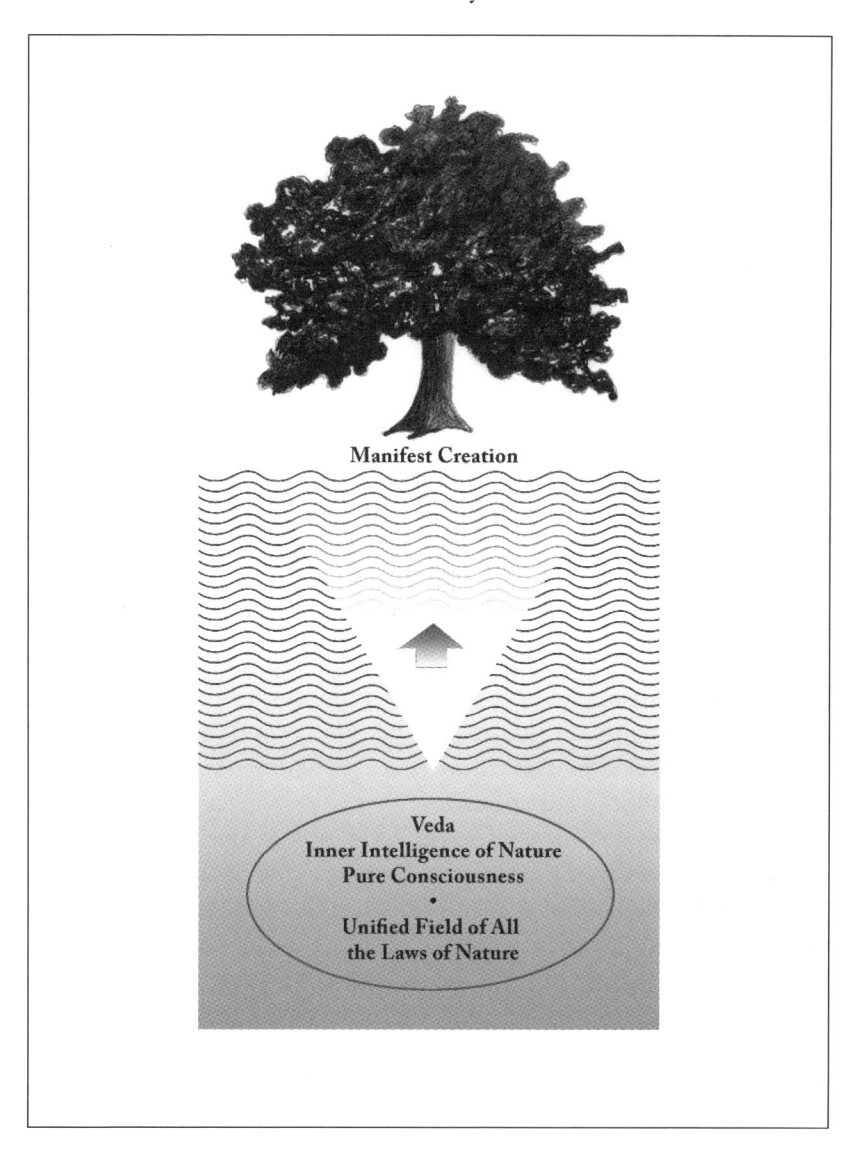

Manifest Creation

Veda
Inner Intelligence of Nature
Pure Consciousness
·
Unified Field of All the Laws of Nature

damental level, then the whole body and mind will function normally, in a healthy way. All the treatments of Maharishi Ayurveda aim to wake up this fundamental level.

To extend the analogy, when the ocean rises, all the boats rise with it. In the same way, when the fundamental level of consciousness is enlivened, then all the body's systems are enlivened and rejuvenated. Any system of health care that ignores this fundamental level of life is incomplete and will only scratch the surface. It could even create harm.

Another name for this fundamental level of natural law is *Veda*. The laws of nature that govern the human body are the same laws of nature that operate in nature. Veda, in fact, encompasses all the laws of nature that uphold the universe.

Another way to understand Veda is in terms of DNA. At the basis of the physiology is the language of DNA, which contains the laws that structure every cell in the body. In the same way, Veda (which you could also call consciousness, or the unified field) is at the basis of the mind, body, and all aspects of life. See the Unified Field Chart for Physiology on the following page, which demonstrates the connection between consciousness and the physiology.

The Veda contains all the laws of nature that structure the body and the entire universe. From the perspective of the quantum field theory of modern physics, all matter is ultimately vibration. Your child's body is a complex waveform, made up of many smaller waves or vibrations. These fundamental frequencies are excitations of universal fields, and all of these fields are in turn the expression of one single underlying field, called the unified field. In quantum physics, this unseen, underlying field that gives rise to all nature and to the human body is called the unified field of all the laws of nature.

What this means on a practical level is that the infinite power, beauty, and diversity of the entire creation is found in the human body. If the vast intelligence of the stars and galaxies and the millennia-old universe is inside us, then surely we have the means to keep ourselves healthy.

In my experience, Maharishi Ayurveda offers profound and far-reaching benefits for my patients, both children and adults alike. In Maharishi Ayurveda, no aspect of life is disregarded. It takes into account the whole child: consciousness, mind, body, behavior, and

NATURE KNOWS BEST

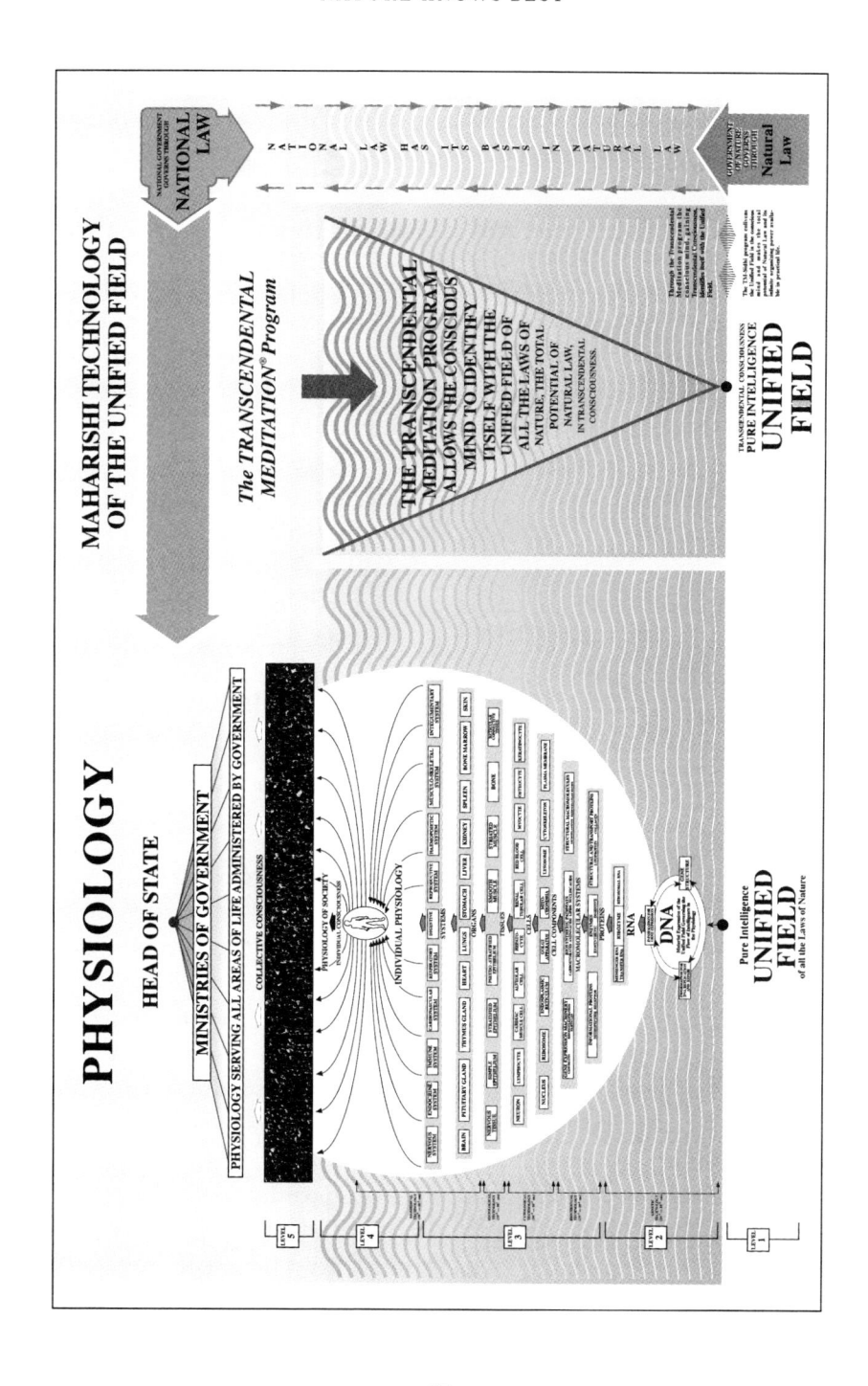

environment. By using such a comprehensive approach, the benefits for health are enormous. In the next chapter, you'll see how this power of the body's inner intelligence is expressed in your child.

The Role of the Mind and Emotions in Creating Health

Consciousness is unseen and invisible; yet it is expressed in the mind as thoughts and feelings. When nature's intelligence, or consciousness, is fully enlivened and balanced, then the mind is also balanced. Creativity and intelligence are signs of a balanced mind, while happiness, generosity, and love are signs of balanced feelings.

The role of the mind in health is now widely recognized. It is said that 90 percent of disease is psychosomatic, meaning that it is caused by or aggravated by psycho-emotional factors. Yet in Maharishi Ayurveda we would say it somewhat differently. We'd say that all disease has physical, mental, and emotional components. There is no one who suffers a physical disease who does not experience a corresponding effect in the mind and emotions. As to which creates the other, it's a moot point. Both are created at a more fundamental level—a breakdown in the connection with nature's intelligence.

Commanding the Switchboard of Nature

If your child has within him the perfection of nature, what is it, then, that causes disease? According to Maharishi Ayurveda, disease is caused by the violation of natural law. In other words, if your child could enjoy the full development of his consciousness, make the right choices, and never go against his own nature, he would always be healthy.

That, of course, sounds like an impossible task. You can't warn your child of every situation that may come up—though surely some parents have tried it!. And how many parents feel that they themselves know the right thing to do or say in every situation?

Yet if there were a way to get to the switchboard, to open the awareness to the control panel of all the laws of nature, then it might be possible to cultivate the ability to act in accord with those laws and avoid making mistakes.

One of the most profound insights offered by Maharishi Ayurveda is that through your own human consciousness, you can open your awareness to nature's intelligence. All the therapies and techniques of Maharishi Ayurveda help remove the stress, impurities, and other blocks to directly experiencing this field of nature's intelligence, the home of all the laws of nature. It is this infinitely powerful intelligence of nature that is awakened through Maharishi Ayurveda.

This is the most important difference between Maharishi Ayurveda and other systems of health care: all of the treatments evoke the power of nature itself to heal disease from within, rather than using drugs to treat the superficial symptoms. Like a river cut off from its source, a person with a disease needs to be reconnected with the Self, with nature's intelligence inside. In the following chapters of this book, you will see how the power of nature can be employed to heal your child and keep him healthy and happy throughout life.

CHAPTER THREE
Treating Individual Differences

No mother needs to be told that her child is unique. Even within the same family, one child might excel in sports, while another might shine in social skills. One might have a voracious appetite, while the other may eat lightly. One may find it easy to keep his room neat, and the other may have to work harder to keep his environment orderly.

In Maharishi Ayurveda, a child's nature, or *prakriti*, is considered to be especially important to identify, because once you understand your-child's nature, you can also predict the kinds of imbalances and the kinds of diseases he or she might be prone to. This is an extremely valable insight that all parents need to master in order to help prevent illness in their children. For no matter what individual differences exist in children, every child can live a life of balance, and unfold his or her full potential.

In the previous chapter, you saw how each child holds the power of the universe inside him, and has the potential to live a life of energy, bliss, intelligence, and happiness. In this chapter, you'll see how this innate intelligence is expressed differently in each individual, giving rise to the particular bundle of energy that is your child.

Three Streams of Nature's Intelligence

To understand your child's basic nature, you first need to identify the basic building blocks of nature itself, called the five elements: space, air, fire, water, and earth.

Interestingly enough, these five building blocks of nature are found in the same proportions in nature as in your child. For instance, if you consider the vast universe, it is mostly space. Your child's body, too, is mostly space. Fire is found in the digestive juices, and water is found in all the fluids. Air is found in the breath, and the bones and muscles of the body correspond to the earth element.

Maharishi Ayurveda makes it even simpler: the five elements are condensed into the three mind-body operators, or *doshas*. The doshas are *Vata*, *Pitta*, and *Kapha*. Each governs different functions in the human body. These are the three streams of nature's intelligence in the body, the three key principles in understanding the Consciousness-Based[SM] model of health.

Vata is composed of space and air. It governs movement in the mind and body, anything from a thought moving across your mind to blood pumping through your veins. It governs all the channels of communication and transportation in the body, all the empty channels and spaces that information, fluids, and nutrients flow through.

Pitta is composed of fire and water. In your mind and body, it governs the processes of digestion, metabolism, and transformation. The acidic digestive enzymes, which break down food, are governed by Pitta, as are all catalysts and hormones.

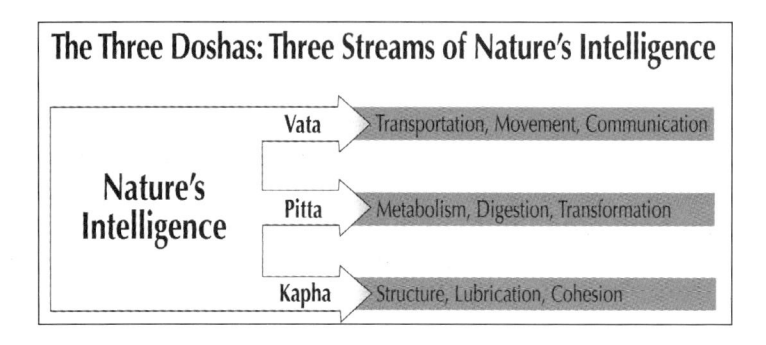

The Three Doshas: Three Streams of Nature's Intelligence

Nature's Intelligence
- Vata → Transportation, Movement, Communication
- Pitta → Metabolism, Digestion, Transformation
- Kapha → Structure, Lubrication, Cohesion

Kapha is composed of earth and water. It governs the physical structure—the muscles, flesh, and bones of your body.

The doshas have different qualities. Vata dosha, for instance, being made of space and air, is dry, rough, cold, light, subtle, moving, clear, and coarse.

Pitta dosha, being composed of fire and water, is slightly oily, hot, sharp, liquid, sour, flowing, and pungent.

The elements of earth and water form Kapha dosha, so it is heavy, cold, soft, moist, oily, sweet, stable, and sticky.

The Connection Between Your Child's Body and the Body of the Universe

You can see evidence of the three doshas all around you. Some plants and foods are more Vata (the dry, spindly ones) and some are more Kapha (the lush, watery ones). With regard to the weather, the cold, windy, dry winter is when Vata predominates. Pitta governs the hot, humid summer. And Kapha dosha is evident in cool, rainy springtime.

It's thrilling to see that the same streams of nature's intelligence that govern all of nature are also in your child's body—the same five elements, the same three doshas. In Maharishi Ayurveda, the connection between the individual and the universe is not only recognized, but forms its basic operating framework. The Vedic texts state that the individual is an epitome of the universe, because all the phenomena in the universe are present in the individual, and all those present in the individual are also contained in the universe.

The three doshas also predominate in different times of life and in different times of the day. For instance, the Kapha time of day, time of the year, and time of life is characterized by the heavy, slow, solid, structure-building qualities of Kapha dosha. Kapha dosha is evident from 6:00 a.m. to 10:00 a.m., and again from 6:00 p.m. to 10:00 p.m. It also governs the spring season, and the time of life from birth up to thirty years. Childhood, then, is governed by the Kapha time of life, when the structure of the body—the muscles, bones, and cells—are growing rapidly.

The Pitta time of the day, which occurs at noon when the sun is at its zenith, is characterized by increased heat and increased digestive power in the body. The Pitta season (which corresponds to the hot summer months) and the Pitta time of life (age thirty to sixty) also reflect the hot, sharp, metabolic qualities of Pitta dosha.

The dry, cold, moving qualities of Vata dosha are reflected in three ways: 1) the Vata time of day (2:00 to 6:00 a.m. and p.m.), 2) in the winter season, and 3) in the Vata time of life—above age sixty.

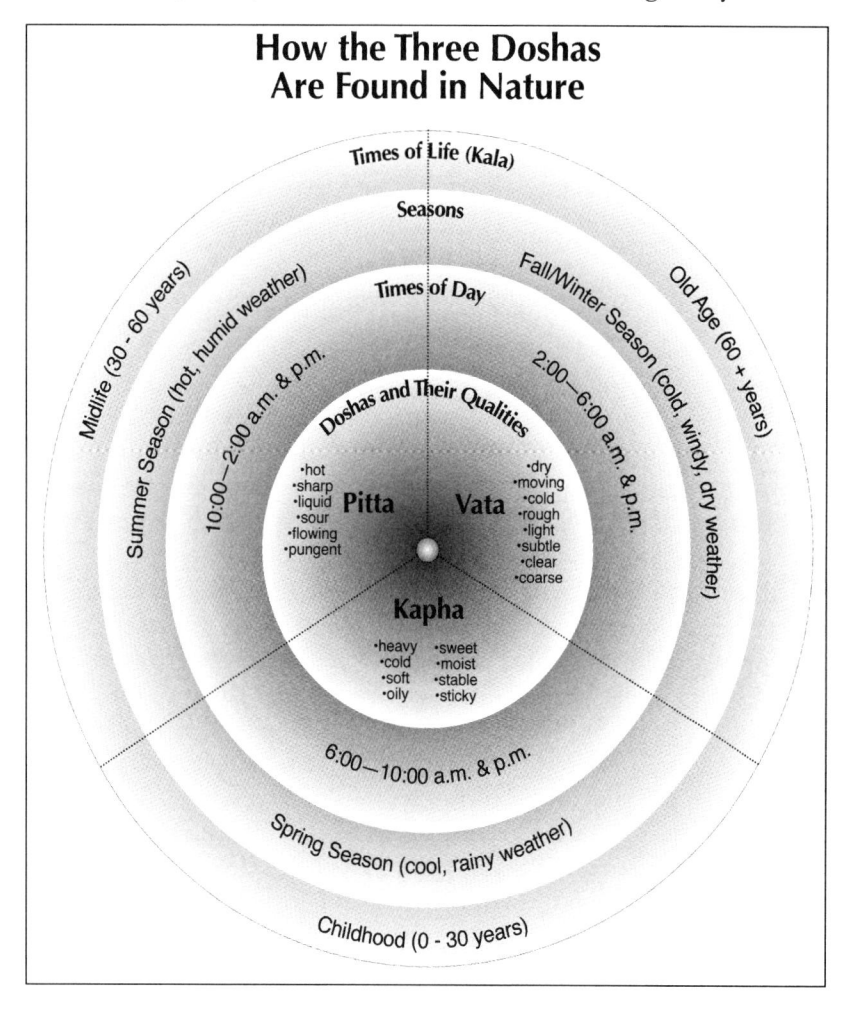

How the Three Doshas Are Found in Nature

- Times of Life (Kala)
- Seasons
- Times of Day
- Doshas and Their Qualities

Pitta: hot, sharp, liquid, sour, flowing, pungent
Vata: dry, moving, cold, rough, light, subtle, clear, coarse
Kapha: heavy, cold, soft, oily, sweet, moist, stable, sticky

- Midlife (30 - 60 years)
- Summer Season (hot, humid weather)
- 10:00–2:00 a.m. & p.m.
- Fall/Winter Season (cold, windy, dry weather)
- Old Age (60 + years)
- 2:00–6:00 a.m. & p.m.
- 6:00–10:00 a.m. & p.m.
- Spring Season (cool, rainy weather)
- Childhood (0 - 30 years)

A Child with a Vata Imbalance

Each of the doshas, the three basic mind-body operators, has an essential function in the body. So all three are always present as long as a person lives. Yet they are not always present in equal quantities. They differ from person to person, and they fluctuate throughout life. They can be in balance or out of balance. When they are out of balance, they can cause disease.

Let's look at the case of Emily, an active and intelligent four-year old. Emily, it seems, has trouble sitting still. She is an imaginative, talkative child with a big vocabulary for her age. A picky eater, she is thin and willowy, sensitive to criticism, and she tires easily. Her parents worry because even though Emily is often tired, she can't fall asleep at night. She also seems anxious and bites her fingernails.

From her symptoms, Emily displays a classic case of Vata dosha imbalance. remember that Vata dosha is moving, quick, dry, light, subtle, and coarse. These qualities give rise to certain qualities in the mind and body. When it's in balance, Vata is expressed in imagination, cheerfulness, clarity of thinking, liveliness, ease in movement, and a slender, light body build.

Qualities of Vata in Balance	Qualities of Vata Out of Balance
Vibrant, lively	Restless, unsettled
Clear, alert	Light, interrupted sleep
Flexible, resilient	Easily fatigued
Imaginative, sensitive	Anxious and worried
Cheerful, optimistic	Underweight
Energetic	Constipated
Regular elimination	

When it's out of balance, it can cause loss of weight, insomnia (the mind whirling too fast), fatigue, constipation (too much internal dryness), and anxiety.

A Case of Pitta Imbalance

Emily's nine-year-old sister, Amy, has a very different temperament. she has strawberry blond hair and freckles, is of medium build and weight, and has a voracious appetite. She is somewhat of a leader with her friends at school, and ice skates in competitions. At home she is usually sociable and loving, but she can also be intense, irritable, and even fiery when she's under pressure. She has a persistent problem with eczema that won't go away.

Amy displays many qualities of Pitta dosha. remember that Pitta's qualities are hot, oily, sharp, liquid, sour, and flowing. When it is in balance, Pitta expresses itself in children as contentment, a strong appetite, and a sharp intellect. When it is out of balance, it can flare up as anger, a critical attitude, or skin rashes.

Qualities of Pitta in Balance	Qualities of Pitta Out of Balance
Warm, loving, contented	Skin rashes
Enjoys meeting challenges	Irritability, anger, impatience
Strong digestion	Demanding, critical, and excessively perfectionist behavior
Efficient in activity	
Articulate and precise in speech	Heartburn, digestive problems
Sharp intellect	Finds hot weather unbearable

The Kapha Friend

You may think that the two girls could not be more different, yet their friend Sanjaya is different still. He is ten years old, but he looks twelve or older. Big-boned and athletic, he is easygoing and relaxed. Nothing seems to get under his skin. When it's no longer basketball season, he tends to put on weight easily. He gets frequent colds, and has occasional bouts with asthma.

Qualities of Kapha in Balance	Qualities of Kapha Out of Balance
Strong, vital energy	Complacent, dull, lethargic
Affectionate, generous, kind, forgiving	Oily skin, allergies, congestion
Solid, powerful build	Slow digestion, tendency to gain weight
Natural resistance to disease	Possessive, emotionally attached
Good memory	Intolerant of the cold and damp
Courageous	Inability to accept change

You'll remember that the qualities of Kapha dosha are heavy, cold, soft, oily, sweet, stable, and sticky. When in balance, these qualities can be expressed as a generous and stable nature, a strong body, and a good memory. When out of balance, Kapha dosha can cause dullness, lethargy, slow digestion, obesity, and problems with congestion.

Treating Children as Individuals

Emily, Amy, and Sanjaya each display different proportions of the three doshas. Thus each has a different nature, or *prakriti*. It is easy to see which doshas predominate in their minds and bodies. Emily has more Vata in her nature, Amy more Pitta, and Sanjaya more Kapha.

These three children represent the three major *prakritis*: Vata, Pitta, and Kapha. In these examples, the three *prakritis* are simple to recognize because the children are each *mono-doshic*, meaning that only one dosha predominates. But most people are more complex. They might be a combination of Vata and Pitta, or Kapha and Pitta. They might have a *tri-doshic* makeup, with all three doshas—Vata, Pitta, and Kapha—equally present in their minds and bodies.

Maharishi Ayurveda recognizes these inherent differences in every child, and the physician takes those differences into account when diagnosing illness and prescribing treatments and therapies.

These tendencies also come into play in preventing disease. As a parent, you can learn to recognize these characteristics and learn how to give your child the foods, exercise, and lifestyle that will bring health and balance to his or her life.

An Example of How Maharishi Ayurveda Balances the Doshas

Let's look at how Emily's, Amy's, and Sanjaya's imbalances could be caused, and how they could be treated. In Emily's case, she is by nature a person who has more Vata dosha. Because Vata predominates, she must be careful all her life to balance Vata. Things that can aggravate Vata are going to bed late or at irregular times, eating at irregular times, eating foods that are cold, dry, and rough (like too many cold sodas, popcorn, and crackers), and traveling a lot.

The Causes of Vata Imbalance	Ways to Keep Vata in Balance
• Irregular routine • Staying up too late • Cold, dry weather • Excessive mental strain • Traveling • Accident or injury • Eating too much dry, cold, rough food • Eating too much astringent, bitter, and pungent food	• Maintain a regular daily routine, with meals and bedtime at the same time every day. • Do an Ayurvedic oil massage (abhyanga) every day. • Go to bed by 8:00 p.m. and get more sleep early in the evening. • Eat three warm meals a day. • Drink plenty of warm liquids, avoiding stimulants. • Dress warmly, taking warm baths. • Live in a calm, quiet environment. • Eat more warm, oily, moist foods. • Eat more sour, salty, and sweet foods.
The Causes of Pitta Imbalance	**Ways to Keep Pitta in Balance**
• Excessive heat or exposure to the sun • Time pressure, stressful deadlines • Too much activity • Skipping meals • Alcohol, smoking • Eating too much sour, salty, and spicy food	• Maintain a moderate schedule, not too structured. • Avoid sports that require exercising in the hot sun. • Eat largest meal at noon. • Eat more cooling foods. • Eat more bitter, astringent, and sweet tastes.
The Causes of Kapha Imbalance	**Ways to Keep Kapha in Balance**
• Oversleeping, especially after 6:00 a.m. • Overeating • Eating too much salty, sour, and sweet tastes • Eating too many cold, heavy, or oily foods • Insufficient exercise • Cold, wet weather	• Don't oversleep. • Don't overeat. • Include more pungent, bitter, and astringent tastes in your diet. • Eat more light, easily digestible, warm foods. • Enjoy a variety of stimulating activities. • Exercise regularly and vigorously. • Stay warm and avoid feeling cold and damp.

Emily would benefit from a soothing, quiet, and low-stimulus environment at home, especially in the evening. Television is stimulating, so for Emily I would suggest avoiding it at night, and watching it for only limited times during the day. An Ayurvedic oil massage (abhyanga) would soothe and relax her before bed, and also would help her build up her strength and immunity. I would give her a special Vata-pacifying diet, with foods that are warm and rich, such as hot milk and rice, to soothe and nourish her and help her to sleep. Emily would benefit from a regular daily routine, so I would advise her mother to schedule Emily's meals, bedtime, and wake-up time at the same time each day. In addition, I would diagnose the underlying cause of her insomnia, and would probably prescribe some herbal compounds to help bring balance.

Consulting a Physician or Expert Trained in Maharishi Ayurveda

While this book will provide many new insights into your child's health, it cannot be used to diagnose or treat your child. For one thing, diagnosing the doshas and their imbalances takes skill and expertise. When you bring your child to be diagnosed, the physician trained in Maharishi Ayurveda will take into account all aspects of your child's life: his or her body size and shape; muscular development and fat distribution; skin color and texture; hair, nails, and facial expressions; walking and talking speed; the quality of voice and gestures; sleep and eating patterns; food choices; mental habits; emotional makeup; and reaction to stress.

The physician will also use a subtle but effective technique, called pulse diagnosis, to assess the underlying doshic imbalances. Pulse diagnosis, a gentle, noninvasive technique that involves taking your child's pulse at the wrist, helps determine the causal imbalance for any disease or discomfort. This is very important, because often the underlying cause is not evident. A headache, for instance, could be caused by a Vata dosha imbalance, as in the case of a tension headache. But it could also be caused by a Pitta imbalance (as in some migraines) or by a Kapha imbalance (as in some sinus headaches). Or it could be caused by some combination of the three doshas. It does not do any good to

> **Primary Location of Vata, Pitta, and Kapha in the Body**
>
> VATA—colon
> PITTA—small intestine
> KAPHA—stomach

just treat the symptom. In Maharishi Ayurveda, the underlying doshic imbalance must be detected and then brought into balance through natural means. That way the cause of the disease or discomfort can be eliminated completely.

This is one of the things I like best about Maharishi Ayurveda. A physician trained in Maharishi Ayurveda never treats every headache the same, nor every case of insomnia the same. Nor do I ever treat two children alike. The treatment will be different depending on what the underlying imbalance is that caused the headache or insomnia—and what the child's individual body type is.

Pulse diagnosis determines not only the origin of the disease, but also the location. This is because each of the doshas corresponds to a specific part of the body. The primary location of Vata is in the colon, of Pitta the small intestine, and Kapha, the stomach.

Analysis can be specific and precise, because the three doshas have five components, called the *subdoshas*, each with their own locations in the body. When a physician feels an imbalance in any of the fifteen subdoshas, he knows precisely where the source of the problem is located, even if the symptoms are showing up in a different part of the body than the source of the problem.

The cause of fever, for instance, is not really hot skin. Fever results from a quantitative increase of Pitta in the circulation when Pitta dosha, which governs digestion in the stomach and intestine, cannot flow out of the area because the passages are blocked by impurities. Pitta dosha then starts to accumulate in the stomach and intestines, causing increased heat. A secondary cause of fever is when the heat accumulating in the body cannot flow out through sweat in the skin, due to blockage of the skin pores by impurities.

So if a physician trained in Maharishi Ayurveda diagnosed your child, he or she would be able to locate the cause of the illness and treat that underlying imbalance, rather than the superficial symptoms. In the case of fever, the physician would recommend treatments to dissolve the impurities that caused Pitta dosha to build up in the digestive tract, rather than giving pills to bring down the fever, which would only mask the symptoms and not cure the actual cause of the imbalance at its source.

Treating Diseases Before They Arise

How many times has your child said, "I just don't feel good"? If you brought your child to me with that complaint when I practiced Western medicine, I would have asked him or her to try to locate some area of pain, some part of the body where the disease was manifesting, so I could diagnose and hopefully cure the disease. If nothing physical could be located, I would have to recommend plenty of rest, and wait for the symptoms to emerge.

Yet the fact is, when your child "just doesn't feel right" for a long period of time, it's probably due to a real imbalance. Children are more attuned to their bodies and have not learned to brush aside the warning signals of ill health the way adults have.

A "not-so-good feeling" may be due to emotional or physical factors. Your child might have trouble focusing or keeping his attention on one thing at a time. He may feel restless and his mind might feel cloudy, he may feel isolated and rejected, or his stomach might feel like it's tied in knots.

Today, as a physician trained in Maharishi Ayurveda, I would consider these mental and emotional factors to be equal in importance to physical symptoms. Usually, if the body is ill, the mind and emotions are also disturbed, and vice versa. This is because the mind and body, in fact, are so closely interconnected that they are one.

By using pulse diagnosis, it would be possible for me to discover the underlying doshic imbalance before it became a chronic disease. This is precisely the right time to visit a doctor, for by the time the illness shows up as a full-blown symptom, it has already progressed quite far and is more difficult to treat. That's why we recommend that children have a checkup with their physician trained in Maharishi Ayurveda every four months, at the change of seasons. The families who do this are able to head off disease before it ever happens, and this is far more useful to life and good health, and beautiful for me to see.

If you consult a physician trained in Maharishi Ayurveda early on, you can help your children conquer disease at an early age and avoid further complications later in life. Then as your children reach maturity, they can reach their full mental and physical potential. As a parent, your motive is to take your children out of the cycle of disease and discomfort. If you work closely with a physician trained in Maharishi Ayurveda, then the treatment quickly begins to show its worth.

Different Learning Styles

It's important to recognize that different children learn in different ways. There are many different learning styles, and these are often associated with the doshas. Children whose nature is more Vata learn better by hearing information spoken (and thus often do well at school). Children who have more Pitta might relate more to visual knowledge, as when it is written down or drawn in a picture.

Kapha-predominant children learn more slowly, but tend to remember everything they learn. They need to be given the time to systematically study new things at their own pace, and then they will do quite well.

If a child is having trouble at school, check to make sure his routine is balanced and his diet is healthy. In addition to consulting your child's pediatrician, it would be advisable to see a physician trained in Maharishi Ayurveda, to see if there is an imbalance in the doshas that could be causing the learning problem. Attention Deficit Hyperactivity Disorder (ADHD), for instance, can be caused by a Vata imbalance, and many children have been helped with the natural treatments of Maharishi Ayurveda.

Every Mother Should Learn Self-Pulse Diagnosis

It's so important for a mother to understand her child's doshas, strengths, and weaknesses. When the mother understands which dis-

TREATING INDIVIDUAL DIFFERENCES

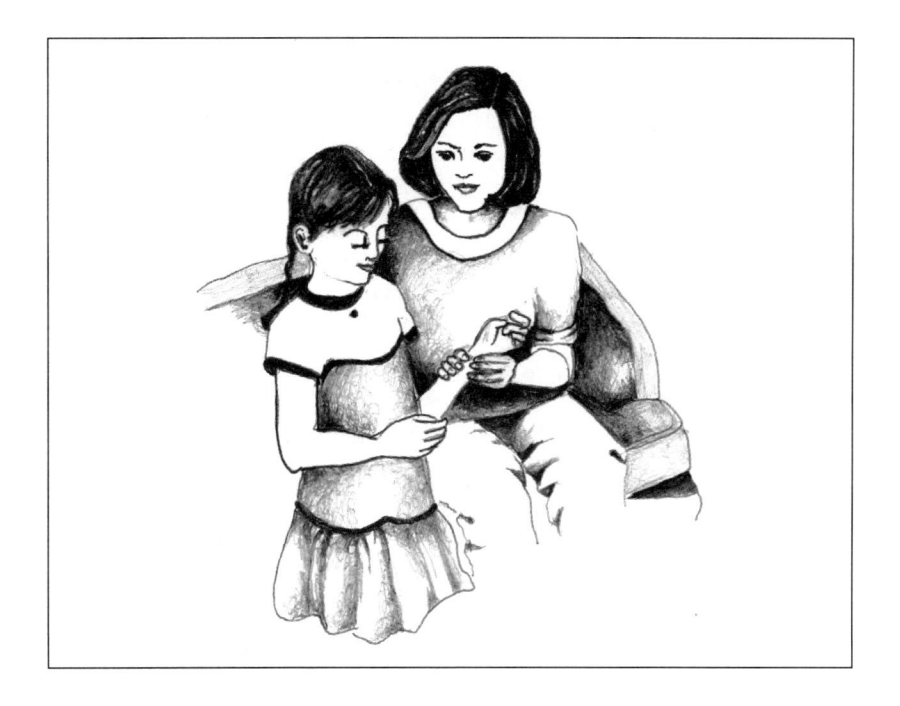

eases her child may be prone to, she can prevent disease by adjusting the diet and routine to correct imbalances before they become symptoms.

But how can you detect your child's imbalances before they become symptoms? A simple, noninvasive diagnostic technique, called Maharishi Ayurveda pulse diagnosis (Nadi Vigyan), is surprisingly effective for this. Once you are trained in pulse diagnosis, you can place your three fingers on your child's radial pulse at the wrist and detect whether she is experiencing a state of balance or imbalance. And you can determine which doshas are causing the imbalance.

Imagine that after your daughter wakes up tomorrow morning you feel her pulse. It becomes clear immediately that Vata dosha is out of balance. You know this because you take your child's pulse on a regular basis, and thus are acutely aware when there is a sudden change. You also know that almost every time your daughter has fallen sick with a cold, it has been preceded by a Vata imbalance in the pulse. So you're anxious to bring the doshas back into balance to prevent her from getting sick.

Once you detect the imbalance, you can look at her diet and routine to see how to adjust it. You're not surprised that Vata is out of balance. She is a Vata type, with a light, thin build, and thus is more susceptible to Vata disturbances. She excels in ballet, and has been practicing for a performance several evenings a week, and the extra activity and pressure could be causing the imbalance.

So you immediately decide to take precautions to help her to balance Vata dosha. You give her an extra abhyanga at night to help her sleep better, and prepare Vata® Tea, a mixture of spices that balance Vata dosha, for her to drink before bed. You also make sure that her diet has a balancing effect on Vata dosha. Within a few days after making these simple adjustments, her pulse is back to normal.

This is an example of a temporary imbalance that is easily corrected because the child is basically healthy. Of course, there may be deeper imbalances that should be treated by a physician trained in Maharishi Ayurveda. But whatever the starting point, whatever the predispositions to different imbalances and diseases—it's important to realize that every child's mind and body can be brought into balance. How fast this happens depends on the basic immunity of the child and also how deeply the imbalance is embedded in the system.

Every mother can learn to feel the pulse of her children and in this way prevent many illnesses and problems. By learning pulse diagnosis, the mother can detect her child's imbalances at an early stage, before they manifest into disease. There is a special 16-lesson course in Maharishi Ayurveda Pulse Diagnosis (see appendix).

Even children can learn to practice Maharishi Ayurveda pulse diagnosis. In some schools in the U.S., the children learn how to feel their own pulse. In this way they start to take responsibility for their health, and see the connection between the choices they make and the way they feel. Through self-pulse reading, the child's attention enlivens his own pulse, his own inner intelligence. This stimulates natural balancing mechanisms in the body and helps to rectify any growing imbalance. A child who learns to take his own pulse has an opportunity to stay in touch with his own body, and can begin to align his individual pulse with the pulse of the universe.

Once you understand your child's strengths, weaknesses, and predispositions to imbalance, you can help your child become a more healthy person. If you don't understand your child, that ignorance becomes the

TREATING INDIVIDUAL DIFFERENCES

basis for making mistakes. You may feed your child the wrong foods for his constitution and may encourage him to be on a routine that is actually harmful for him.

I'd also like to clarify that understanding your child's weaknesses does not mean excusing. You can't say, "Oh, he's a Kapha child, so he can be obese," or "She's Vata so she can be disorganized," or "He's Pitta so he can have a temper tantrum." The important thing is to understand your child's unique makeup, help him to understand himself, and then outline the steps to restore balance and good health. Even if your child has temper tantrums, that can be changed early on. He has only to learn to modify his daily routine and eating habits.

Every child can live in a state of ideal health. As a parent you naturally want to give your children what they need and protect them from harm. But you also want to make it possible for them to develop their full consciousness, live life without mistakes, and experience the perfection of nature within. As a parent, you can help your children become the healthy, self-realized individuals that they were born to be.

CHAPTER FOUR
Why Kids Get Sick and How to Prevent It

Julie brought her son Tyler to my office when he was two years old. Tyler suffered from an acute upper respiratory infection and bronchitis. For the past six months, he had taken many rounds of antibiotics, which weakened his immune system. Each time he took antibiotics he did get better at first, but then immediately afterward he would relapse into bronchitis again.

The child was miserable and looked unhealthy. His breathing was labored and difficult, and he was underweight for his age.

In discussing the family history with Julie, I found that with her first child she had only worked part-time during pregnancy and was able to take care of herself. Her first son was born a robust nine pounds and remained healthy.

During her pregnancy with Tyler, on the other hand, she had just started a challenging and stressful full-time job that required her to work seven days a week. She didn't have the time or the insight to eat regular, balanced meals, or to rest enough. She felt that taking prenatal vitamins and making regular visits to the obstetrician was enough to produce a healthy child.

But Tyler weighed only six pounds, six ounces at birth, and from the start faced constant health problems. He suffered from infections, frequent gas and colic, and difficulty sleeping. In general, Julie felt that he was much more unhappy than his brother. Understandably, it's hard for a child to be happy when he's feeling miserable inside. What Julie was seeing on the outside was a reflection of Tyler's inner state of ill health.

A few days after applying the treatments of Maharishi Ayurveda—which included changes in diet, Maharishi Ayurveda herbal food supplements, and changes in daily routine—Julie reported that Tyler's symptoms were subsiding. He was much more happy and energetic. He took more interest in his toys and games. As the treatments progressed, he and his brother started to get along better.

Within six months, Tyler grew two inches, his coloring became normal, and he looked much healthier. He had broken through the vicious cycle of constant coughs and colds and the weakening rounds of antibiotics. Today, Tyler behaves like any other happy, healthy child.

"I never thought he'd escape from the cycle of sickness," said Julie. "It's wonderful to see him so happy."

This is a common scenario that I see in my office. A child gets sick with a cold, cough, fever, or the flu. The mother consults a Western physician. The child is prescribed antibiotics along with antihistamines, decongestants, and cough medicines. These provide temporary relief for the infection, but are treating symptoms only, because these prescription drugs don't address the underlying imbalance that is causing the child to be prone to congestion in the first place. Worse, the antibiotics actually weaken immunity by destroying helpful organisms in the digestive tract. Antihistamines also break down immunity and disrupt digestion, throwing the child's system further off balance. The next time he is exposed to an infectious disease, his immunity is weaker and he succumbs more quickly, bringing on another round of antibiotics and antihistamines. The child is constantly falling sick to colds, coughs, and sinus problems—and the treatments become part of the problem.

Sadly, there are many American children who end up in pediatricians' offices once a week or several times a month. Then it becomes a chronic problem. The child loses his liveliness and becomes depressed and irritable. He also becomes more prone to other diseases.

Maharishi Ayurveda provides a new model for breaking out of this routine and creating health for a child who is locked in the cycle of sickness.

A Different Concept of Immunity

According to the traditional view, children are more prone to flu, colds, upper respiratory infections, and other illnesses because their immune systems are untested. As they grow up, the conventional wisdom goes, they develop resistance to disease and thus don't get sick as frequently. The only thing the conventional doctor has to offer to boost immunity is immunization shots for major infectious diseases, and later, when a child succumbs to illness, antibiotics.

Maharishi Ayurveda presents a different concept of immunity. Immunity is the internal strength, or *bala*, that comes from the doshas being in balance, the digestion and metabolism functioning normally, and the tissues growing properly. Immunity comes from the inside, from eating a healthy, balanced diet, from having a strong digestion, and from following a healthy daily routine. Prevention of disease results from strengthening immunity, which essentially means strengthening digestion.

In Western medicine, the focus is on chasing the germs and then killing them. Maharishi Ayurveda focuses on strengthening the body so the germ is no longer a threat. You probably have noticed that even though several children may be exposed to the same virus or flu bug, only some of them get sick. The difference lies in how balanced the children's doshas are, their level of vitality, and their internal immunity.

But why, then, are children more susceptible to certain childhood diseases than adults? The answer from Maharishi Ayurveda is that children are in a unique stage of life, called *Kapha Kala*. You'll remember from the last chapter that there are different stages of life associated with the three doshas. In the Kapha Kala (from birth to age thirty), Kapha dosha predominates. This is when the child builds strong bones, muscles, organs, and the brain—and this formation of the physical structure of the body is largely a function of Kapha dosha.

Kapha dosha predominates in many ways during this period. For instance, very young children display the qualities of Kapha; they have a higher percentage of body fat than adults, spend longer periods in sleep, and display a slower reaction time. If a small child falls down, often there is a delay before he or she starts crying or even comprehends the hurt.

At the same time, children are also more prone to Kapha imbalances than adults. When Kapha dosha is out of balance, its heavy and sticky qualities can lead to slow digestion and excess mucus production in the body. Thus children are more prone to certain Kapha-related diseases, such as respiratory disorders, colds, flu, and childhood diseases such as chicken pox, measles, and mumps.

By understanding this one point—that Kapha imbalance and slow digestion is at the basis of most childhood illness—you can shape your child's diet and daily routine to avoid excessive Kapha. Throughout this book, you'll learn various ways of doing this. For example, you can reduce "Kapha-increasing" foods in your child's diet. Excessive sweets (especially candy, heavy pastries, chocolate, and ice cream), ice-cold soft drinks, aged cheeses, and packaged, canned, and processed foods can be dramatically decreased without depriving him of needed nutrients. The daily routine can also be adjusted to avoid Kapha imbalance. Sleeping late in the morning, for instance, can increase Kapha and diminish digestive power for older children, as can lack of exercise. These are just a few of the many simple but practical recommendations that can increase your child's health dramatically.

Strong Immunity Means Strong Digestion

Immunity depends on healthy and vibrant digestion during the Kapha stage of life and beyond. This is a central principle of Maharishi Ayurveda.

The digestive juices are likened to a fire, called *agni*. In fact, the word *agni* refers to the sun and fire, and to the digestive and metabolic transformations that take place in the body. *Charaka Samhita* (one of the forty aspects of Veda and the Vedic Literature, an ancient text that expounds the principles of Ayurveda) states that strength, health, and longevity all depend on the power of agni.

Agni also refers to the digestive enzymes and secretions in the stomach and small intestines. Called *jatharagni*, the main agni, these digestive enzymes and secretions are responsible for breaking down food and turning it into chyle, or nutrient fluid. When jatharagni is healthy and strong, the nutrient fluid is formed correctly and easily reaches the cells to create and nourish healthy tissues.

After the process of digestion breaks down the food you eat into nutrient fluid, the various tissues of the body are metabolized through a series of transformations. These tissues include plasma, hemoglobin, muscle, fat, bone, bone marrow, the central nervous system, and the reproductive tissue including semen and ovum.

The creation of tissue, called *dhatu*, requires a brightly burning digestive fire, or metabolic process. This is because the dhatus are formed in a sequence, starting with the nutrient fluid in the blood and ending with the reproductive tissue. If there is any block or abnormality at any point in the digestive process, then there will be a weakness in that tissue, and in all the tissues that follow in the chain of transformation. So you can see how very important a strong digestion is to children, who are growing so rapidly and need to develop healthy blood, bones, organs, and brain. This chart outlines the seven dhatus with their Sanskrit names.

The Seven Dhatus (Body Tissues)

Rasa—Blood plasma, chyle, nutrients
Rakta—Blood cells, hemoglobin
Mamsa—Muscle
Meda—Fat and adipose tissue
Athi—Bone
Majja—Bone marrow and the central nervous system
Shukra—Reproductive tissue, including semen and ovum

This process of forming nutrient fluid into new tissues takes place in the cells—thus agni also resides in each cell. In fact, there is a metabolic process (agni) associated with each tissue (dhatu) cell, to transform that tissue into the next tissue in the sequence.

Thus *rasa agni* transforms nutrient fluid (*rasa*) into blood (*rakta*). Once that transformation is complete, *rakta agni* transforms blood into muscle (*mamsa*). *Mamsa agni* transforms muscle into fat, and so on. A disturbance in mamsa agni could cause the muscle to be weak, and because the dhatus are formed in a sequence, all the subsequent

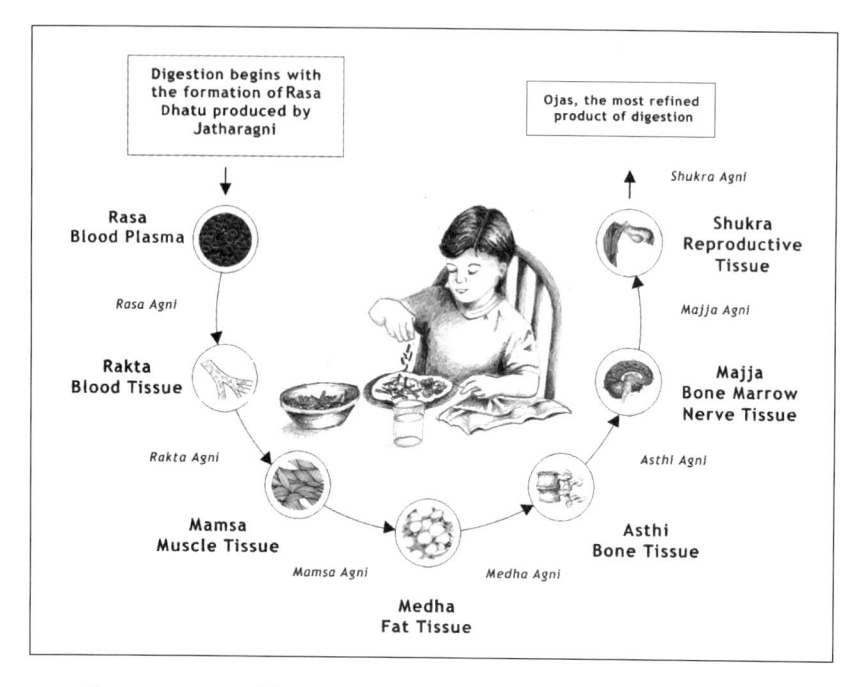

```
         ┌─────────────────────┐
         │ Digestion begins with│
         │ the formation of Rasa│      ┌──────────────────────┐
         │ Dhatu produced by   │      │ Ojas, the most refined│
         │     Jatharagni      │      │ product of digestion │
         └──────────┬──────────┘      └──────────────────────┘
                    ↓                            ↑ Shukra Agni
        Rasa                                          Shukra
    Blood Plasma                                   Reproductive
                                                      Tissue
        Rasa Agni                                  Majja Agni
        Rakta                                          Majja
     Blood Tissue                                  Bone Marrow
                                                   Nerve Tissue
        Rakta Agni                                 Asthi Agni
        Mamsa                                          Asthi
    Muscle Tissue                                  Bone Tissue
           Mamsa Agni              Medha Agni
                         Medha
                       Fat Tissue
```

transformations—of fat to bone and bone to bone marrow, and so on—would also be weakened.

In order for the nutrient fluid to be completely healthy, and in order for each dhatu agni to complete its transformation in each cell, the jatharagni, or digestion, must be functioning smoothly. You can see how healthy food and healthy digestion are essential for your child's blood, muscles, fat, and bone tissues to be properly formed.

Agni also exists in every cell as the metabolic or transforming function, and thus maintains the proper functioning of the RNA and DNA.

Agni is responsible for keeping the body's cellular function vibrant. Each of the billion cells in the body has its own function, its own mechanisms. One may be concerned with seeing, one with hearing, one with digesting. Each organ and each cell has its own mechanisms. And in a healthy child, they're all vibrant.

Types of Digestive Imbalance

When digestion, or agni, is imbalanced, it leads to weakened immunity and disease. There are different types of digestive imbalance, and often these are correlated with the different doshas. Too strong or too sharp agni can cause the nutrient fluid to become charred, just as food gets burned if the stove is turned up too high. A dull agni can cause food to remain undigested, and an irregular agni can create a mix of digested and undigested food.

All three of these are imbalances. If your child has either a weak, sharp, or irregular digestion, the physician trained in Maharishi Ayurveda will recommend a change in diet to correct the imbalance. A natural state of balanced digestion creates immunity, strength, and health.

If the dhatu agni is weakened and the transformation from one tissue to the other is not complete, then it becomes a source of future disease in the child. First, it could manifest as a myriad of physical, behavioral, and emotional problems, including tiredness, lethargy, lack of appetite, indigestion, constipation, lack of luster in the skin, irritable

---

Four Qualities of Agni
Sharp (associated with Pitta imbalance)
Dull (associated with Kapha imbalance)
Irregular (associated with Vata imbalance)
Balanced (balanced Vata, Pitta, and Kapha)

---

behavior, temper tantrums, lack of focus, lack of enthusiasm, frequent fights with siblings and friends, and susceptibility to colds and other illnesses.

Later, if the digestion is not brought into balance, even more serious problems can develop. Long-standing indigestion and elimination problems can be the cause of serious diseases: irritable bowel syndrome, diverticulitis, polyps, peptic ulcers, skin problems, obesity, arteriosclerosis, and even mental problems such as anxiety and depression. In fact, most disease starts with a weak digestion.

Toxins in the Digestion

When digestion is weak or irregular, a sticky, toxic, waste product of digestion forms, called *ama*. Ama is the result of undigested food. It collects in the stomach first, but if it is not eliminated, it can spread to other parts of the body through the nutrient fluid and cause disease.

When digestion is weak and the nutrient fluid does not metabolize properly, it gets mixed with ama. Ama blocks the channels that carry nutrients to the cells, resulting in undernourishment, and if left unchecked, weakness and disease in the tissues. Ama also causes blockage in the channels of circulation and elimination, resulting in fatigue, lack of energy, lethargy, and a heavy, dull feeling. It can cause the flow of Vata to reverse itself, which results in constipation, indigestion, excessive belching, bloating, gas, heartburn, bad breath, or regurgitation of food. In general, ama can cause dullness in the eyes and skin and a dull mind.

Ama creates a fertile environment for bacteria, thus contributing to disease. It also provides a breeding ground for free radicals, the reactive oxygen molecules that many scientists believe cause 90 percent of disease.

Signs of a Healthy Digestion

You've now seen how a weak digestion can affect your child's health. On the bright side, a healthy digestion can create a state of health that is so invincible that disease rarely, if ever, happens. When digestion is balanced, the body produces greater quantities of the vital material called *ojas*. Ojas is the end-product of digestion, the essence of the dhatus, created from the proper transformation of each of the agnis. It is always present in the body, as it resides in the gaps between the body tissues and also in the heart.

The healthier a child is, the more ojas, and vice versa. When ojas is lively, it creates contentment, enthusiasm, vitality, bliss, and clear thinking. It is reflected in a sparkle in the eyes and luster in the skin. You could say that ojas is the material form of bliss in the body. It is also the expression of immunity, or bala. Ojas helps prevent disease and maintains the balance of the doshas and dhatus.

Ojas is the finest material form of consciousness, and exists at the junction point between consciousness and matter. It is similar to balanced Kapha dosha in quality: heavy, soft, smooth, thick, sweet, stable, clear, and unctuous.

You can see that ama and ojas are exact opposites. When digestion is balanced, then food gets digested without excess waste, ojas is created at each transformation, and the tissues are properly nourished and infused with vitality. When digestion is weak, toxins (ama) mix with the nutrient fluid, are transported throughout the body, obstruct the channels, diminish ojas, and create weakened or abnormal tissues.

In this chapter you have seen how Western medicine does not effectively address the problem of boosting immunity in children. Giving immunization shots to prevent infectious disease is not enough. Even the practice of prescribing multiple vitamins to improve immunity is limited in its effectiveness, because vitamins are often not absorbed properly and can weaken the liver and kidneys.

I am not denying that Western drugs and antibiotics are effective in checking infections and treating many symptoms. But unfortunately antibiotics can also cause imbalance in the body, disturbing its normal functioning. They severely disrupt the digestion, the elimination, and the metabolism of the child.

Worse, they are not addressing the root cause of the health problems the child is facing. Western medicine offers little to improve the bala, the strength, the immunity, the digestive agni, and the individual agni of every cell. There is no modality or protocol in Western medicine to improve the child's health on this fundamental level. Treating the symptoms with antibiotics is like applying a bandage to a boil. Nothing is being done to purify the blood, to eliminate the source of the boil.

When immunity is fostered with proper health care, then each cell functions to the best of its capacity. Then there is perfection at the basic level of the cell—perfection in digestion, perfection in metabolism, and perfection in the RNA and DNA. Immunity is at its peak in every cell—whether in the brain, the muscles, or the skin. The immunity and strength in the body create vitality, a happy smile, and the vibrant health of youth. And more importantly, they wipe out disease.

This is the primary goal of Maharishi Ayurveda: to create total health in mind, body, and emotions throughout life. You could say that conventional medicine is treating at the level of the wave, while Maharishi Ayurveda treats the level of the deep ocean, at the source. When immunity is based on the strength of the deep ocean, then germs are like little waves on the surface, and do not pose a problem.

They come and go and are not disturbing. If there is enough bala or immunity in the body, the child doesn't get the flu so easily. After all, the germs will always be there—whether your child succumbs to the infection or not depends on his immunity. If bala is strong, various physical, emotional, and environmental changes won't affect the child's basic stability and strength.

Throughout the rest of this book, you'll see how to improve your child's immunity through a variety of natural means. These include meditation, daily and seasonal routine, proper diet, proper rest, herbal supplements, and restorative therapies known as *rasayanas*.

PART 2
Reconnecting with the Source

CHAPTER FIVE

How to Eliminate Stress and Restore Immunity

In the recent years of my practice, I have noticed a marked increase in childhood stress. This was something that was not heard of much twenty years ago, yet now the mainstream child-care magazines carry stories on how your child can cope with stress—at age four.

Part of the reason for this is increased stress in the home. With both parents working, more parents suffer from fatigue than in the past.

I am a working mother myself, so I don't want to say that working mothers are not good mothers. However, it does add its own tensions and stresses that parents must learn to manage.

In a recent survey by the Families and Work Institute in New York City, more than 1,000 children were surveyed on a number of issues. One question asked was, "What do you feel about your mother working?" The answers surprised many adults. The children did not seem to mind the fact that their mother worked outside the home: 67 percent felt that they had enough time with their mother, and 60 percent felt time spent with their father was enough. What was surprising was that 34 percent replied that they wished their parents weren't so stressed and tired. They were worried about their parents. More than 10 percent said they did wish they had more time with their mother, and 15 percent with their father.

Surprisingly enough, parents are not the only ones who are tired. Fatigue is a problem among children today. Sometimes this is due to a chronic illness, but other times it is due to an irregular routine, not enough sleep at night, and too much television. Lack of harmony in the home also creates stress in children.

Unfortunately, I meet many children who are facing difficulties sleeping, performing well in school, or getting along with their friends and families—all due to too much tension and stress.

While many experts blame the structured lifestyles of two-wage-earner families, in which children are shuffled from one structured activity to another with no time to just "be a kid," few offer any real solutions other than counseling. Yet this is an area that Maharishi Ayurveda has focused on for thousands of years. Dealing with stress is not a new phenomenon—but it's the first time that modern scientists have recognized the link between stress and childhood health.

A Case of Eliminating Stress

I recently treated eight-year-old Miguel. His mother said that he had difficulty concentrating in school and complained of boredom. Miguel said that he felt anxious in any new environment. He found it challenging to make friends and he was also teased by other children, which resulted in frustration and temper tantrums. He had been diagnosed as having borderline ADHD.

Although he had been on medication for ADHD for the last three months, his mother felt that it was not helping him much. She was concerned because the medication destroyed his appetite and gave him constipation; he was moving his bowels only once a week. Due to the medication, Miguel also experienced a sleep disorder. He would wake up at the slightest sound, or when a light was turned on in the hallway. Waking up frequently throughout the night, he would toss and turn, and feel as though he never slept. Understandably, his mother wanted to take him off the medicine.

After diagnosing Miguel's pulse, I found that his problems were predominantly caused by an imbalance in several subdoshas of Vata, although there were other imbalances as well. I recommended that he add pure and wholesome foods—such as milk, ghee, raw honey, grains, sweet fruits, herbs, fresh fruits, and cooked vegetables—to his diet to balance Vata dosha. I also recommended Ayurvedic oil massage, especially for the head. This immediately helped him sleep soundly through the night. Maharishi Ayurveda herbal formulations were given to balance other subdoshas, to help him feel more emotionally stable.

Almost immediately, his anxiety and fear subsided. At this point I advised Miguel's parents that they should introduce him to the Transcendental Meditation (TM®) technique. I explained the benefits of the Transcendental Meditation technique in reducing stress, improving focus, and providing the deep rest that he needed. I advised the parents to also learn the Transcendental Meditation technique so the child would feel supported by the whole family.

Another month passed before I met with him again. Miguel had learned the Transcendental Meditation technique and was already experiencing good results. His sleep disorder was completely gone, and he looked more calm and happy. He told me, "I experience less anger and I'm more friendly with people." He also had improved in his class work.

Although at this point not all of his problems were completely resolved, both Miguel and his parents felt that he was on the right path and that there was enormous benefit in continuing the program. They were especially encouraged that their child was not experiencing negative side effects, and was only feeling ease and happiness. After just a month of practicing the Transcendental Meditation technique, Miguel's parents were able to take him off his medication.

Thousands of children like Miguel have enjoyed enormous benefits from the Transcendental Meditation technique, as have their parents. Research published in *Current Issues in Education*, 2008, indicated that children with ADHD who practiced the Transcendental Meditation technique showed significant improvements in working memory, attention, organization, and behavior regulation.

In Chapter Two you learned about the vast field of nature's intelligence that is at the basis of all the healing modalities of Maharishi Ayurveda. In this chapter, you'll learn how the Transcendental Meditation technique opens human consciousness to the field of nature's intelligence within. It is a simple, natural procedure that allows the mind to settle down to its quietest, least-excited state, to contact the infinite field of happiness, tranquility, energy, silence, power, and bliss that is found inside everyone. More than any other treatment, the Transcendental Meditation technique cultivates the ability to act in accord with natural law. This happens spontaneously by becoming established in pure consciousness on a daily basis.

How It Works

Because the mind is able to settle to a silent and tranquil state during the practice of Transcendental Meditation, the body also experiences a deep state of relaxation. When experiencing deep rest, the body is able to throw off stress. Having reviewed the research, I can say without a doubt that the Transcendental Meditation technique is the most effective, clinically proven method for relieving stress available today.

You and your child can learn to meditate together. If you were to watch your child meditate, he would be sitting in a comfortable chair or on the floor or sofa, his eyes closed and his face and body relaxed. While adults meditate for twenty minutes twice a day, children meditate a shorter time.

Having grown up in India, I was exposed to many meditation techniques. But I have found the Transcendental Meditation technique, as taught by Maharishi Mahesh Yogi, to be the most effective. It is different from other techniques, because it is so completely natural and effortless. It does not include any concentration or contemplation. It does not involve the active thinking part of the mind. It allows the mind to transcend thought and reach the unbounded, silent, full potential of human ability that is hidden within.

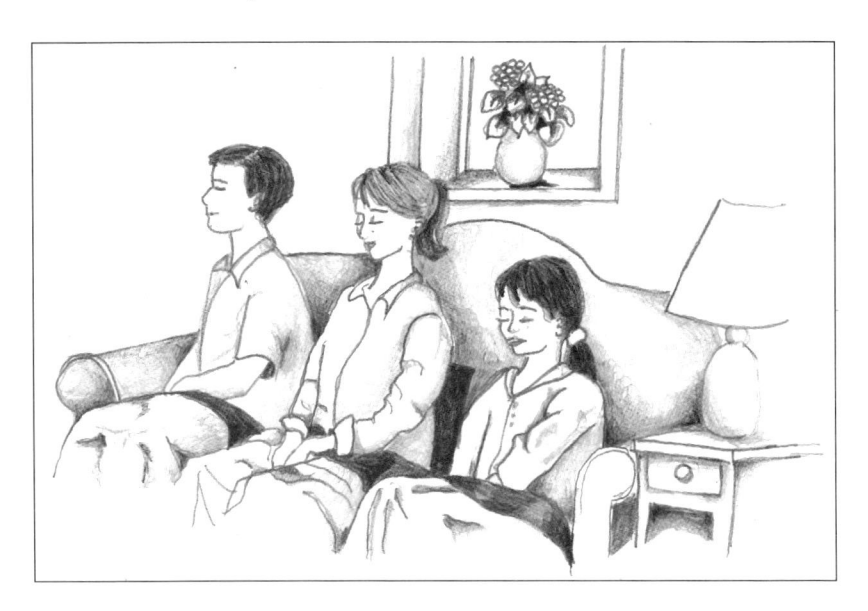

Because it does not involve any strain or effort, it is completely safe for children and free of negative side effects. It simply makes use of the natural tendency of the mind to seek greater happiness and fulfillment.

My daughters recently showed me a magazine article that professed to teach young people how to meditate. It said that basically all you need to do is find a candle and some incense, sit cross-legged, and choose some relaxing word to think about. It also said that all relaxation techniques are alike.

First of all, it is not possible to learn to meditate correctly from reading a magazine article. The Transcendental Meditation technique is based on a long tradition of teachers who have all taught the authentic technique in a prescribed, step-by-step manner. Research has shown again and again (over 600 studies at 250 research institutes in 30 countries) that the Transcendental Meditation technique, when taught by a qualified, specially trained teacher, has brought remarkable benefits to the mind, body, behavior, and the environment to more than five million people in the last five decades.

Second, a great amount of research shows that all self-development techniques are not equal. Many other techniques have not been researched at all.

Let me give you just one example of how the Transcendental Meditation technique compares to other forms of meditation. A study conducted at Stanford University compared 146 techniques of self-development and found that the Transcendental Meditation technique was more than twice as effective in reducing anxiety as techniques involving concentration, contemplation, or muscle relaxation.

Time is so precious. If you and your child are going to practice meditation each day, be sure that your time is not wasted.

Benefits for Children

Children enjoy practicing the Transcendental Meditation technique, and research shows that they gain many benefits, including increased IQ, better relationships with parents and teachers, and better health.

For Children Four to Ten Years of Age. There is a special meditation that is especially suited for the developing nervous system. The children

Reduced Anxiety

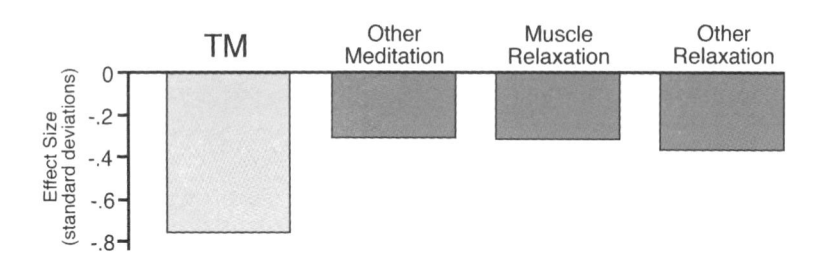

[Bar chart showing Effect Size (standard deviations) on y-axis ranging from 0 to -.8, with bars for TM (approximately -.7), Other Meditation (approximately -.3), Muscle Relaxation (approximately -.3), and Other Relaxation (approximately -.3).]

A statistical meta-analysis conducted at Stanford University of all available studies (146 independent outcomes) indicated that the effect of the Transcendental Meditation program on reducing trait anxiety was much greater than that of concentration and contemplation or forms of physical relaxation, including muscle relaxation. Analysis showed that these positive results could not be attributed to subject expectation, experimenter bias, or quality of research design.

References: 1. K. Eppley, A. Abrams, and J. Shear, "Different Effects of Relaxation Techniques on Trait Anxiety: A Meta-analysis," *Journal of Clinical Psychology* 45 (1989): pp. 957–974.
2. Michael C. Dillbeck, "The Effect of the *Transcendental Meditation* Technique on Anxiety Level," *Journal of Clinical Psychology* 33 (1977): pp. 1076–1078.

learn their Word of Wisdom℠ technique when they are old enough to keep a secret. They do not sit down to practice the technique, but practice it while they are naturally active, such as when they are moving about their room or the house.

This special technique does not help children release stress or transcend (younger children naturally release stress in sleep), but it does help the mind to focus, so the whole day goes better. Many parents notice that their children are more settled, creative, and happy after learning to practice their Word of Wisdom technique. Teachers of the Transcendental Meditation technique are also qualified to teach the Word of Wisdom technique.

Mean IQ Scores Over a One-Year Period for New Students Grades 4–11 at Maharishi School of the Age of Enlightenment

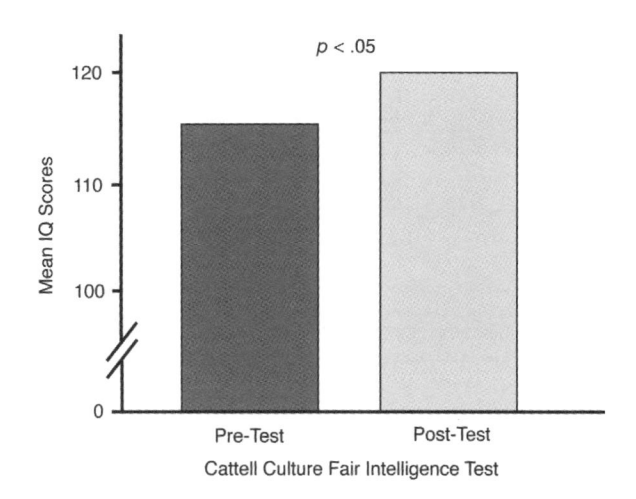

IQ scores for new students at Maharishi School of the Age of Enlightenment, grades 4 through 11, significantly increased over a one-year period. During this period an average increase of 5 IQ points was found. The norm for IQ is 100.

Reference: S.I. Nidich and R.J. Nidich, "Holistic Student Development at Maharishi School of the Age of Enlightenment: Theory and Research," *Modern Science and Vedic Science* 1 (1987): 433–470.

For Children Age Ten and Above. At age ten, children are sufficiently developed to be able to start the Transcendental Meditation technique. They practice it for shorter periods than adults, but otherwise it is the same technique. The research mentioned throughout the book refers to this technique of Transcendental Meditation.

Mean Creativity Scores for Students in Grades 5-8 at Maharishi School of the Age of Enlightenment Compared to Controls

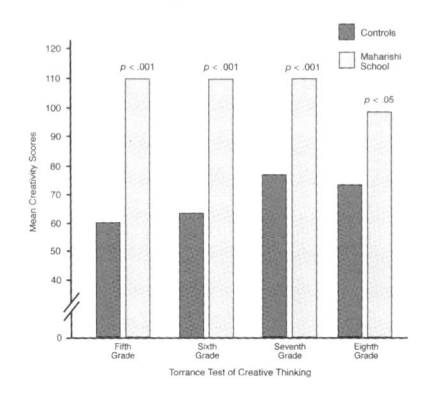

This study found differences between the mean creativity scores of students at Maharishi School of the Age of Enlightenment and controls selected from Torrance's data bank. Maharishi School of the Age of Enlightenment students at each grade level exhibited a significantly higher degree of creative thinking than controls.

Reference: S.I. Nidich and R.J. Nidich, "Holistic Student Development at Maharishi School of the Age of Enlightenment: Theory and Research," *Modern Science and Vedic Science* 1 (1987): 433–470.

By handling the most fundamental level of life, the field of natural law, the Transcendental Meditation technique develops all aspects of the healthy child, from self-concept to mind-body coordination.

Mind: Children who practice the Transcendental Meditation technique are found to improve in school achievement, clarity of thinking, creativity, IQ, concentration, moral reasoning, and field independence.

Body: One study found that people who practice the TM technique reduce doctor's visits and hospitalization by 87 percent.

Emotions: When stress is less, anxiety, depression, and negative self-image become problems of the past.

Behavior: A child's behavior is usually a direct mirror of how he or she is feeling. Children who are unhappy due to stress, fatigue, or ill health often have behavioral problems as well.

Decreased Hospitalization and Doctor Visits

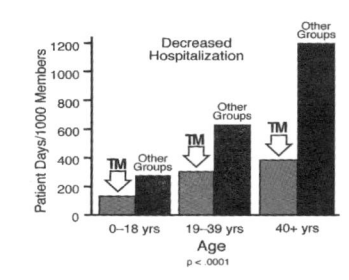

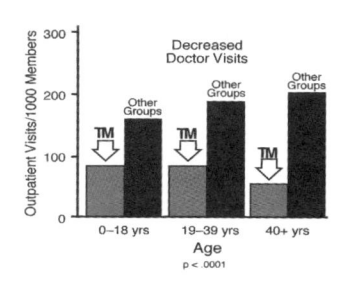

A five-year study of medical care utilization statistics on 2,000 people throughout the U.S. who regularly practice the Transcendental Meditation program found that their overall rate of hospitalization was 56% lower than the norm. The group practicing the Transcendental Meditation technique had fewer hospital admissions in all disease categories compared to the norm— including 87% less hospitalization for cardiovascular disease, 55% less for cancer, 87% less for diseases of the nervous system, and 73% less for nose, throat, and lung problems.

References: 1. *Psychosomatic Medicine* 49 (1987): 493-507.
2. *American Journal of Health Promotion*, (1996).

Healthier Family Life
1. *Psychological Reports* 51 (1982): 887–890.
2. *Journal of Counseling and Development* 64 (1986): 212–215.

Benefits for Parents

As a parent, I have found the Transcendental Meditation technique to be invaluable. I have led a busy life, returning home from my practice late in the day and facing a full evening with my family. I started the habit of meditating at my office before I returned home. This worked beautifully, because I could leave the stress of the workday behind. I found that I could create a much happier environment for my children and husband when I was more relaxed, more rested. I could really be the "two hundred percent parent" that I wanted to be: one hundred percent mother and one hundred percent professional woman.

Children enjoy meditating and find that it is an important part of the routine. They also like to remind their parents to meditate. They like to see their parents more rested and relaxed. One teenager I know remembers, "Whenever my mother was tired or unhappy or upset, I'd ask her, 'Have you meditated yet?' Then she'd laugh and do her meditation and she'd feel a lot better."

I regularly recommend the Transcendental Meditation technique to my patients. Time and time again, I have seen it resolve problems that the parents thought could never be resolved. It has a remarkable effect on all aspects of family life, and creates a healthy family environment for raising children.

The Foundation of Ideal Health

The TM technique is one of the most important techniques to unfold the full potential of the individual, and to activate the body's healing power. By enlivening nature's intelligence, it allows children and parents alike to live a more healthy life.

Although the Transcendental Meditation technique is the cornerstone treatment, all the other preventive guidelines in this book also awaken nature's intelligence. That is the beauty of this health-care system. In the following chapters you'll learn about the powerful effect of your child's food and diet on his total well-being.

PART 3

Healthy Foods, Food Supplements, and Eating Habits

CHAPTER SIX
Six Keys to a Healthy Diet

"When my daughter was two years old she had a rash on her forearms and I noticed that she kept scratching it," remembers Aisha's mother. "I put diaper rash powder and herbal creams on it, and I covered it with sterile gauze bandages. After a few weeks, I realized it wasn't getting any better. I would avoid that area during her daily Ayurvedic oil massage. It was starting to bleed when she scratched it—that's how uncomfortable she was."

Aisha's mother took her to see a health expert at a Maharishi Ayurveda Health Center, and he recommended a Kapha-Pitta reducing diet and a Maharishi Ayurveda herbal preparation.

"Within a week the eczema was gone and has never come back," she says. "Now when I see children who have eczema, my heart goes out to them because I know how uncomfortable and annoying it is. I was so happy when Aisha's rash went away with just a change in diet and some herbal supplements. It was dramatic."

Food is considered one of the pillars of Maharishi Ayurveda. If children eat the right foods, very little illness will occur. Yet there is so much controversy about food today that it is difficult to even know what foods to feed your child. Many well-meaning parents would like to do the right things, if only they knew how.

Maharishi Ayurveda takes the guesswork out of menu planning. Not only does it outline the healthiest foods for all children, but it also identifies the healthiest foods for your child as an individual. Food becomes a powerful medicine that can bring balance to the body, mind, emotions, and behavior of your child. In this chapter, you'll learn what foods bring balance to your child's individual physiology.

Creating Balance with the Six Tastes

When a child looks at a banana, he doesn't think of the calories and nutrients that it contains. Nor does he think of the food groups. These are learned behaviors that adults employ in reacting to food. A child responds to food in the most natural and healthy way. He responds to taste.

Taste is the most specific way to classify food. Maharishi Ayurveda does not categorize food by calories or food groups. Rather, it recognizes six tastes: sweet, sour, salty, bitter, astringent, and pungent. The six tastes are a very natural way to think about food, because they are derived from the five basic elements found in nature: earth (*prithivi*), water (*jala*), fire (*agni*), air (*vayu*), and space (*akasha*).

Sweet foods include not only sugar and raw honey but also rice, milk, wheat, and sweet fruits. Because they are composed of the heaviest elements, earth and water, sweet foods are heavier in nature and are grounding. Sour foods, composed of earth and fire, include lemons, grapefruits, and cheeses. Salty foods (from water and fire) are self-explanatory, but you may be surprised to learn that many vegetables also have natural salts. Pungent foods are hot and spicy, being composed of fire and air. They include chilies, cayenne, black pepper, and any spicy foods.

The sweet, sour, and salty tastes are all a common part of the modern American diet. Astringent tastes are less common. They are drying (derived from air and earth) and include legumes and dried fruits. Bitter foods, composed of air and space, are very light and include bitter salad greens and cooked, leafy greens such as spinach, Swiss chard, and kale. Most vegetables are in the bitter or astringent category.

The Six Tastes: Keys to a Healthy Diet

It's important that every meal contain a variety of foods with all six tastes. Yet within that framework of all six tastes, in the Ayurvedic diet certain tastes are increased, depending on the child's constitution, his imbalances, and the season of the year.

Taste	Elements	Food
Sweet	Earth/Water	Sugar, milk, butter, rice, breads, pasta, sweet, fruits, juicy vegetables such as squashes
Sour	Earth/Fire	Yogurt, lemon, cheese
Salty	Water/Fire	Salt and salty foods
Pungent	Fire/Air	Spicy foods, ginger, chilies, cumin, cayenne, black pepper, radishes
Bitter	Air/Space	Bitter greens (endive, parsley), leafy green vegetables (kale, spinach, chard, collard greens), sprouts, bitter gourd
Astringent	Air/Earth	Beans, lentils, pomegranate, persimmons, spinach, cabbage, broccoli, and cauliflower

How Food Creates Balance or Imbalance

As a parent, you're highly aware that children have specific likes and dislikes. You're there on the front lines every day, trying to get your child to eat what is good for him or her. You'll probably be relieved to know that Maharishi Ayurveda explains these individual preferences and makes use of them to help bring balance.

Every food will either increase or decrease balance in your child. This is because the same five elements and the same three doshas are found in food, in the human body, and in everything in nature. There are plants that are more dry and spindly, and thus are more Vata. Plants that are more succulent and moist display more Kapha. Plants that are hot and spicy contain more fire, or Pitta.

There is a major principle in Maharishi Ayurveda: "like increases like." In other words, eating Kapha-increasing foods increases Kapha dosha in the body. At the same time, the opposite quality will bring a decrease in Kapha dosha. So warm, spicy foods, which are the opposite of the cool, heavy Kapha, will decrease Kapha dosha in the body.

Let's look at an example. If your daughter has a predominance of Pitta dosha, then she has more heat in her body. With a predominance of Pitta dosha, she may exhibit a sharp intellect, leadership abilities, and excellent speaking skills. These are all the result of balanced Pitta.

But if she makes a habit of eating foods that increase Pitta (foods with more fire: spicy foods, pizza, cheese, yogurt, etc.), heat may increase too much and eventually cause health problems such as skin rashes, cold sores, or irritability. Eating a steady diet of heating foods could cause Pitta dosha to go out of balance, which, if it's untreated, could create more severe health problems such as ulcers, hypertension, and eczema.

On the other hand, you may have another child who is more Kapha, and therefore is more cool and slow by nature. He could benefit from eating more heating, spicy foods. These energizing foods could help balance his body, making him more alert and stimulated.

Here is a chart to explain how different foods affect the doshas.

How to Choose the Right Foods for Your Child

There are several factors to consider in choosing foods to bring balance.

Tastes and Qualities that Decrease Vata	Sweet, sour, salty, heavy, oily, moist, warm
Tastes and Qualities that Increase Vata	Pungent, bitter, astringent, dry, rough, light, cool
Tastes and Qualities that Decrease Pitta	Bitter, astringent, sweet, dry, soft, cool
Tastes and Qualities that Increase Pitta	Pungent, sour, salty, moist, warm, sharp, oily
Tastes and Qualities that Decrease Kapha	Pungent, bitter, astringent, dry, rough, warm
Tastes and Qualities that Increase Kapha	Sweet, sour, salty, moist, oily, cool

One is the nature of the food, another is the seasons, and another is the digestive capacity and habits of your child. Let's see how these three factors combine to bring good health to your child.

Nature of the food. This refers to the six tastes, as you have already learned. Some tastes increase Vata, Pitta, and Kapha. Other tastes decrease them.

Vata-Increasing Foods Include:	Rough, dry, hard, cold, light
Pitta-Increasing Foods Include:	Hot, sharp, sour, pungent
Kapha-Increasing Foods Include:	Cold, soft, oily, smooth, sticky, sweet

Besides tastes, there are other qualities to consider. Foods take on the quality of the environment, or habitat, that they are grown in. Foods grown in the desert, for instance, are very light. Depending on where they are grown, different foods can be heavy or light, oily or dry, soft or hard, rough or smooth, hot or cold.

Crackers are dry and rough, which means that they have more Vata. Popcorn and cold, raw vegetables are other foods that increase Vata. Bananas, soups, and white bread are soft and moist. Softness and moistness are qualities of Kapha, so these foods would increase Kapha. Hot foods increase Pitta, so hot drinks increase Pitta.

Once you know the six tastes and the qualities of food, you can add all different kinds of foods to your menu. You'll know which foods are heavy, which are light, which are Vata-aggravating, and which are Pitta- and Kapha-aggravating, etc.

The Vedic texts mention several other factors to take into account when choosing foods. One is the changing quality of food during the preparation process. Raw apples, for instance, can be quite Vata-aggravating, due to their dry and rough qualities. But when they are cooked they become soft and moist, and thus are no longer Vata-aggravating. Heating, diluting, churning, storing, maturing, flavoring, and preserving food can affect its qualities.

Another factor to consider is the combination of foods. There are a few foods that do not combine well with others. Milk, for instance, digests better when you drink it apart from other tastes. Milk is primarily a sweet taste, and combines well with other sweet foods such as cereal grains, toast, or cookies. It also is easily digested when you drink it separate from a meal, for a snack or before bed at night. Maharishi Ayurveda recommends that you avoid combining it with salty, sour tastes (especially fish), as that combination makes it indigestible. This becomes especially important for older people.

While it's ideal to boil the milk first and serve it separate from meals as a snack by itself, it's also important not to skip serving your child milk just because it's too hard to prepare. These precautions are more important if your child has trouble digesting milk or is getting frequent colds due to congestion. Many other children can digest milk with the meal even if mixed with other tastes, and this is a better solution than leaving milk out of the diet.

Foods for the Seasons

One of the most important factors to consider in choosing foods is the seasons. Children are very sensitive to the changes in weather, and their health often reflects that. In winter, most children require more food and nourishment to keep their bodies warm, and thus they need heavier, warmer, more substantial food. They can eat more ghee (clarified butter), oil, and richer foods as long as the digestion is good.

In summer, digestion often decreases in an attempt to cool the body. In this season we crave cooling, light foods. In spring, the cool and rainy weather can cause agni to be less active, and thus warming and light foods help to build up the digestive fire again. In spring, it's best to serve less heavy, oily, sweet foods that produce mucus, as children are more prone to coughs, colds, and flu then.

Foods for Kapha Kala

From birth to age thirty, children are in the Kapha Kala, and tend to have more mucus and congestion. For this reason it's especially important that they eat warm, cooked foods rather than cold foods straight

Foods to Avoid or Reduce
For Kapha Season (Spring) February–June and for Kapha Imbalance
- Cold foods and drinks
- Sweet, sour, and salty tastes
- Large quantities of food at night
- Oily and fried foods
- Ice cream or heavy desserts
- Aged, salty, hard cheeses such as cheddar, Swiss, Roquefort, and Jack
- Tofu
- Sweet potatoes, potatoes
- Yogurt in large quantities (lassi, a drink made with 1 part yogurt and 4 parts water, is fine)
- Cream, butter (ghee in moderate quantities is fine)
- Nuts
- Salt
- Avocados, bananas, pineapples, oranges, melons, plums, prunes, mangos, coconuts, apricots
- Rice and wheat that has not been aged

Foods to Avoid or Reduce
For Pitta Season (Summer) July–October and for Pitta Imbalance
- Spicy, pungent foods
- Oily foods
- Sour and vinegary foods (mustard, ketchup, salad dressings with vinegar)
- Aged, hard cheeses such as cheddar, Swiss, and Jack
- Caffeine and chocolate
- Tomatoes, hot peppers, radishes, beets, onions, and garlic
- Salty foods
- Sour cream, salty butter, yogurt (except in lassi, a drink made from 1 part yogurt and 4 parts water)
- Chili powder, cayenne, black pepper, mustard seeds, cloves, celery seeds, fenugreek
- Grapefruits, sour oranges, sour pineapples, cranberries, papayas, peaches

Foods to Avoid or Reduce
For Vata Season (Winter) November–January and for Vata Imbalance
- Light, dry, cold foods and cold drinks
- Pungent, bitter, and astringent tastes
- Raw vegetables and sprouts
- Carbonated beverages
- Barley, corn, millet, rye, buckwheat, raw oats
- Beans (except mung dhal, a legume similar to lentils) and red lentils
- Cauliflower, cabbage, broccoli, celery, green leafy vegetables, potatoes, peas

from the refrigerator. You can explain to them that warm foods are healthier for children.

Heavy foods are also a problem for children. French fries and other deep-fried foods are difficult to digest and can lead to the formation of digestive impurities (ama). Aged cheeses are also hard to digest, which is why Maharishi Ayurveda recommends fresher cheeses such as cottage cheese, cream cheese, farmer's cheese, or panir (a recipe for making this homemade cheese is given in the next chapter).

Also, refined sugar and store-bought sweets of all kinds can overwhelm the digestion. Every doctor is aware of this, especially around holiday times when sweets are eaten in greater quantities. The number of children being treated for flu, colds, and bronchitis soars right after Halloween and Easter, for instance.

Yet children certainly love sweets and should not be deprived of them. In the next chapter, you'll learn about two types of sugar, jaggary and rock sugar, that are wholesome and healthy for children because they are easy to digest and do not create ama.

Remember that Kapha dosha is the basis of most sickness in childhood. All the frequent earaches, colds, coughs, flu, allergies, sinus problems, and sore throats can be prevented by one simple principle: no cold food, no heavy food, and no refined sugar.

As soon as parents understand and apply this principle, they will have happy, healthy children. When agni is dull, it dulls the mind, body, and emotions. It manifests as lack of energy, weak digestion, constipation, and fatigue. It affects the entire child.

And it is progressive, because it leads from one stage of illness to another, more serious one. Let's say the child is not digesting what he eats. Then digestive toxins (ama) are formed and diarrhea, a cold, or a cough starts. It becomes a loop. Antibiotics and other treatments further weaken him. For some children it may not be so dramatic or traumatic, but gradually the disease builds and shows up in later years.

Foods to Avoid during Kapha Kala
Cold foods and drinks
Heavy foods
Refined sugar

Using the Six Tastes to Bring Balance

In general, it's best to feed your children a balanced, healthy diet that includes all six tastes. Children need a variety of foods, and if given the choice, will often choose foods that are best for them, unless toxins (ama) have accumulated and are distorting their body's natural signals.

At times a child will have an imbalance (*vikriti*), or perhaps by nature has one of the doshas predominating (*prakriti*). Both vikriti and prakriti will guide you in choosing the right foods. Also, during the various seasons you should adjust the diet.

One mother explains, "I generally feed my son all six tastes, but whenever he starts coming down with a cold, it really helps knowing that he should avoid sweet, heavy, Kapha-aggravating foods. If I don't let him eat rice when he has a cold, some people wonder why. But it is heavy to digest when the digestion is weak. I avoid feeding him cheeses or milk when he's sick or is starting to get sick, as these also increase Kapha. Consequently, he gets over colds very quickly. I also try to prevent colds by adjusting the diet during the cold season. In Pitta season, I definitely don't serve him hot, spicy foods like tomato sauces. I give him more cooling foods, as he has more Pitta dosha by nature and is prone to Pitta imbalances."

If your child is ill and receives a health assessment from a physician trained in Maharishi Ayurveda, he or she may recommend a Vata-pacifying, Pitta-pacifying, or Kapha-pacifying diet to bring your child's system back into balance. Let's say you have a child who is congested all the time. By looking to the nature of the child (prakriti), the physician may find that by nature he has more of the slow, heavy, Kapha qualities. Then the physician will modify the diet and recommend foods that are more Kapha-pacifying. That doesn't mean that you completely restrict your child from eating oil, or take away salt in his diet. That would be too extreme, and children need balance. But your child could decrease refined sugars, heavy sweets, ice cream, and hard cheeses, and include more astringent, bitter, and pungent tastes in his diet.

Or you may have a child who has temper tantrums and becomes angry easily, has a reddish complexion, and is always hungry. This child may need more Pitta-balancing foods (sweet, bitter, and astringent). He should avoid foods made with vinegar, such as ketchup, mustard, and pickles.

Another child might be having trouble with irregular digestion and constipation, falling asleep at night, and wildly fluctuating energy levels; for this child's needs, Vata-pacifying foods (sweet, sour, and salty) may be emphasized. Vata-related digestive problems, such as constipation, are often accepted as a natural part of childhood. Yet they are signs of an imbalance that could lead to disease if left uncorrected.

In general, to prevent disease, children with Vata disorders should avoid eating raw, heavy, hard-to-digest foods; children with Pitta predominant should avoid eating sour foods such as vinegar, mustard, ketchup, and tomato sauces; and children who are more Kapha should avoid eating too many heavy, rich foods. You can also follow the seasonal dietary recommendations to avoid seasonal illnesses.

Three Case Histories of Changed Diet

Serena, age seven, had a severe red rash on her outer ear that had started to ooze. The pulse diagnosis indicated that there was too much heat in the pulse along with an imbalance in the subdosha of Pitta associated with the blood. Her mother was advised by the physician trained in Maharishi Ayurveda to avoid feeding Serena pungent spices such as cayenne and mustard seed, as well as sour foods such as vinegar and tomatoes. Instead, he advised her to season Serena's food with spices that would help improve her digestion, such as cumin, coriander, mint, and cilantro. She also was advised to give her daughter Liver Balance™ tablets to reduce toxins in the liver and to apply an Ayurvedic oil on the affected area. By the third day, she reported that Serena's rash had completely disappeared.

Andrew, age ten, was Kapha by nature and was experiencing dullness, tightness in the stomach, gas, heaviness in the head, lack of appetite, lethargy, and a tired feeling for more than two hours after eating a meal. His pulse diagnosis revealed that Kapha dosha was disturbing the Vata functions, making the pulse heavy, dull, and sluggish. That was why Andrew was feeling dull and lethargic even three hours after a meal.

When examining his diet, the Maharishi Ayurveda health expert found that Andrew was eating large quantities of peanut butter, salty cashews, unripe bananas, cheese, and meat. The boy also did not drink much water and was not getting exercise.

For this situation, the Maharishi Ayurveda expert recommended that Andrew drink five to eight glasses of warm water each day; to stop eating bananas, nuts, and nut butters; to drink Kapha® Tea and cumin-ginger tea; to try to develop the habit of moving the bowels in the morning after rising; to follow a Kapha-pacifying diet; to exercise daily, and to take Digest Tone™ tablets (a mild herbal laxative) before bed. He also recommended that Andrew's mother add digestive spices to the food while cooking, such as Stimulating (Kapha) Spice Mix, cumin, ginger, fennel, black pepper, cinnamon, bay leaves, and parsley. After a few days, when the digestive impurities (ama) were dissolved, the black pepper was discontinued except for small amounts for seasoning.

Andrew's elimination became regular after one day, due to the Digest Tone tablets, and in one week he reported more energy, freshness, and an interest in sports. He also had a healthy appetite and was able to digest his food. The tiredness after eating was gone. After three months, he was able to discontinue the use of the Digest Tone tablets and still maintain regular elimination.

Twelve-year-old Leroy had such severe acne that it covered his whole face and even was forming into abscesses. His diet included large amounts of salsa, vinegar, ketchup, and other sour foods. He also was very constipated. His medical doctor wanted him to take antibiotics, but the mother hoped to cure it without drugs and therefore consulted a physician trained in Maharishi Ayurveda. The Maharishi Ayurveda physician identified excessive heat and heaviness in the pulse, weak digestion, accumulated ama, and an imbalance in the subdosha of Pitta that regulates the skin.

She also recommended that Leroy drink more water throughout the day, up to eight glasses, and to prepare it in a special way by bringing a quart of water to a boil and adding one teaspoon each of coriander, fennel, cardamom, and chopped fresh cilantro. Drinking this herbal water throughout the day helped to stimulate Leroy's digestion and clear away toxins (ama) without increasing Pitta dosha and the heat in his body.

The physician trained in Maharishi Ayurveda also recommended avoiding pungent spices—such as cayenne, mustard seed, black pepper, and ginger—because these aggravated Pitta dosha. Leroy was advised to stop eating sour foods, such as mustard, ketchup, and vinegar.

At the same time, Leroy's mother was advised to add mild spices to his food, such as cumin, coriander, mint, and cilantro, that would help his digestion and reduce toxins. It was also recommended that Leroy take the Maharishi Ayurveda herbal formulas Elim-Tox®-O and Aci-Balance®, which help remove toxins, reduce acidity, and improve digestion and elimination. Leroy's skin started to clear up after one week. After two weeks, his skin had completely cleared.

In this chapter, you have learned some of the principles of dietetics. It's important to first understand these fundamental principles of Maharishi Ayurveda, and then it becomes easier to apply them. If you understand that certain foods aggravate Vata, Pitta, and Kapha, then you can adjust your child's diet according to the prakriti of the child, his imbalances, the seasons, and the time of childhood.

As a parent, it's a good idea to master these simple taste principles of Maharishi Ayurveda. Once you learn them, it is easy to choose the right foods to bring balance.

The principles of Maharishi Ayurveda are universal. It doesn't matter where you live in the world; the principles remain the same. They're also very flexible, as they take into account the fluctuating doshas of the individual, as well as the seasonal, geographical, and even planetary changes. In New Mexico it's hot and dry in summer; in Iowa it's hot and humid. The winter in Miami is far different from the winter in New York. Therefore, diet and lifestyle need to be adjusted to accommodate these differences. There is no rigid schedule, no rigid protocol. The knowledge of Maharishi Ayurveda is flexible and universal.

The six tastes—the factors that determine the usefulness of food—can be found anywhere on earth. They are the same the world over. Once you understand the basic principles and structure of Maharishi Ayurveda, then you have the means to prevent future disease in your child.

CHAPTER SEVEN
Foods That Build Immunity and Foods That Destroy It

"You are what you eat" is a common expression. Yet it contains a great deal of truth. For it is through food that your child imbibes the energy and intelligence of nature. If the food is of good quality, it will create a healthy body and strong immunity. If it is of poor quality or of the wrong type, it will create ill health. Quite literally, the food your child eats today becomes his body tomorrow. Food has consciousness, and it is this vital energy that gets transformed into matter.

Public health officials recognize the importance of food for mental functioning, which is why children who do not receive breakfast at home are served it in schools. It is very difficult for a hungry or undernourished child to focus. Lack of proper proteins and nutrients can cause dizziness, anger, anxiety, apathy, and lack of focus.

Maharishi Ayurveda takes this idea a step further, recognizing that a wholesome, happy, healthy child is quite literally a product of a wholesome, happy, healthy diet. Wholesome food is not only nourishing to the body, it is nourishing to all aspects of life: mind, body, emotions, senses, and spirit. The entire brain and body are built from the nutritive material created by digested food, and their quality depends on the quality of the food eaten. Different foods affect mood and emotions in different ways. Too much sugar can cause some children to feel hyperactive, while it causes others to become more dull and sleepy. Spicy foods can increase anger. The right foods can make a child happier, more contented, more relaxed. Good food is healing; it balances the doshas and prevents disease.

How a Wholesome Diet Can Heal a Child

I can't emphasize enough how important it is that children eat a wholesome diet. Nadia, an eight-year-old girl with eczema, comes to mind. Her eczema usually would get worse during the winter months. Since she was involved in sports, her skin would break out every time she sweated and the rash would remain for weeks at a time. It was very ugly, all over her arms, and was becoming a continuous occurrence. She was treated by several dermatologists and with various prescription medications without much relief. When she first came to me I realized that she was eating a number of foods that were contributing to her eczema. She often ate french fries, hamburgers, peanut butter sandwiches, soda, and ketchup. That was her staple diet. She also had very dry skin.

The first visit was really about changing the diet and educating Nadia and her mother about foods that would tend to cause eczema. I recommended that Nadia start coconut oil massage and herbal salves to stop the itching and dryness. She was also given Maharishi Ayurveda herbal formulas to bring balance to her doshas and eliminate toxins (ama) from the blood and the skin.

Nadia responded quickly, within a few weeks. The diet alone made a difference. And even at such a young age, she was able to recognize which foods really aggravated her problem—for example, the ketchup, mustard, tomato sauces, and cured meats. She gradually became symptom-free.

After a six-month period of remission, Nadia's symptoms started to recur, because she had reverted to the same eating mode as before. Also, she was experiencing stress in school, which aggravated her outbreak. I advised her mother that she follow up with regular checkups, because skin disease like eczema is chronic and whenever there is an opportunity, the disease will show up in the skin. Since that time Nadia's parents have brought her to me every three months and for the most part she has been in remission. Even if she gets a rash on occasion, it is very mild and lasts only one or two days.

Immunity-Boosting Foods

Nutrition plays an important role in the developing human immune system. This is especially true during gestation. Undernourished, low-birth-weight babies show persistent immunological impairment for several months, even years.

Food is especially vital for the growing child. Every day your child is building bones, muscles, and brain cells at a rapid rate. You'll remember that in Chapter Four we described how food gets converted into the seven dhatus, and becomes the flesh, bones, blood, and muscles of the body. The more fresh the food is, the more consciousness it has, the more quickly it is converted into ojas. And remember, ojas is directly related to immunity. The more wholesome the foods your child eats, the greater his immunity will be.

Because the amount of ojas is directly linked to the level of immunity, offering children ojas-producing foods should be the highest priority for parents. Here are five ways to increase the amount of ojas in your child's diet to boost immunity.

1. Choose fresh foods.

In order to create ojas, food must be fresh to start with, the fresher the better. In Maharishi Ayurveda, there is the concept of *prana* or "life force." Some foods contain more prana than others, and these are the foods that nourish both the body and mind.

Frozen, canned, packaged, and processed food has very little prana, and is therefore difficult to digest. If your child eats a steady diet of these foods, the result will be ama.

As a physician, it is easy for me to see which children are eating fresh, home-cooked meals and which children are eating processed, frozen, or canned foods. Signs of digestive toxic buildup (ama) in children include drowsiness, fatigue, a pale color, and lack of enthusiasm. Children who eat fresh foods tend to have rosy cheeks, sparkling eyes, and buoyant energy, not to mention less sickness and disease. Just by converting your child's diet to fresh foods, you can increase his health and vitality immeasurably.

Foods that are packaged are not only old and lacking in prana, but they likely have many harmful additives and preservatives. A rule of thumb for choosing food: the more natural, whole, unprocessed, and unadulterated the food is, the healthier it will be for your child.

2. Serve regular meals of warm, cooked food.

Raw food is difficult to digest and can cause a Vata imbalance. Although many people believe that there are more vitamins in raw foods than in cooked ones, the problem is that the raw foods are hard to digest and assimilate. A preliminary study presented at the American Chemical Society showed that the antioxidant beta carotene—which exists in carrots, broccoli, and spinach and has been found to combat tissue damage and plaque in arteries—is absorbed 34 percent more easily in cooked and pureed carrots than in raw ones. The researchers concluded that cooking vegetables softens the plant tissue, allowing antioxidants to be released.

It's better to serve children warm, delicious, attractive, and wholesome meals that have been cooked by someone who loves them. The warmth is essential for proper digestion, and helps avoid the buildup of ama. Children, being in the Kapha time of life, find warm foods especially soothing and helpful to the digestive process.

Avoid serving your child food straight from the refrigerator. It's better to serve warm drinks or warm water, fresh-cooked foods, and room-temperature fruits. Fresh salads made with grated carrot, ginger, fresh parsley, and cilantro are fine in small quantities to tone the appetite before the meal, if the child has strong digestion. (Grating makes vegetables more absorbable.)

3. Whenever possible, provide home-cooked meals for your child.

There is no better medicine than mother's home-cooked meals. Just as fresh food has more prana, so does food that is lovingly prepared without rushing. And the most important element of food is preparing it with love. As a mother, you put so much love into a meal. The mother's love is pure ojas to the child. A mother's food is, for that reason, recognized as the most nourishing in every culture in the world.

I'm sure many of you are thinking, "but I don't have time to cook elaborate meals using all natural ingredients!" Many of you are working mothers, and as a working mother myself, I know how difficult it is to prepare a hot supper after a long day on the job.

I would suggest that you start by adding just one more home-cooked meal a week. If you already cook twice a week, try cooking three times. If you don't cook at all, try just one meal. Instead of picking up food at a restaurant, instead of popping a frozen pizza in the oven, try to cook a simple meal of fresh vegetables, grains, and legumes. The next chapter contains some menus, recipes, and ideas.

Then see how your family reacts. Do they appreciate your efforts? Are the children more satisfied, more settled after eating? How do you feel when you eat fresher, more lovingly prepared foods? How do your children feel? Are they more relaxed, more focused?

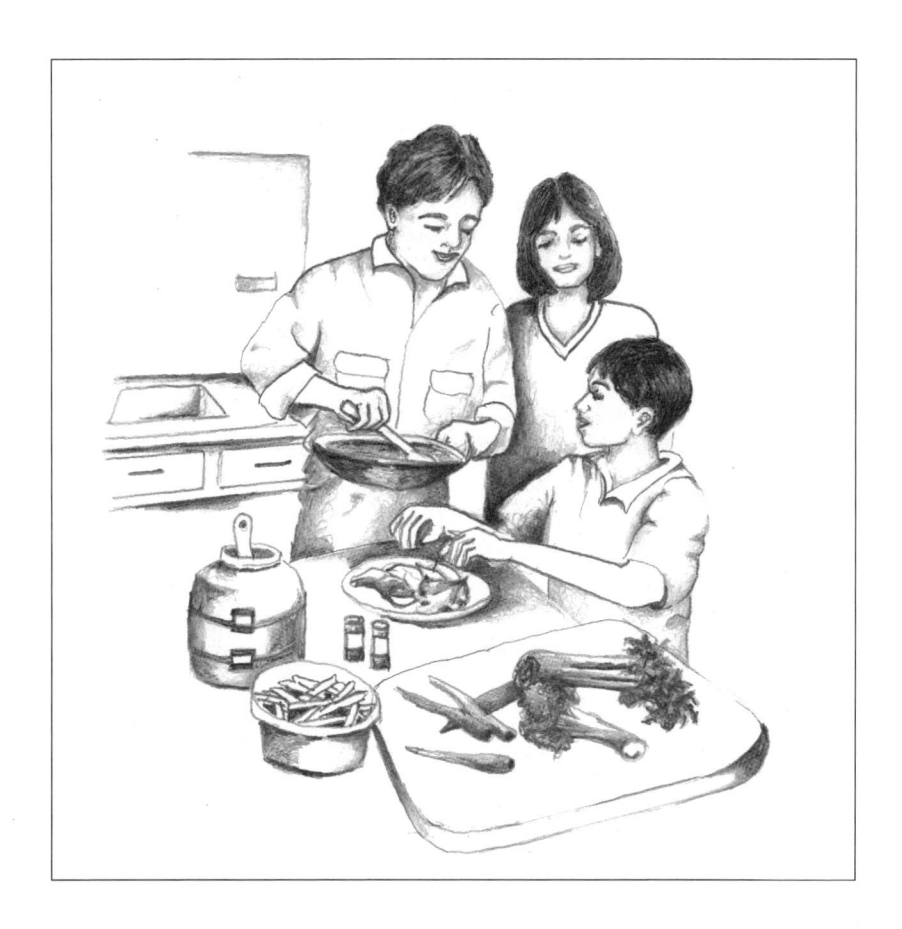

Then gradually add another home-cooked meal, and another. One thing I know about cooking—the more you do it, the easier it gets. If you just have in your mind that you are committed to cooking more, you will find ways to do it. Once you are committed to the idea, then it just becomes a matter of finding the easiest way to carry out your plan. For instance, you can enlist your older children and husband to help. Some families enjoy cooking together, and make the preparation of meals a family project.

The other problem is school lunches. If your child is eating institutionally prepared meals at school, the fact is that he or she is eating food that is not fresh. It may even be harmful. School cafeterias are notorious for using canned, frozen, and packaged foods, which are often laced with preservatives and other chemicals. Children usually complain about such food, calling it all sorts of unpleasant names. Most adults would not eat the food that is served in many school cafeterias.

I am not bringing this problem up to make you feel guilty. I am bringing it up because I know that if parents get passionate enough about something, they can do amazing things. You can band together with other parents and get the food in your child's cafeteria changed. Or you can try to provide your child with a thermos of nourishing soup or other hot food from home. The main point is to first recognize the problem. The solution will make itself known.

4. Include sattvic foods in your child's diet.

In Maharishi Ayurveda, certain foods are known to convert more quickly into ojas. These are called *sattvic* foods, sattvic meaning "pure." These ojas-producing foods nourish the growing child's tissues, organs, and brain. It's a good idea to include these in your child's diet, because they help build the physiology and enhance immunity.

Sattvic foods also encourage sattvic tendencies in the personality. There is an Ayurvedic saying, "As is the food, so is the quality of one's mind." Maharishi Ayurveda identifies three gunas, or qualities, in nature: sattva, rajas, and tamas. Sattva is the creative quality, rajas spurs and maintains activity, and tamas is the destructive quality.

A sattvic nature is one that is more creative, more positive, more contented, and happier. Sattvic foods cultivate these qualities. Sattvic foods create energy, rosy cheeks, sparkly eyes, and immunity to disease.

Here are some of the most sattvic, life-enhancing foods for children.

Milk: In Maharishi Ayurveda, milk is considered to be the most healthy, wholesome, and essential food for children. Milk contains all six tastes and quickly converts to ojas. Of course, today there is a huge controversy concerning cow's milk for children. Many pediatricians are concerned with milk allergies.

It's possible that many of the problems modern children face when drinking milk are due to the hormones injected in the cows who give the milk and the additives added in processing. For this reason, it's best to drink organic milk. Many children who have milk allergies find organic milk easy to digest.

Boiling milk with fresh ginger also helps make it more digestible and removes some of the Kapha-creating qualities. You could add a small amount of cardamom or powdered ginger to make it easier to digest. It's best to drink milk separate from sour, salty, or spicy foods, because these make the milk curdle in the stomach and impair its digestion. Milk is more digestible when served alone, as a snack, or with sweet foods such as cereals or cookies.

One mother says, "When my son was younger, he had a milk sensitivity. So it really helped to boil his milk with ginger, as then he could digest it. One simple key from Maharishi Ayurveda—to boil the milk with mild spices—can really make a difference."

Milk builds strong bones and bodies. A recent report by the American Academy of Orthopedic Surgeons notes that one of the best protective factors for osteoporosis is drinking milk and eating other dairy products such as yogurt regularly during childhood. Ninety to 95 percent of bone mass is formed before the age of twenty, so children need to eat plenty of calcium and exercise regularly to build up a reserve of bone mass to last throughout life.

Unfortunately, many children today are deficient in calcium, perhaps because they drink more juice and soda instead of milk. Research shows that most children under five years of age get only about 46 percent of the recommended daily allowance amount of calcium.

Even though they have much smaller body mass, the daily serving of calcium recommended for children is almost the same as for adults, which amounts to two or three servings of milk per day. Besides milk and milk products, green leafy vegetables such as broccoli, kale, turnip greens, and Chinese cabbage, as well as kidney beans, almonds, and sesame seeds are good sources of calcium. Vitamin D is also important to enable calcium to be absorbed properly. It can be obtained by getting plenty of sunshine or by drinking milk fortified with vitamin D. Maharishi Ayurveda recommends whole milk for children unless your child has weak digestion or a weight problem.

Everything should be done in moderation, of course. If your child has a Kapha imbalance and is developing colds and mucus, you may need to add a small amount of water to his milk or he should drink less of it than other children for a while. And to reduce Kapha dosha, avoid serving ice-cold milk in any season.

Ghee (clarified butter): This healthy cooking oil and spread for breads is highly recommended by Maharishi Ayurveda for its ojas-producing qualities. Ghee helps digestion and elimination and makes the complexion clear and bright. It is considered the supreme cooking oil because of its health-giving qualities.

Even though ghee is technically a saturated fat, its molecular structure differs from other animal fats, because it is a short-chain fatty acid (easily assimilated by the body) rather than a long-chain fatty acid (not metabolized by the body and leading to cancer and blood clots). It is much more nourishing and, if used in moderation, does not raise cholesterol.

Ghee is especially important for children to eat because it nourishes the developing brain. It's also a carrier. When you sauté healthy spices in ghee, their nutritional qualities are carried to the cells by the ghee.

Ghee has the following remarkable qualities:
- Contains 8 percent lower saturated fatty acids than any other edible oil or fat. This makes it the easiest fat to digest.
- Has no protein casein (it is removed during the preparation of ghee). Studies on animals have shown that protein casein raises cholesterol levels.
- Contains antioxidant vitamins A and E. Ghee is the only edible vegetarian fat that contains vitamin A (for meat eaters, fish oil also contains vitamin A). These antioxidants in the fat help prevent the formation of lipid peroxides, which trigger the process of arterio-

sclerosis and cause damage to DNA in the cells. According to one study, ghee does not contain cholesterol oxidation products.
- Contains 4 to 5 percent linoleic acid, an essential fatty acid that promotes growth and development of the body's tissues and organs. "Essential fatty acid" means that the body cannot produce the fat itself, and must ingest linoleic acid in foods in order to function properly.
- Remains fresh for three or four months when stored at room temperature, removing the risk of rancidity and oxidation.
- Contains high levels of conjugated linoleic acid (CLA) isomers, which may have anticarcinogenic properties.

Ghee is made by boiling butter and removing the solids. Once the solids are removed, the clear, purified substance that remains is ghee. Ghee is healthy because unlike butter it doesn't burn when heated, and thus is safe for preparing sautéed spices and vegetables. You can also use the ghee like butter to spread on toast or sandwiches. You do not need to refrigerate ghee. It will be semisolid at room temperature.

To make ghee, you simmer organic, unsalted butter until the milk solids sink to the bottom. What is left is a clear, golden liquid.

Here's a recipe. You can also purchase ghee at Indian groceries or at many health food stores.

Ghee

1. Place one or more pounds of unsalted, organic butter in a deep stainless steel or glass pan. Melt the butter on medium-to-low heat.

2. Keep simmering the butter for thirty to forty minutes on medium-to-low heat until the water boils away. Milk solids will appear on the surface and eventually sink to the bottom of the pan.

3. As soon as the milk solids turn golden brown at the bottom of the pan, remove the pan from the heat. You can often tell it's ready because the ghee smells like popcorn and tiny bubbles rise from the bottom and burst on the surface. Be alert so the butter doesn't burn.

4. Pour the hot liquid through a cheesecloth or fine-mesh strainer into a heatproof bowl or another stainless steel pan. Be careful not to splash yourself with the hot ghee.

5. Pour the ghee into smaller, condiment-size jars and store at room temperature. Keep a jar handy by the stove to use as cooking oil.

Fresh yogurt: This is another sattvic food that you can make at home. Yogurt increases digestive strength and helps foster friendly bacteria (acidophilus) in the digestive tract.

Yogurt becomes fermented and ama-producing when it is old, so it's best to make it fresh. You can make yogurt easily in a thermos, or you can purchase an electric yogurt maker at a kitchen supply store.

Lassi: Yogurt has some heavy and sour qualities, and may aggravate Pitta or Kapha dosha when eaten regularly. It becomes suitable for balancing all the doshas if you make it into a drink called lassi (pronounced lah-see).

Lassi is an excellent digestive aid after meals, and children like its frothy, creamy texture, especially when flavored with raw honey.

Fresh Yogurt

It works best to start the yogurt the night before you're going to eat it, after the evening meal. To make yogurt, bring the desired amount of organic, unhomogenized milk to a boil and let it boil for 10 minutes with a few slices of ginger. Then let the milk cool until it is slightly warmer than body temperature (around 40° C or 99° F). Pour the milk into a thermos or a yogurt maker. Add 1 tablespoon of yogurt culture per 1 cup of milk (you can purchase a plain, natural commercial brand of yogurt at the store for this). Do not stir.

If you use a thermos, just seal the top and the yogurt will be solid by morning. If you use a yogurt maker, plug it in, and the yogurt should be ready by morning. Save a small amount of yogurt as starter for the next day's batch.

> **Lassi**
>
> To make lassi, put 1/4 cup yogurt with 1 cup water in a blender and blend. Add cumin, ginger, and salt if you want a Vata-pacifying lassi. For a Pitta-pacifying lassi, add a small amount of Rose Petal Preserve™ or raw honey, cardamom, and rose water. Add ginger and raw honey for a Kapha-pacifying lassi. For any lassi, keep the proportion of water to yogurt about 4:1.

Panir: Panir is a fresh cheese you can easily make at home. It is an excellent source of protein, and because it is fresh and not aged, it is a sattvic dairy food.

> **Panir**
>
> 3 quarts whole or low-fat milk (organic if possible)
> 2 cups plain, natural-style yogurt or 1/4 cup fresh lemon juice
>
> Pour the milk into a large 4-quart saucepan. Turn the heat to medium high. When the milk begins to boil lightly, add 3 tablespoons of lemon juice or 1 and 1/2 cups of plain yogurt. Stir in well. Then monitor the mixture, stirring occasionally as it begins to curdle. You'll know when the milk curdles, as the white curds will visibly separate from the whey (a clear, yellow liquid). If after three to five minutes the milk has not curdled, make sure that the heat is high enough for the mixture to be slightly boiling. If it still does not curdle, add another 1/2 tablespoon of lemon juice or another 1/2 to 2/3 cup of yogurt.
>
> Once the curds form, pour the curdled milk through a cheesecloth or fine wire sieve. Save the whey for soups or rice. You can hang the cheesecloth from your faucet to drain for an hour, or else you can squeeze the excess whey through the cheesecloth once the curds are cool enough.

One way to eat panir is to cut it into cubes and sauté it in ghee. Add it to spiced vegetables or rice. Or, you can just crumble it into salads, add it to casseroles, or use it on pizza.

Split mung dhal soup: Split mung dhal (also spelled dal), available in Indian grocery stores, is a good source of protein, and is easier to digest than other beans. (Note that these are not whole mung beans, which come in their green skins, but are peeled, split, and yellow in color.)

Mung Dhal Soup
(Serves a family of 4)

1 cup organically grown split mung dhal
5 cups water
1 teaspoon salt
1 teaspoon ground turmeric
1 tablespoon ghee
1/2 teaspoon black mustard seeds
1/2-inch fresh ginger, peeled and grated
1 teaspoon cumin seeds
1 teaspoon ground coriander
1 tablespoon fresh cilantro leaves
1 teaspoon lemon juice

Rinse dhal. Place dhal in 5 cups of water. Add the salt and turmeric. Bring to a boil. Watch that it doesn't boil over. A foam will rise to the top; remove the foam and lower the temperature to a low boil. Cook for 20 minutes or more if you would like a thicker consistency. In a separate frying pan melt the ghee. Add black mustard seeds, cumin, and ginger. When the mustard seeds begin to pop, remove the pan from the heat or they may burn. Add the coriander and stir. Add the spice mixture to the dhal. Garnish with lemon juice and cilantro leaves.

Serve over rice or plain with a chapati (flat bread). You can also add a variety of diced vegetables to make a hearty vegetable soup.

Rice and whole grains: Food digests more easily if the taste buds are stimulated (the aroma of tasty food actually starts the flow of digestive juices in the stomach, aiding digestion). Rice, wheat, fresh fruits and vegetables, whole grains, ground almonds, and sweet herbs and spices are other nourishing, healthy, sattvic foods recommended by Maharishi Ayurveda. These foods are light and easy to digest, yet are nourishing and healthy.

Barley, bulgur wheat, rye, amaranth, and quinoa are ancient grains that have energizing, nutrient-packed properties. Quinoa even contains some protein. These grains can be cooked similarly to a rice pilaf, by sautéing the grain in melted ghee and spices, and then adding two parts water to one part grain. Bring to a boil for ten minutes, then cover and continue cooking at low to medium heat for twenty more minutes. The ghee is important, as otherwise the grain will be too drying.

Spices and herbs such as turmeric, cumin, coriander, cilantro, basil, mint, fresh ginger, and fennel aid digestion, energize the body, and make the food more appetizing—and thus should be included in the daily diet. For these reasons, Maharishi Ayurveda recommends spicing vegetables rather than just steaming them and serving them bland. For instance, you can sauté spices in a little ghee and then add steamed veggies and sauté them with the spices. Cooking the spices first in ghee is recommended even if you are adding them to soup, as this releases their energy and enhances flavor. Calming (Vata) Spice Mix, Cooling (Pitta) Spice Mix, and Stimulating (Kapha) Spice Mix are delicious spice mixtures that contain all six tastes, balance the doshas, and make cooking delicious vegetables easy.

Jaggary, rock sugar, or raw honey as sweeteners: In general, cold, heavy desserts like ice cream should be avoided because these foods put out the digestive fire. It's also best to make desserts without refined sugar, because it's difficult to digest and causes ama. Use jaggary or rock sugar instead. Jaggary, unrefined cane sugar, is best because it creates some heat in the body to stimulate the digestion. Rock sugar is also good, because it is balancing to all three doshas. You can purchase jaggary and rock sugar at Indian groceries. Another more easily available sweetener is Sucanat, which is an unrefined form of sugar cane with some heating qualities similar to jaggary. It's available in health food stores.

Honey is a sattvic food and a wonderful sweetener on toast or cereal. However, Ayurvedic texts recommend that honey be eaten raw. It should not be cooked as it becomes toxic when cooked. For cooking you can use raw sugar, barley syrup or rice syrup, but not honey. Also, honey should not be combined in equal quantities with ghee, as that makes it indigestible. For this reason, it's better not to serve ghee and honey together on toast.

Remember that it is the heavy, cold, indigestible foods that give rise to many of the common childhood illnesses, including colds, coughs, tonsillitis, adenoiditis, ear infections, and flu. They block the srotas (micro-channels of communication) and cause manda agni (weakness) in the digestive tract. They cause manda agni at the cellular level as well, which results in weakened metabolism and disrupts the healthy formation of body tissue. Sugar contains no vitamins, minerals, or fiber. Its "empty calories" take up the stomach space your growing child needs for healthy foods. It also causes tooth decay. Research indicates that sugar suppresses the immune system, which is explained in Ayurvedic terms by the extra production of toxins (ama).

5. Feed your child healthy fats.

Some parents are confused about fats, thinking that they should limit fats even in very young children in order to keep their cholesterol down. This can be very damaging to the child, and can even cause "wasting disease." The brain itself is over half fat by weight. At birth a newborn's brain contains only 30 percent of the billions of brain cells that it will need as an adult. Your child's brain acquires 95 percent of its brain cells by age eighteen months—a phenomenal rate of growth.

This shows how essential a diet rich in fat is for the growing infant, and why fat-rich breast milk is perfectly programmed by nature to provide exactly the right kind of fat and the right proportion to fulfill this need. It also shows why infants and toddlers need more fat than adults, with infants twelve months and younger needing half their calories in fat, toddlers from one to three years needing 35 percent of their calories in fat, and from three to six years, 30 percent of their calories in fat. In contrast, adults need less than 30 percent of their diet to contain fat. Thus infants and children under three years of age need high-fat diets to grow properly, and this is best provided through mother's milk, cow's milk, and ghee.

Besides feeding your child's growing brain, fat is essential for building the bones and muscles. Fats help membrane development, cell formation, and cell differentiation. Fat protects against mutations in the cells and contains antioxidants.

But it's essential to choose healthy fats that do not raise LDL cholesterol or create other imbalances in the body. As we mentioned above, Maharishi Ayurveda recommends ghee as the most healthy and sattvic cooking oil and as a spread to replace butter. Here are some other healthy oils to use.

Olive Oil: Extra-virgin, first cold-pressed olive oil is also recommended. Other types of olive oil are heated, which destroys nutrients and increases free radical content. To prevent free radical damage, olive oil should not be heated above 302° F when cooking. This is why, in many parts of Italy, olive oil is traditionally added to pasta and vegetables after cooking to flavor the food. Olive oil can be used in bread recipes, as baking only raises the temperature inside the bread to 221° F. This is low enough to avoid destroying its positive properties.

Extra-virgin, first cold-pressed olive oil is the only commercially produced, mass-marketed oil available that has not had its properties destroyed by heat, chemicals, and refining. One of the advantages of olive oil is that it stores well in a cool, dark place, and does not lose its nutritional properties unless overheated or exposed to light.

Extra-virgin olive oil is especially good for Kapha types, because it is lighter and less fattening than other oils and fats such as ghee. It is a monounsaturated fat, does not raise blood cholesterol, and has been shown to lower cardiovascular risks. Olive oil also tastes good in salad dressings.

Other healthy oils: Essential fatty acids are fats that the body cannot produce and must obtain from food. These are essential in the sense that without them, the body cannot function properly. Flaxseed oil, hemp-seed oil, safflower, sunflower, and sesame oils all contain varying amounts of essential fatty acids. However, flaxseed and hemp-seed oils are extremely fragile, and their essential fatty acids are destroyed when exposed to heat, light, or air. They must be stored in the refrigerator, cannot be used at all for cooking, and should be used within three weeks of opening. Flaxseed oil is not recommended in Maharishi Ayurveda because of its heating effect on the liver. Instead, grind fresh golden flaxseed in a spice grinder and add a teaspoon to the food.

Safflower, sunflower, and sesame seed oil are polyunsaturated oils, which are low in cholesterol but create excessive free radicals, which is why they are not often recommended in Maharishi Ayurveda.

Unfortunately, most of the safflower, sunflower, and sesame oils you buy commercially (and even in health food stores) have been prepared using heat, light, harmful solvents, and chemicals, and thus are not nutritionally sound. If you do use them, make sure they are pressed mechanically without heat, light, or chemical processing and are organic and pesticide-free. Because oil becomes rancid easily, oils should be stored in opaque containers in a cool, dark place.

You may be able to find unheated, unrefined, organic oils in your health food store. Check to see if the different oils are all the same color; if so, then they have been over-processed and are harmful to the body. When processed mechanically without heat, chemicals, or light, the oils of different seeds take on different colors and hues.

Canola oil is a monounsaturated fat, but unfortunately, much of it is now genetically engineered and therefore not recommended, especially for children, unless it is organically grown (which means the seeds are not genetically modified) and processed mechanically, without heat.

Whole seeds and nuts: Healthy sources of oils and essential fatty acids for children are whole nuts and seeds. Sesame, sunflower, and pumpkin seeds are delicious, as are blanched almonds, walnuts, and organic soybeans (in the form of tofu, flour, or oil). They are also a good source of protein. (Cashews tend to be fatty and constipating, and should not be eaten in large quantities. Peanuts are not recommended.) Nuts are more digestible when soaked overnight, then ground and added to dishes.

Vegetables: Dark-green vegetables such as spinach, parsley, and broccoli also contain small quantities of essential fatty acids. Actually, all whole, fresh, unprocessed foods contain some amount of essential fatty acids.

Avocados, for instance, are a good source of essential fatty acids. Herbs such as rosemary and thyme also contain essential oils.

Foods to Avoid

Just as there are foods that boost immunity, there are foods that create the opposite effect. Called tamasic foods, these contain very little life force (prana) or nutrition. Rather than increasing ojas, these foods are hard to digest and create ama, the sticky waste product of digestion. Eating a diet heavy in these foods could cause a decrease in immunity and eventually result in disease.

Tamasic foods are those that are not recommended for any body type because they have negative effects on everyone. These include foods that are fermented (such as alcohol) and foods that are old, such as leftovers and packaged, canned, and frozen foods. They also include foods such as vinegar, mushrooms, red meat, aged cheeses, and charred or burned foods.

A Vegetarian Diet Is Healthier

The health benefits of a vegetarian diet have only recently become widely known in America. Yet a high-fiber, low-animal-meat diet has been the norm for most of the world's population throughout time, and is the diet recommended by Maharishi Ayurveda for most people.

There are several reasons for this recommendation. One is that red meat is difficult to digest, and often creates ama, which collects in the colon as undigested waste material. In fact, eating a diet high in red meat is recognized today as a major risk factor for colon cancer. The National Cancer Institute pinpoints wrong diet as the cause of one-third of all cancer deaths and the cause of eight out of ten of the most common cancers. In one study, vegetarians were 40 percent less likely to die of cancer than a control group of people with a similar lifestyle but meat-eating diet. Other diseases linked to eating red meat include osteoporosis, kidney stone formation, and kidney disease. Beef, pork, and chicken raised in the U.S. is often injected with harmful hormones and antibiotics. This makes it unsafe and unhealthy for children.

> **Health Benefits of a Vegetarian Diet**
> Lower rates of cancer, especially colon and lung cancer
> Lower rates of heart disease
> Lower blood pressure
> Less risk of diabetes
> Fewer gallstones
> Less kidney disease and kidney stones
> Less colon disease
> Less osteoporosis
> Less obesity

According to Maharishi Ayurveda, the effects of eating meat may be even more widespread. Because it is difficult to digest, meat often creates ama, the cause of a wide range of diseases.

There are many other advantages to the vegetarian diet. Vegetarian children eat more high-fiber foods, more nutrient-rich fruits and vegetables, and less saturated fat than nonvegetarian children. While fat is certainly essential for the growth of young children, vegetarians eat less of the harmful cholesterol-causing saturated fat and consequently have lower cholesterol levels and less of a problem with obesity. A diet high in saturated fat and cholesterol has been cited as a risk factor for diseases such as diabetes, cardiovascular disease, and cancer. The death rate from cardiovascular disease of vegetarians is only one-fourth that of meat-eaters.

Vegetarians also consume more antioxidants and phytonutrients—the biologically active, nonnutritive plant components that exist in plant foods and help boost immunity and are thought to help protect the body against diseases such as cancer.

Eating Enough Protein, Iron, and Other Nutrients

Many parents worry that their children will not get enough protein with a vegetarian diet. Yet some of the healthiest cultures in the world eat a diet that is low in animal protein and high in complex carbohydrates and fiber (a diet which has been shown to protect against cancer, high cholesterol levels, and heart disease). Children who eat well-balanced vegetarian diets grow at the same rate as nonvegetarian children. Research shows that vegetarian children are similar in height to meat-eating children, being on average one-third-inch shorter, and less obese. One study on Seventh Day Adventist vegetarian children showed that these children were taller than nonvegetarian children.

However, modern vegetarian mothers do need to focus on providing enough protein, iron, and B vitamins in the child's diet. First of all, let me clarify that the traditional diet recommended by Maharishi Ayurveda is lacto-vegetarian, which means that it includes dairy products. These are an important source of protein, calcium, and vitamin B12 for the vegetarian child. The parents in my practice who are raising their children as lacto-vegetarians find it possible to meet their child's protein needs with milk and dairy products, soy proteins such as tofu and tempeh, and a variety of legumes such as garbanzo beans and lentils. Soup can also be made with a variety of legumes, such as split mung beans, channa dhal, split peas, and others. Nuts and seeds such as almonds, cashews, pecans, walnuts, and pumpkin, sunflower, and sesame seeds are also good sources of protein.

The key is serving a wide variety of protein sources, because then even if one protein source does not have all the amino acids, over the course of a day your child can eat a combination of all the amino acids from a variety of foods. Each day, a child should have at least three servings of dairy plus legumes, nuts, and seeds. (Peanuts and peanut butter should be avoided, as they aggravate all three doshas and are considered tamasic foods. Many children also have severe allergic reactions to fungus on peanuts.)

Another area of concern to many parents is obtaining enough iron with a vegetarian diet. Iron is essential for developing motor skills, IQ, and athletic endurance. Even a short bout of mild anemia can have a detrimental effect on young brains, and one in seven American children suffers from iron deficiency. Vegetarians can obtain enough iron from dried beans, dried peas, mung dhal, soybeans and soy products, whole grains, wheat germ, iron-enriched breads, cream of wheat, cream of rice, oatmeal, prune juice, dried apricots, and leafy greens such as spinach and Swiss chard. Again, the key is serving a wide variety of whole grains, vegetables, and legumes. Cooking food in cast-iron cookware also increases iron in food.

Vitamins B12 and B6 are difficult to obtain in a vegetarian diet. Normal levels of vitamin B12 can be obtained from three servings of dairy per day. Vitamin B6 is found in whole grains, whole-grain cereal, sunflower seeds, prunes, hazelnuts, walnuts, potatoes, bananas, dried apricots, currants, soy, raisins, spinach, broccoli, and other vegetables and fruits.

If you are concerned that your child is not eating enough of these foods, consult your physician to make sure that your child is receiving enough protein, iron, and B vitamins from his diet.

As for other vitamins and minerals, you can see that in many ways, by eating a balanced vegetarian diet, with a wide variety of fresh vegetables, fruits, dairy products, whole grains, and nuts and seeds, it is actually easier to fulfill most of your child's nutritional needs than if a child is eating a meat-rich diet, or is eating a lot of empty calories in junk food or packaged foods. Vitamin C and beta-carotene, a precursor to vitamin A, for instance, can only be obtained from plant sources.

How to Make the Transition to a Vegetarian Diet

If you want to make the switch to a vegetarian diet, it's better not to do it all at once. Changing a habit takes time. You can start by introducing vegetarian meals several times a week. When you do serve meat, try serving chicken and fish instead of red meat. Chicken or fish is more digestible when served in soups. Gradually reduce the amount of chicken and fish in dishes, adding more vegetables until you are serving no red meat and no chicken or fish.

In making the transition, you can watch out for the vegetarian foods your children like, and serve those foods. Start by finding recipes for favorite American foods, such as veggie burgers, french fries, and vegetarian pizza (see recipes next chapter).

Explain to your children why these new foods are more nutritious. You can tell them why you think a vegetarian diet is healthier. This is true for all dietary changes that you make. Don't just say "white bread is bad for you." Children respond better when you explain that whole wheat bread has more fiber and more nutrients, and that refined foods have been altered to the point that they contain no fiber or nutrients and are difficult to digest. If your children still crave meat, let them order a burger when the family goes out to eat. If you don't force them, and take care to make the vegetarian meals appealing and delicious, they may soon find that they like the new diet better than the old one.

The Vegetarian Diet Is Recommended but Not Required

Even though the vegetarian diet is ideal, it is not necessary to be a vegetarian to benefit from Maharishi Ayurveda. You may not feel comfortable feeding your child a vegetarian diet, or your child may still crave meat. That is all right. But, in general, it is better to avoid a steady diet of red meat and instead substitute more chicken, turkey, or fish. How suitable chicken or fish is for the child depends on his doshas. A steady diet of fish is not recommended for Pitta and Kapha imbalances, for instance, because it is oily and increases Pitta and Kapha dosha. If you do serve meat, try to obtain organic meat.

Avoid Packaged, Frozen, Leftover, or Canned Foods

As you have already learned, packaged, canned, and frozen foods are old and devoid of prana. They are difficult to digest and create instant ama. It is important to make a habit of feeding your children fresh fruits and vegetables as much as possible.

Processed and packaged foods have another disadvantage. They contain chemical additives and preservatives that can be harmful to health. Also, labels can be misleading. Foods that are labeled "low in cholesterol" often contain indigestible trans-fats such as hydrogenated vegetable oil. Another label to watch for is "natural flavoring," which is often a pseudonym for MSG (monosodium glutamate), a powerful chemical that can cause allergic reactions in some children.

Food that has been cooked the previous day and stored in the refrigerator is also ama-producing, because it is not fresh. Ideally, food should be prepared fresh each day.

Children can only eat so much before their stomachs get full. It is important that they fill their stomachs with wholesome foods that will build their dhatus and nourish brain development. The rule of thumb is: natural is better. And natural means unprocessed, unpackaged, and fresh.

Another problem with packaged foods is the high amounts of sugar and sodium contained in them. Some commercial breakfast cereals contain as much as 40 percent sugar and are also high in sodium.

You can teach your children to appreciate the taste and feel of whole foods. You can also explain that homemade desserts are healthier. Try to have them on hand, so your child won't be attracted to unhealthy packaged sweets.

Avoid Unhealthy Fats

Eating a steady diet of packaged sweets, snacks, and other foods is not recommended for another reason—they contain unhealthy, indigestible types of fats.

During the past twenty years, the average American diet has become substantially higher in saturated fats and trans-fats, and deficient in fruits, vegetables, and whole grains. Meals, snacks, and fast foods consumed by children reflect this trend. For instance, a typical serving of french fries contains more than 13.2 percent hydrogenated oil, and a serving of potato chips contains 39 percent partially hydrogenated fat. Government school lunches have been found to contain more than one-third of their calories in fat, and it's usually the unhealthy type of fat.

These unhealthy fats are taking a toll on the health of American children. Forty percent of five- to eight-year-olds show at least one heart disease risk factor, such as elevated cholesterol, hypertension, or obesity. In the past, arteriosclerosis rarely appeared until after age thirty. Now it is showing up in some children as young as age five.

There is a tremendous amount of controversy about fats, and unfortunately all fat has gotten a bad name. It might be useful to take a few minutes to sort out the bad from the good fats.

Avoid Artificial, Synthetic, Altered Fats and Trans-Fats

Unhealthy fats such as trans-fats, contained in almost all packaged foods, have been shown to increase cholesterol, decrease the good (HDL) cholesterol, clog the liver's waste-removal system, and block the assimilation of essential fatty acids. In many foods, trans-fatty acids make up 60 percent of the food, yet they contain less than 5 percent essential fatty acids. Trans-fats are made from hydrogenating (adding a hydrogen molecule) to vegetable oil to make it solid. This process of hydrogenation changes the molecular structure of the fat, making it literally indigestible by the human body. Hydrogenated fats in packaged foods may be a major contributor to the high cholesterol levels found in American children today. These fats also create toxins (ama) in the body, since they do not fit the body's molecular framework and cannot be digested. They disrupt the natural balance of body, because they do not fit the specific requirements of the digestive system.

Hydrogenated and partially hydrogenated vegetable oils are found in almost all packaged goods available at your grocery store, including shortening, margarine, baked goods, candies, chocolate, crackers, chips, cookies, soup mixes, and breads. It's also contained in deep-fried foods, convenience foods, and fast foods such as french fries.

Just because a package is labeled "low in fat" doesn't mean that's so. Many foods labeled "low in cholesterol" contain hydrogenated vegetable oils, and thus are actually high in cholesterol and indigestible to humans. Avoid buying these foods. If you must buy packaged breads or other foods, try your local health food store. Many of the foods sold there will contain fats that are not hydrogenated. Be sure to check the labels.

Avoid Foods with Oxidized Fats, Animal Fats, Saturated Fats, and LDL Cholesterol

Aged, processed foods contain oxidized cholesterol, oils, and fats, which means that air has been pushed into them during their processing. These foods include meats, sausages, aged cheeses, fried convenience foods, and stored foods. Especially because they are lacking in the antioxidant minerals and vitamins that fresh foods contain, these are the foods that build up fatty wastes in the arteries and create damage. Also, if you serve your child fresh, whole foods you will avoid serving him oxidized fats altogether.

Saturated fats, found in large proportions (up to 60 percent) in animal meats, are associated with heart disease, arteriosclerosis, and other health problems later in life. With a vegetarian diet, these harmful fats can be avoided.

Remember that when it comes to children, they will be more influenced by what you do than what you say. If you eat foods that are wholesome, sattvic, and fresh, your child will be much more likely to eat a healthy diet, too.

A Formula for a Sattvic Diet

Greater variety
+
Fresh vegetables, fruits, grains, and vegetarian protein
−
Tamasic food
=
Sattvic diet

Children Want to Eat Healthy Foods

One thing that makes a parent's job easier is that most children want to eat healthier foods. A Gallup poll sponsored by the American Dietetic Association and the International Food Information Council found that when 410 children between the ages of nine and fifteen years were surveyed, 97 percent agreed, "a balanced diet is very important for health." More than half the children were aware of the Food Guide Pyramid.

They also were aware that it is important to eat a variety of foods. Nine out of ten children agreed, "trying new foods is good for you." Almost all said they like to eat a lot of different foods. Eighty-seven percent also said, "it's best to eat smaller amounts of many different foods and not too much of one food."

Two-thirds of children thought their own eating habits were good to excellent. More than half rated their habits and their parents' habits at the same level, showing that their parents were their role models for eating. Schools and teachers were the source for nutritional information for 90 percent of the children, although more than three-fourths reported that their parents were a source of nutritional information; friends were cited only at 19 percent. Again, this demonstrated that children are open to instruction from their parents.

That same poll also found that children didn't always find that healthy foods were their favorite ones, and felt that "foods that are good for you don't taste good." In the next chapter, you'll learn different menu suggestions for children of all ages, and some recipes for healthy fun foods as well.

If you feed your children healthy and sattvic foods, they will grow up with that as their standard. There is nothing more important that you can do for their health than feeding your children nourishing foods.

One mother says, "I definitely feel that the reason my twelve-year-old son is so vibrantly healthy, smooth in his emotions, and radiating such silence from within is that he has always eaten holistic, organic, sattvic, home-cooked meals. We stay away from fast foods, so there are no chemicals or additives in his diet, or any unhealthy foods to irritate his system. This allows him to function from an even and solid foundation. His cells are balanced from eating pure, balanced foods, and he really notices the difference when he eats foods that aren't sattvic. It gives him a tremendous basis for his teen years."

CHAPTER EIGHT
Foods for Different Ages

Every mother knows that children have different needs at different stages of growth. Maharishi Ayurveda takes those nutritional needs into account when recommending foods for different ages—and these guidelines are contained in this chapter. You'll also find recommendations and recipes for making food more appealing to children, and ways to help children who have cravings to eat more healthy foods.

For all ages of children, Maharishi Ayurveda recommends warm, cooked meals with no ice-cold foods or drinks, and no carbonated drinks, as these disrupt digestion. Maharishi Ayurveda has recommended a wide variety of fresh, organic vegetables, fruits, whole grains, and vegetarian protein for thousands of years.

Today, researchers are recommending a similar diet as prevention and treatment for a wide variety of chronic diseases. For example, a recent study of 42,000 women showed that eating a balanced diet of fresh fruits, vegetables, whole grains, and low-fat protein reduced risk of cancer, heart disease, and stroke. While in the past nutritional research often focused on certain foods that reduced disease (broccoli to reduce colon cancer, for instance), now researchers are realizing that it's the balanced diet as a whole that creates health. And if it is important for adults, it is even more essential for children, who are turning food into bones, muscles, and brain cells.

During the First Year

Maharishi Ayurveda recommends breast milk as the ideal food for infants. It contains all the nutrients a child needs as well as fats and antibodies. Research shows that the benefits of breast-feeding include stronger immunity, greater self-confidence, stronger teeth, and better bonding between mother and child. If at all possible, it's ideal to continue breast-feeding your child for the entire first year. Recent research has found that teenagers who were breast-fed for even a few weeks showed higher IQs, better school grades, and half the risk of quitting high school early than other teenagers who were fed formula from birth.

During the first five or six months, your child will start teething. This is taken as a sign from nature that the child is ready for solid foods.

Recommended first foods include the broth of long-grain rice and the broth of mung dhal cooked with a little ghee. Be sure to add eight parts water to one part dhal or rice. As the child becomes accustomed to eating the broth, you can start to make the broth heavier until he can digest the dhal as a soup and the rice as a soft, well-cooked solid. Basmati rice is not recommended for infants because it is aged and Vata-producing. Buy a white, long-grain rice such as Carolina Gold.

After the child gets used to dhal soup and rice, you can add vegetable soups and fresh, juicy fruits such as mango. Bananas should be avoided because they are difficult for infants to digest and can cause mucus. A small amount of freshly prepared yogurt is a good food for morning and noon meals, but it is too heavy at night and may cause mucus if eaten then.

As your child begins to eat solids, your breast milk supply will naturally start to taper off. You can introduce cow's milk (preferably organic) after six months. If your infant can't digest cow's milk, you could try goat's milk until he is one year old. Goat's milk is easier to digest but less nourishing, so it's better to switch to cow's milk when the baby's digestive system is more mature.

Be sure to boil the milk first with a pinch of turmeric or ginger, to make it easier to digest. Serve it to your child when it cools to room temperature. Do not serve your child cold milk, as this will be harder to digest and could cause congestion.

In fact, it's important to avoid feeding your infant any cold foods and drinks. If your child eats cold food, teething becomes more difficult and prolonged, because the root does not grow as strong. The teeth can even become deformed. Cold foods and drinks also contribute to excess mucus. Vata-increasing foods, such as raw vegetables and yeasted breads, are also important to avoid. Refined sugar should be avoided, but it's fine to feed your child foods cooked with small amounts of jaggary or ground rock sugar. For infants, food should be freshly prepared. Avoid refrigerated, canned, frozen, or bottled foods or juices. This is best, but you don't want to create a terrible strain for yourself or your baby.

One to Three Years

For this age group, it's a good idea to introduce a wide variety of new foods over time. Children this age need to eat when they are hungry, so plan to serve several small meals throughout the day. They burn up the calories very quickly as their small stomachs do not hold much and their metabolism runs much faster. At age one you can move gradually toward a schedule of three meals a day with substantial and nutritious snacks mid-morning and mid-afternoon.

Vegetables: Yams, zucchini, carrots, chard, asparagus, and a variety of other well-cooked and seasoned vegetables are good. Asparagus is especially healthy and digestible. Peas and string beans aggravate Vata and are difficult to digest, and should be avoided at this age. Vegetable soups are a light and nourishing choice for the evening meal.

Dairy: Milk, fresh yogurt, lassi, and ghee. Ghee can be used to sauté vegetables and in cooking soups and grains. This is not the time of life to limit healthy fats, and your child will need as much as three cups of whole milk daily. As your child gets older, he will naturally crave less fat.

Cereals and Grains: Hot cereals are ideal for breakfast, such as cream of rice, cream of wheat, or couscous. You can cook them with milk if the child's digestion is good, otherwise with water. Ghee and jaggary can be added. In general, hot rice cereals are the most wholesome. If there is no time to prepare hot cereal, once in a while you might serve cold cereal with warm milk that has been heated to the boiling point and cooled down. Corn cereals aggravate Kapha dosha, and may increase obesity and even contribute to diabetes. Cooked oatmeal is all right, but cold oat cereals aggravate Vata dosha.

For lunch, you can serve upma (a cream of wheat made with spices and vegetables), small chapatis (Indian flat breads), softly cooked rice, or well-cooked, soft pastas.

For dinner, you could serve whole grains such as couscous, quinoa, or bulgur wheat cooked with small amounts of ghee. Vegetable soups that contain grains such as barley or rye are also a good way to serve grains at night. Although plain rice is a bit heavy for evening, rice pilaf with cumin and turmeric is a more digestible combination.

Fruit: Pomegranate is especially good for teething; it prevents diarrhea and colitis. Grapes balance all the doshas. Mangoes and ripe, sweet oranges are also healthy for children this age. Introduce a wide variety of fruits, but serve bananas only occasionally, as they are heavy. They should also be ripe, as greenish bananas are constipating.

Protein: Mung dhal soups or red lentil soups are an ideal source of protein. Crushed almonds and soft, fresh cheeses such as cottage cheese, farmer's cheese, and panir are also recommended.

Desserts: At the noon meal children can eat fresh, homemade cookies and freshly made puddings, pies, and pastries (made with jaggary, Sucanat, or rock sugar). At night sweets are too heavy to digest and should be avoided.

Avoid: Ice cream is better left out of the diet for babies up to one year and served only occasionally during the summer months for all children. Remember that you generally want to avoid feeding children cold, heavy desserts made with refined sugar because they put out the digestive fire and cause ama. For the same reason, avoid packaged desserts.

Age Three to Twelve Years

At this age it's a good idea to establish three regular meals of fresh, warm, light foods. It's important not to let children skip meals, and it's best if the meals are served at the same time every day. Light snacks mid-morning and afternoon are ideal for three-to-six-year-olds, and after-school snacks are also recommended for school-age children if dinner is served late.

Breakfast: Cooked cereals, warm milk with cold cereal, cream of rice or cream of wheat with a little ghee and jaggary is a healthy breakfast for this age. Depending on their preferences, children might also like toasted bread with raw honey or sugarless preserves (most grocery stores today carry fruit-juice-sweetened preserves), along with warm drinks such as Maharishi Ayurveda Vata, Pitta®, or Kapha Teas. Milk brought to a boil with a pinch of cardamom, ginger, or turmeric is also a good breakfast drink when it cools to room temperature.

Sometimes children don't have much appetite at breakfast, since they are in the Kapha time of life and since it's the Kapha time of day. If that's the case, try feeding him or her fresh juice or a piece of fruit. Over time, with the Ayurvedic diet and routine, your child's digestion will improve and he will be able to eat a more substantial breakfast. A light breakfast works especially well for younger children if they are served a mid-morning snack in preschool or kindergarten. Warm water with lemon and a teaspoon of raw honey is a great morning drink for children, as it tastes good and also stimulates the digestion, which can get sluggish during Kapha season. If your child drinks it after waking, he or she may be hungry for a bigger breakfast before school.

Lunch: Lunch should be the main meal, since the digestive fire is highest at noon. You can serve any combination of freshly cooked and seasoned vegetables, cooked whole grains such as couscous, quinoa, or bulgur wheat, and light dairy products such as lassi and panir. A light salad of shredded carrots, fresh ginger, and parsley or other fresh herbs is good in small quantities at the beginning of the meal.

This is the best time to serve homemade desserts such as pie, pudding or cookies made with jaggary or rock sugar, since the digestion is strongest at noon and children can digest them more easily. Many times children want to eat their dessert first. And actually, this is considered the best way to start an Ayurvedic meal, with the heaviest food first. You'll be surprised to find that once children start with something sweet, usually they go on to eat more vegetables and grains than usual because their craving is satisfied. It's a good idea to have a portions already measured out on small plates, so the child just eats one cookie or a small piece of pie and then goes on to the rest of the meal.

It's always best to end the meal with light foods such as fresh, ripened, sweet fruit. Lassi is also recommended, as it is light, contains healthy bacteria that aids the digestive process, and can be made sweet to satisfy the urge for sweets at the end of the meal.

Supper: It's best to serve light foods, such as vegetable and dhal soup served with toasted flat bread. Another suggested meal includes cooked vegetables and light grains such as amaranth and quinoa. Pasta and fresh vegetables without cheese is also a good evening meal. These foods are light, and your child can eat as much as he needs without feeling overloaded.

Avoid serving your child red or white meat, chicken, fish, sour cream, yogurt, tofu, or cheese at night. These will only overload the liver and the digestive system, creating digestive toxins (ama) and excess mucus.

Snacks: If children want a snack, most of the time they really need to eat. Your school-age child may be hungry after school, especially if dinner is not served until 6:00 p.m. Suitable snacks include warm milk spiced with cardamom, cinnamon, ginger, or turmeric; freshly made cookies; crackers; chapati with cinnamon and raw honey; fresh fruit; dried fruits (such as figs, dates, and raisins); fresh juices; fruit balls made with ground dates, coconut, and ground, blanched almonds; and any freshly cooked foods. The preschool child will also need a mid-morning snack of fruit, milk, or juice.

A small amount of warm milk with ghee before bed balances Vata and Pitta doshas and provides sound sleep. If the child has much Kapha dosha by nature, or if it is Kapha season, you could dilute the milk with a little water.

Protein: Milk, milk products, beans, dhal, lentils, nuts (except peanuts), and sesame seeds are all healthy sources of protein at this age. Three glasses of milk daily is a healthy amount.

Foods to avoid: Eggs, red meat, sausage, hot dogs, bacon, and peanut butter are heavy, tamasic, and difficult to digest at any age, and cause indigestion and congestion of the micro-channels (srotas) that carry nutrients to the cells and wastes away from the cells. Avoid these foods to prevent future heart disease, high cholesterol, obesity, and diseases caused by free radicals.

Let Your Children Choose What to Eat

Even though Maharishi Ayurveda offers these guidelines for food, the foremost principle in choosing foods is to respect your child's likes and dislikes. Children tend to be more innocent in following their internal signals. As much as possible, serve foods that your child likes and chooses.

If your daughter says that she doesn't want to eat a certain vegetable, ask her what vegetable she would like to eat, and serve that the next day. Or if she complains about the food, say that you will eat her way one day and then ask if she will eat your way the next. Then she can see which meal makes her feel better.

You can explain the principles of healthy eating to your child. Ask your son how he feels after eating a balanced Ayurvedic meal. Does he feel light and happy? Then ask how he feels after he has eaten some heavy, packaged food. Does he still feel as good? In this way you can teach your child to be attuned to the good effects of wholesome food.

Variety is important. If you offer a variety of foods with all six tastes, your children will surely find something that they like. It may take time, though. One researcher found that you might have to introduce a two-year-old to a new food up to fifteen times at intervals over a period of several months before he will accept it. For older children who are reluctant to eat vegetables, serving more than one vegetable at a meal may increase the total amount of vegetables that they eat. Offering more than one vegetable at each meal can also increase the likelihood that at least one will be eaten. It's the same principle used in offering a plate of different kinds of cookies; people will eat more if there is more than one type of cookie on the plate.

In general, as toxins clear away and your child becomes more attuned to his body's needs, he will spontaneously start to choose healthier foods. This is the beauty of Maharishi Ayurveda. The more attuned to nature's intelligence, the more self-aware your child becomes through all of the methods described in this book, the more he will truly want the things that are healthiest for him. Thus, implementing these natural guidelines is not a burden for parents, but a great help.

Sometimes it may seem overwhelming to the mother to provide the different tastes needed by each person in the family, especially if they need different tastes to balance their doshas. The mother could prepare foods with minimal spices and let each person add Calming (Vata) Spice Mix, Cooling (Pitta) Spice Mix, or Stimulating (Kapha) Spice Mix to the food at the table.

Spices that enhance digestion and balance all three doshas include cardamom, cinnamon, fennel, turmeric, fresh ginger, cumin, coriander, and salt.

Cravings for Chocolate and Candy

Children often have cravings for specific foods. If you don't keep candy and chocolate around the house, your children will be less likely to beg for it. Children learn by imitation and if they see you eating healthy foods, they will be more likely to respect their bodies, too.

Food cravings can be caused by not eating a diet that includes all six tastes at each meal. Children who eat a steady diet of sweet, sour, and salty tastes, for instance (as found in packaged sweets, sour condiments such as ketchup and mustard, and salty french fries), may have strong food cravings because they rarely get to eat the astringent, bitter, and pungent tastes, and thus are always craving more balance. The wild cravings for refined sugar and chocolate will start to fade once a diet with all six tastes is introduced.

Also, when the digestion is clogged with toxins and impurities, this can cause the body's natural desire for healthy foods to break down. As you start feeding your child healthier foods and he starts following better eating habits, the digestive fire will increase and your child will no longer be guided by distorted impulses. Rather, your child's desires will be more in tune with his body's true needs.

You can also try to motivate your children by pointing out that if you don't spend money on chocolate, then you can take them swimming (or some other activity they like) more often. You can also ask them if their muscles and joints feel stiff. Do they want to get rid of that feeling? Explain that chocolate creates a lot of mucus, and leads to headaches and a dull, stiff feeling. So rather than forbidding them to eat chocolate, let them try it occasionally. Help your child to substitute a food that has a similar quality but won't make him feel bad (such as milky, fresh puddings or licorice, which pacifies Vata and Kapha) if it is made without artificial colors or flavors. Teach your children to play with choices.

Ice cream is another difficult-to-digest dessert that children crave. Unfortunately, it creates mucus in the mouth, and cools down the agni, causing the digestion to shut down. Gas, indigestion, and the formation of digestive toxins (ama) are the results. It can greatly contribute to childhood illnesses such as runny nose, colds, and flu, especially if eaten in the winter or when the digestion is weak.

Again, it's best to point out the connection between sickness and diet. You could allow your child to eat small portions of ice cream when the weather is hot. If the child's digestion is strong, he may be able to digest ice cream more often. Also, you can try to serve more creamy desserts, such as rice pudding or cake with whipped cream topping to help satisfy the craving for ice cream.

How to Change a Habit

It takes time to change a long-standing habit. Don't try to change your family's diet overnight. It could even be harmful to shock the body with a sudden change. It's better not to force a child to give up bad habits; slowly and gradually substitute different foods that he likes instead. Find some flavor that he could adopt.

Charaka Samhita gives wise advice for changing a habit. It states, "A wise person should gradually give up unwholesome practices to which he is addicted and he should simultaneously adopt those which are wholesome." By offering your child healthy, delicious foods with all six tastes, it will be easier for him to stop eating empty calories and junk foods that aggravate the doshas and bring on ill health.

Serve Fun, Tasty, and Healthy Foods

When trying to feed your child healthy foods, it's important to make the food attractive and fun. You eat with your eyes as much as your stomach, so a good meal should look appealing and colorful. In fact, according to Maharishi Ayurveda, the food will not digest smoothly and provide nourishment if it doesn't taste good to the person eating it.

In the Gallup poll mentioned earlier, 64 percent of the children surveyed said foods that are good for you do not taste good. Three-fourths said they were tired of hearing what foods are good and bad for them. Seven out of ten said their favorite foods are not good for them.

One idea is to cook foods that your child perceives as "fun" in a healthy way. Potatoes can be tossed in ghee and baked in the oven instead of deep-fried; pizza can be made with fresh cheeses and breads, and burgers can be made of grated vegetables. You can prepare almost any food in a healthy way.

The sooner you start educating your children in healthy eating habits, the more they will start appreciating healthy foods. And it's always a good idea to give them more choices, so they will see for themselves that certain foods make them feel better. They will start choosing the meals that you cook rather than junk foods.

Baked French Fries

4 organic Idaho baking potatoes
3 tablespoons olive oil or ghee
1/2 teaspoon turmeric
1/4 teaspoon ground ginger
1/2 teaspoon ground cumin
1/3 teaspoon ground coriander
salt and pepper to taste

Preheat oven to 400° F. Peel and cut like french fries. In a large bowl, add potatoes and sprinkle with oil, spices, salt, and pepper. Stir until well coated. Place potatoes on cookie sheet and bake for 45 to 60 minutes. Turn with a spatula after 25 minutes.

Ayurvedic Pizza
(Makes 3 individual pizzas)
6 organic whole wheat flour tortillas or chapatis
2 cups freshly made pesto sauce or fresh pizza sauce
1 jar of organic pizza sauce or pesto
3/4 cup broccoli florets
1/2 lb. organic tofu
1 1/2 cups fresh organic mozzarella cheese
1/2 cup olives
1/4 teaspoon turmeric
1/4 teaspoon ground ginger
1/8 teaspoon black pepper
1/8 teaspoon ground coriander
1 tablespoon olive oil
oregano to garnish

Steam broccoli and tofu until tender and salt to taste. Blend in blender until smooth. Set aside. In a separate frying pan, dry roast the whole-wheat tortillas about 40 seconds on each side over a medium heat.

Make fresh pizza sauce with the spices. Set aside.

Place three tortillas on a baking pan. Spread a thin layer of cheese over each tortilla and then place another tortilla on top. This makes a thicker crust and makes it easier to eat. Brush the top tortilla with olive oil. Then spread a layer of pizza sauce. Next comes the tofu mixture. Spread a thin layer of it over the sauce. Spread the cheese over the tofu mixture. Garnish with olives and a pinch of oregano.

Place in a 350° F preheated oven and bake about 10 minutes or until the cheese is melted.

Veggie Burgers
1 cup grated carrots (steamed)
1 cup pinto beans or black beans cooked and mashed
1 cup cooked short-grain rice
1/4 cup ground almonds that have been soaked overnight
1/4 teaspoon salt
1/4 teaspoon pepper
1/8 teaspoon cinnamon
1/4 teaspoon ground cumin
ghee or olive oil for frying
grated organic mozzarella cheese for garnish (optional)

Blend all ingredients together to form a thick mixture. You can use a food processor, and if needed add more ground nuts to make a thicker mixture. (Be careful not to process too much, as the batter will become too thin to form patties.) Form thin patties and fry in ghee or olive oil, about 7 minutes each side. Melt fresh mozzarella cheese over one side and serve on a bun. You can also serve it in a pita pocket bread with lettuce.

CHAPTER NINE

Ten Healthy Eating Habits for Powerful Digestion

According to Maharishi Ayurveda, how you digest your food is just as important as the actual food you eat. And there are certain things you can do to improve your child's digestion. If you set up the proper conditions for good digestion, your child will gain more value from the food he eats. Remember that a healthy digestion creates ojas and immunity, and an unhealthy digestion creates digestive toxins (ama) and sickness. That is why keeping the digestion healthy is one of the central goals of Maharishi Ayurveda.

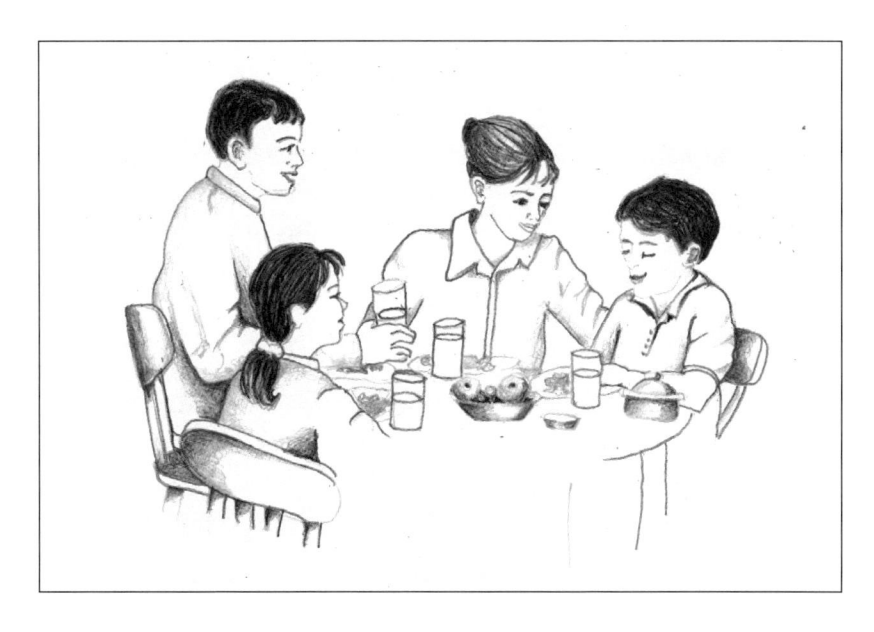

One of the most important ways to cultivate smooth digestion is to create a settled, quiet environment so the child can pay attention to the food he is eating. Just having some attention on the food will help him or her to digest it. If the television is turned off, if there is an unhurried feeling, if the conversation is easygoing and relaxed, the food will digest much better. If there is an atmosphere of rushing and commotion, the digestive process could actually be disrupted and toxins could be created. This could happen even if the food is nourishing and wholesome.

Making the family meal a happy, settled daily event could also improve your child's eating habits. A recent study by Harvard Medical School has shown that children who eat with their parents eat less junk food, eat more fruits and vegetables, and ingest more of the nutrients needed for their developing nervous systems and to fend off heart disease and cancer in later life. The old-fashioned family meal is good for your child's health.

Eating Habits to Cultivate in Your Child

1. Schedule three hot meals and serve them at set meal times each day. The digestion gets accustomed to a schedule. If habituated to operating at the same time every day, the digestive juices will increase at that time, enhancing digestion. Irregularity can cause even a good digestion to become weak.

2. Serve the main meal at noon, when the digestion is at its peak. Just as the sun is strongest at noontime, so your child's internal fire is strongest then. Between twelve and one o'clock is the time to serve the heaviest meal. Fresh cheeses, lassi, yogurt, or fresh desserts should be served at the noon meal, because the optimum flow of digestive enzymes is present in the body at this time. If your child is not a vegetarian, this is the time of day to serve chicken or fish (and if served in the form of soups, it is even more digestible).

Evening is a time to eat lighter, both in quantity and quality, because the digestive fire is weaker in the evening. If a large, heavy meal is sitting in the intestines at bedtime it will not digest. Instead, it will create indigestion and restless, disturbed sleep. Children who go to sleep on a full stomach wake up with puffy eyes and a pale face. For this reason, do not serve your child heavy foods, such as yogurt, tofu, panir, cheese, meat, poultry, fish, or heavy, oily foods at night.

Also, try not to serve supper too late. Give your children dinner by 6:00 p.m., so there are two full hours to digest the food before bedtime.

While this certainly creates a challenge when your child is at school during the day, you can at least try to maintain this pattern on the weekends and holidays. If your child comes home for lunch, serve the main meal then.

3. Be sure your child has finished digesting the previous meal before eating a snack or new meal. The amount of time it takes to digest a meal depends on the child's strength of digestion. It takes at least two-and-a-half hours to digest a meal, and for a large meal, three to six hours. As mentioned in Chapter Eight, preschool children and toddlers take much less time to digest and therefore need to eat much more often.

Children usually know when they are hungry. Do not weaken this natural signal by forcing your child to eat when he's not hungry, especially if there hasn't been enough time to digest the meal before. Eating fresh food on top of food that is still being digested is somewhat like cooking bean soup for an hour and then adding raw beans to the pot. It could create a sour, gluey mess.

4. Serve small amounts of room-temperature or warm water with the meals. According to Maharishi Ayurveda, the stomach should be filled with one-third liquid (including soups), one-third solid food, and one-third space (to allow room for digestion).

5. Do not encourage your child to overeat. By following the Ayurvedic guideline of filling the stomach to two-thirds of its capacity with solids and liquids, the digestive process will have the space it requires to mix the food with mucus and other gastric juices.

If your child feels bloated after eating, it may be that he has eaten too much. A light, comfortable feeling should be the norm after meals. You can roughly judge what two-thirds your child's capacity is by having him cup his hands and estimating how much food would fill the open hands. This is a guide everyone can use for himself or herself.

It's also important to consider the digestive strength of the child in determining the quantity of food he can digest. You'll remember from Chapter Four that there are four different types of digestion (agni). The child's digestive capacity might be sharp, it might be slow and sluggish, it might be irregular (i.e., sometimes he wants to eat and sometimes he doesn't), and it might be very balanced. As a parent, you probably are very familiar with your child's digestive strength. It's important to respect the child's digestive capacity and not to force your child to eat more than he is able. If he's a "picky eater," it's better to consult a physician trained in Maharishi Ayurveda, who will discover your child's needs through pulse diagnosis and, based on the health assessment, recommend individualized changes in diet, lifestyle and behavior to strengthen your child's agni. Then your child will naturally have a healthy appetite.

Children often take more food on their plate than they can actually eat. While this is something you can train children to watch out for—and as they get older they naturally estimate better what they can really eat—it's not a good idea to force children to eat everything on their plates if they say they are stuffed. Some children have a more Vata digestion, meaning that it is irregular and sensitive, and it may make them very uncomfortable to go over their threshold of comfort.

Overeating causes toxins to form in the digestion, and in time it can lead to a buildup of toxins and even disease. It can also lead to obesity. A recent study done at Penn State shows that while children younger than three-and-a-half will stop eating when full, children as young as five will eat past the point of hunger when faced with larger-than-usual servings of food, having already learned to ignore their internal instincts to regulate eating (most likely at the urging of parents).

In general, it's best to respect the child's natural desires. Children are more in tune with their bodies in many ways, and it's healthy to help them respond to their body's signals. Obesity and other digestive problems often result from not paying attention to the body's natural signals.

There is a tendency in Western culture to feel that if a certain food is good, then the child should eat a lot of it. In the past, meat was considered healthy, and children often were forced to eat it in large quantities. The psychology was, "If meat is good, have four big chunks of it."

Or, "Eggs are good, have two of them." That sort of principle, when used on all children equally, can be destructive. You have to know the prakriti of the child; you have to know his digestive capacity and what he can handle. And as the parent, you probably know this better than anyone.

Even if a food is good, if the child is not digesting it, the food will create digestive toxins (ama) and consequently breed free radicals, becoming the basis for disease.

6. Serve your family meals in a quiet and pleasant place without TV, telephone calls, computers, music, or intense conversations. Food digests most easily when the conversation is light and pleasant and there is not a lot of commotion around. If your child is in the habit of watching TV while he eats, explain that his food needs his attention in order to digest properly. Try to turn the message machine on when you eat, to avoid the family meals being interrupted by phone calls. Set a good example by not reading or watching television, by creating a quiet atmosphere, and by not allowing arguments or unpleasant topics at the dinner table.

This is especially important if your child is a picky eater. If he is not rushed, finds the environment settled and nourishing, and he can choose his own foods, he will feel more relaxed and will eat more. The mealtime is when he can regain energy, and it forms the basis for his happiness and success throughout the day.

7. Encourage your child not to eat too quickly or too slowly. Try to explain to your child that by eating too fast, the food might go down the wrong channel and will not enter the stomach by the right door. If he eats too slowly, the food will become cold and the digestion will be held up, perhaps creating a stomachache.

It's important to teach your children to chew their food carefully without rushing. Chewing the food allows the saliva to do its job in breaking down the food to enter the stomach. This is best learned by example. There is a saying that you should drink your solids and eat your liquids. This refers to chewing. If you chew solids carefully, they will become like a liquid. And if you sip your drinks rather than gulping them down, you will digest them better, too.

8. Ask your child to sit down while eating. This is sometimes difficult for very young children to do, but it's essential in maintaining a smooth digestion. Eating while standing up, or getting up and down several times while eating, can disrupt the digestion and put the digestive fire out. Try to set a good example by not jumping up a lot yourself, and try to train your child to sit down first before eating.

Even young children can learn to sit down while drinking, too. This is important to avoid digestive disturbances and gas.

9. Cultivate a habit of sitting quietly for a moment at the beginning of the meal and for a few minutes at the end. Many families say a brief prayer before the meal starts, and besides the religious benefits, this also helps the mind and body settle down before starting to eat. If your family isn't in the habit of praying, you could suggest that everyone bow their heads silently for a few moments before digging in. Or some families with younger children like to sing a song of thanks. This creates a transition between the rush of activity and the meal.

It's important to cultivate a relaxed, focused attitude toward food. You can explain to your child that if you eat the food in the proper manner, you gain far more than just nutrients. You gain all the meal's subtle values; you nourish not only the body but also the mind, senses, and consciousness itself. Food eaten without rushing develops good behavior, contentment, happiness, coherence, tolerance, endurance, harmony, intelligence, and compassion in the child. The opposite qualities result from eating in a fast-food restaurant. There the food is wolfed down before the flow of enzymes even begins. The subtle values of consciousness and fine feeling do not get nourished.

At the end of the meal, it's important to rest for two minutes or so to help give digestion a settled start. This is especially important if your child suffers from gas, constipation, or weak digestion.

Even if your younger children finish eating before you do and want to be excused to play, you can ask them to sit still for a few minutes first.

10. Avoid serving food and drinks in the car. You can follow these habits even when you're traveling with the family. Motion is Vata-producing, so eating in the car while driving can increase Vata and cause digestive problems and carsickness. Even drinking in the car is not a good idea, unless you're on a long car trip and need to avoid dehydration.

For short car trips around town, you can set a good example by not drinking or eating yourself. Having that cup of coffee in the car could upset your own digestion and create a Vata imbalance and can teach your child bad habits. Food and drink deserve respect, and should only be consumed when you can devote your attention to them.

Many mothers are in the habit of giving their infants a bottle of juice or milk while in the baby buggy. Because the buggy is in motion, it could create Vata disturbances such as gas or indigestion. It's better to stop strolling while your infant is drinking.

The suggestions given in this chapter may seem simple, but they are powerful. Remember that most diseases start with indigestion, which causes the formation of ama. These simple habits can ensure your child's healthy digestion and constitution throughout life.

CHAPTER TEN
Boosting Immunity and Creating Balance with Maharishi Ayurveda Herbal Food Supplements and *Rasayanas*

Food is the best medicine, because at every meal we have the opportunity to balance our bodies and minds simply by choosing the right foods. As we have seen in the past chapters, by eating balanced and wholesome foods, many diseases can be avoided. Sometimes, however, children need an extra boost. This is especially true if the child is going through a stressful time, has been traveling, or if the doshas are fluctuating due to the change of seasons.

Maharishi Ayurveda offers two types of food supplements to children. One type, called rasayanas, is made of whole herbs, minerals, and foods, which aim to increase ojas and immunity. They are for healthy children as well as those who have some imbalance. They prevent disease and enhance the growth and development of the mind, body, and emotions.

The other type of food supplement consists of whole herbs and minerals that are designed to bring balance to specific doshas. These herbal compounds are especially helpful as a complement to Western medicine in treating a temporary imbalance or sickness, when treating chronic disease, or when treating long-standing minor problems, such as frequent colds, stuffy noses, and rashes.

Many times it's exactly these chronic, irritating, minor problems that detract greatly from a child's happiness and comfort. Because they are not full-blown diseases, Western medicine has little to offer in terms of relief. Maharishi Ayurveda, however, can easily treat the underlying doshic imbalance and produce astonishing results. Let me give you an example.

Cathy, a mother of three, was fed up. All three of her children had chronic conditions that the Western doctors couldn't do anything about. Her oldest daughter, Kristen, age eleven, had a chronic stuffy nose, which had literally bothered her since she was born. It irritated her daily, and often stopped her from breathing through her nose. When she was younger it resulted in occasional ear infections.

Her second child, Ariel, age eight, had been complaining of a frequently upset stomach for nearly a year. And her third child, Angela, who was just an infant at the time, had a red rash all over her.

Cathy had taken all three of her children to her pediatrician, who told her that these were chronic conditions and the children would just have to live with them. Nothing could be done, he said.

So Cathy and her husband packed their children in their van and drove to the Maharishi Ayurveda Health Center in Lancaster, Massachusetts, located a few hours' drive from their home. There the Maharishi Ayurveda health expert (Vaidya) recommended Maharishi Ayurveda herbal food preparations for the two older children along with some small dietary changes. For Angela, he recommended a Maharishi Ayurveda massage oil, infused with healing herbs.

Cathy is still startled by the results. "I'm telling you, within a day all three of them were cured. It was incredible. It was truly amazing."

While not all children respond this quickly, I have found these gentle herbal formulas to be surprisingly effective in my practice. Let's find out why these herbal compounds can be so effective in treating children.

Taking the Whole Child into Account

Most Maharishi Ayurveda compounds are targeted to correct specific imbalances, and are recommended during a health assessment by health practitioners at Maharishi Ayurveda Health Centers or in private practice. The physician or expert trained in Maharishi Ayurveda first conducts a pulse diagnosis to determine the underlying imbalances and health needs, and then chooses from a pharmacopoeia that includes hundreds of herbal formulas. The physician trained in Maharishi Ayurveda takes into account the child's body type, specific imbalance, digestive strength, and other factors.

In other words, if you consult a physician trained in Maharishi Ayurveda because your child is complaining of frequent colds, she will not recommend a blanket remedy for all children with colds. Based on her assessment of your child's health needs she will recommend an individualized home health-care program, including diet, lifestyle recommendations and herbal formulas, for your child. This is the beauty of Maharishi Ayurveda: it is tailor-made for each child.

Different from Western Drugs

Let's establish what we mean by Maharishi Ayurveda herbal compounds. They are very different from Western drugs in several significant ways. They are also quite different from the herbs that you can buy at health food stores.

Defining Qualities of Maharishi Ayurveda Food Supplements

1. Use the Whole Herb, Not the Active Ingredient
Maharishi Ayurveda herbal compounds are made from whole plants, herbs, and fruits, and they sometimes contain minerals. By using the whole plant, the herbal compound creates a holistic, balanced effect on the body.

Western drugs, even if they are derived from plants, contain the isolated, active ingredient. This means that the most potent part of the plant is chemically extracted and used to create a potent effect—to expand the capillaries and end the headache (as in the case of aspirin, derived from willow bark) or to deaden the nerve endings (as in the case of medicinal cocaine, used as a surface anesthetic and derived from the leaves of the coca tree).

Extracting the active ingredient turns plants into drugs. The resulting drug almost always creates powerful side effects. The active ingredient may stop the disease in one area, but because it reaches the whole body, it can have destructive effects on other organs. The harmful side effects of modern drugs are well known and well documented.

By using the whole herb, Ayurvedic herbal compounds contain all the balancing inactive ingredients that nature packaged with the active ingredient. These ingredients act together to protect the rest of the body from the active ingredient. In other words, inactive ingredients, bundled in the same plant with the active ingredient by nature, help protect areas of the body not intended for the active ingredient.

2. Create a Synergy by Combining Several Whole Herbs
Maharishi Ayurveda herbal compounds avoid the unwanted side effects of modern drugs in another way. The preparation of the herbal compounds upholds a long tradition that dates back millennia. The herbs are prepared according to the ancient science of *dravyaguna*, which means literally, "qualities of matter." This precise science of combining whole herbs is extremely effective and safe, and harmful side effects are avoided.

All Maharishi Ayurveda herbs are combined in highly sophisticated compounds, or herbal formulas, that contain more than one herb. The herbal formulas are specifically formulated to use the synergistic effects of the herbs. In other words, Maharishi Ayurveda herbs are combined in precise ways to magnify the desired effect while diminishing the harmful side effects.

Maharishi Ayurveda herbal compounds can contain ten or fifteen or even fifty herbs. In a typical formula, different herbs perform different functions. The primary herbs in a formula enhance the target herb, making it easier to assimilate and increasing bioavailability. A second type of herb helps remove waste matter, thus detoxifying the channels of the body and clearing the way for the target herb to reach the target organ. A third type of herb might balance the effects of the target herb, to ensure that no damaging side effects are experienced, no matter how minor.

Each herbal formula contains a combination of herbs that arrive at targeted cells, pass through the cell membrane, and achieve their intended effects inside the cell itself. The synergism also corrects the specific doshic imbalances and improves digestibility, absorption, and overall immunity. In other words, the synergistic effects of these herbs together create a whole that is more than the sum of the parts.

3. Do Not Create Harmful Side Effects

Because the Maharishi Ayurveda herbal compounds contain such balanced, life-promoting formulas, research has found that they actually create side benefits rather than harmful side effects. My patients notice that they feel more energetic, more balanced, and happier when taking these herbal formulas. This is because each herb has a holistic effect of balancing the entire body as well as targeting a certain area. The clearing away of toxins enhances overall immunity and paves the way for better and better health.

It is remarkable to see children respond to these positive, gentle herbal compounds. Often they come to me with their bodies run down from antibiotics and other drugs. They are sad and tired. They don't have energy to do their schoolwork or to play with their friends.

When I recommend the Maharishi Ayurveda herbal compounds, I explain that they may take more time to work than Western drugs. They are not "magic bullets." They work like nature does, slowly rebuilding the immunity and triggering the body's own healing system. I explain to the mother and the child that they have to do their part, too. The child has to eat healthier foods, be on a healthy routine, and give the body a chance to respond.

Yet what incredible rewards these natural treatments create! Not only does the persistent cold or cough or ailment go away, but the child blossoms as his body becomes vibrant and healthy. There is no greater gift that I can give a child than to help him reawaken his own inner intelligence with these beautiful therapies.

4. Use Time-Tested and Safe Methods of Preparation

Many herbs used in Maharishi Ayurveda are gathered in the wild, in their natural, organic state far from agrichemicals or polluted cities. They are picked at the height of their potency, and then sorted to make sure that only the healthy herbs are used.

The preparation process is exact and uses timeless methods from the Ayurvedic texts. The herbs are never boiled, as that level of heat would destroy their potency. There are many different methods of preparation, including drying for powders and tablets, slow cooking for pastes and jellies, and steeping for syrups and liquids. Depending on the formula, it can take days or even weeks.

In addition to following the traditional methods, Maharishi Ayurveda products are prepared in modern, state-of-the-art facilities with third-party inspections for cleanliness and safety by international safety and quality regulators. Rigorous testing is conducted to screen out residual pesticides, biological contamination, and heavy metals such as lead, cadmium, and mercury. The facilities are certified by the world's leading safety and quality regulators.

These methods have proven effective over a long period of time, having been in use throughout the ages. Many of the formulas are made specifically for children. Their effects are known, having been tested for thousands of years. It is not like giving your child a drug that may be withdrawn from the market a year later due to inadequate testing and flawed research, or a single herb from the health food store that may seem harmless but could, in fact, create imbalanced, even dangerous, side effects.

> **Side Benefits of Maharishi Ayurveda Herbal Formulas:**
> Remove impurities and toxins
> Balance the doshas
> Nourish the dhatus and body tissues
> Restore ojas
> Awaken the intelligence of nature

The Difference between Maharishi Ayurveda Herbal Supplements and Vitamins

Maharishi Ayurveda herbal supplements contain the whole plant rather than just the active ingredient, and thus are much less toxic and much more natural than vitamin supplements. Vitamins are similar to drugs in that they contain only the active ingredients, and they are often synthetically made. They are potently concentrated, can disrupt the digestion, and can overload the liver and cause negative side effects if taken in excess.

Many parents wonder if their children should take vitamins. Vitamins are not usually needed if the child's diet contains a wide variety of fresh fruits, vegetables, legumes, dairy products, and whole grains.

Food should include all six tastes, and should be lively, full of consciousness, and easy to metabolize. Food should be prepared so that it doesn't cause derangement in digestion, block the channels of digestion, or increase toxins or free radicals.

It's much better for a child to eat fresh oranges than to swallow a dose of vitamin C instead. The whole orange contains many nutrients that vitamin C does not. Bioflavanoids, for instance, are found in the whitish inner skin of the orange. These have recently been found to produce antioxidant, anti-inflammatory, anti-allergic effects and other protective factors.

Whole fruits and vegetables are more absorbable, and therefore more effective than supplements. A recent study at the U.S. Food Research Institute examined the effect of carotenoids (which are antioxidants found in carrots, broccoli, tomatoes, and spinach) on the production of LDL (bad cholesterol). The results: a diet heavy in carotenoid-rich fruits and vegetables did indeed decrease LDL production and DNA damage. Carotenoid vitamin supplements, on the other hand, had no effect, or even caused adverse effects on absorption. The researchers concluded that the natural balance of carotenoids achieved from a balanced diet is most effective.

Of course, if there is a nutritional deficiency, vitamins may be needed for a short time. Because our soil has been depleted of nutrients through the use of chemical fertilizers, it's possible that even whole foods today do not have the amount of trace minerals and other nutrients that they normally would. For this reason, some vitamin supplementation may be necessary at times.

It's best not to rely on vitamins to fill in the gaps from an unhealthy diet. Switch your child to a healthier diet as soon as possible, for no synthetic vitamin can replace nature's vitamins in whole food.

Rasayanas for Children

Rasayanas are the most important and powerful herbal food supplements in Maharishi Ayurveda. The word rasayana means "that which supports rasa." Rasa means "the essence," and the first dhatu, which is the essence created from digested food that nourishes all the other dhatus, is also called rasa.

One of the major qualities of rasayana is that it creates ojas, the subtle essence of food. Rasayanas are said to produce longevity, better memory, intelligence, immunity, youthfulness, radiant skin, healthy children, physical strength, strong sensory perception, a clear voice and effective speech, and increased sattva (purity of life). The effects

---

The Most Effective Antioxidant

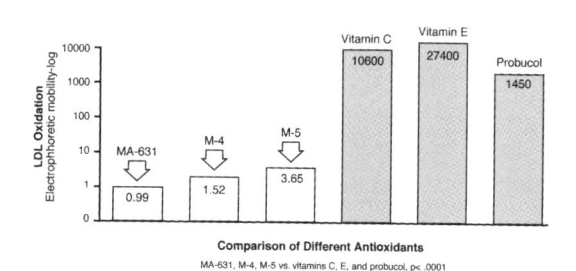

LDL Oxidation (Electrophoretic mobility-log)

MA-631	0.99
M-4	1.52
M-5	3.65
Vitamin C	10600
Vitamin E	27400
Probucol	1450

Comparison of Different Antioxidants
MA-631, M-4, M-5 vs. vitamins C, E, and probucol, p< .0001

Research shows that Maharishi Amrit Kalash is 1000 times more effective than Vitamin C in scavenging free radicals.

References: 1. H.M. Sharma et al., "Inhibition of Human Low-Density Lipoprotein Oxidation in Vitro by Maharishi Amrit Kalash and Maharishi Coffee Substitute," *Pharmacology, Biochemistry and Behavior*, vol. 43 (1992), pp. 1175-1182.

2. R. Waldschutz, "Influence of Maharishi Ayur-Veda Purification Treatment on Physiological and Psychological Health," *Erfahrungsheilkunde-Acta Medica Empirica*, 11 (1988), pp. 720-729.

Increased Resistence to Disease

Research shows that Maharishi Amrit Kalash:
- increases immunity
- prevents atherosclerosis by reducing human platelet aggregation
- reduces LDL (bad) cholesterol
- reduces chemical toxicity

References: 1. "Enhanced Lymphoproliferative Response, Macrophage-Mediated Tumor Cell Killing and Nitric Oxide Production after Ingestion of an Ayurvedic Drug (Maharishi Amrit Kalash)," *Biochemical Archives*, vol. 9 (1993), pp. 365-374.
2. H.M. Sharma et al., "Maharishi Amrit Kalash Prevents Human Platelet Aggregation," *Clinica and Terapia Cardiovascolare*, vol. 8, no. 3 (1989), pp. 227-230.
3. A.N. Hanna et al., "Effect of Herbal Mixtures MAK-4 and MAK-5 on Susceptibility of Human LDL to Oxidation, *Complementary Medicine International*, vol. 3, no. 3 (May/June 1996), pp. 28-36.
4. S.C. Bondy, et al., "Antioxidant Properties of Two Ayurvedic Herbal Preparations (MAK-4 and MAK-5)," *Biochemical Archives*, vol. 10 (1994), pp. 25-31.

of rasayanas enhance not only the body, but the mind and emotions as well. Some rasayanas rejuvenate memory, others are soothing to the emotions, and others promote long life.

Boosting Immunity with Rasayanas

One rasayana that is highly recommended for all children is Maharishi Amrit Kalash®. Maharishi Amrit Kalash increases immunity and overall strength of the mind and body, creating a more balanced and happy life for your child. Besides enhancing vitality, creativity, well-being, and intelligence, it strengthens the body's self-repair mechanisms and normalizes sleep patterns.

Children can take Maharishi Amrit Kalash on a daily basis. If the child's digestion is weak, it's best to take it with some digestive herbs. Your physician trained in Maharishi Ayurveda can recommend the herbs. Children usually take one-fourth or one-half the adult dosage, depending on their ages.

One reason for Maharishi Amrit Kalash's widespread effects is that it has been shown to enhance immunity and destroy free radicals. It has tremendous antioxidant potency. The public has shown great interest in antioxidants lately, and perhaps we should take the time to explain their benefits here.

Antioxidants help prevent the formation of free radicals, the destructive molecules believed to play a major role in aging and disease. Maharishi Amrit Kalash has amazing antioxidant qualities. Researchers at the Ohio State University College of Medicine have found that it is 1000 times more effective in combating free radicals than vitamin C and the major antioxidant drug.

What Are Free Radicals?

Free radicals are unstable, reactive molecules produced by the body as it metabolizes food and produces energy. Free radicals are produced as by-products of energy production. They oxidize fatty substances, contributing to the "bad" LDL cholesterol. While free radicals have a positive function in the body when they are used by the immune system to destroy foreign viruses or bacteria, if they are produced in abundance they can attack the body's cells and organs themselves, causing aging and disease. Free radicals not only occur in the human body; they also are present in nature, causing metals to rust and the ozone layer to break down when it oxidizes.

Free radicals increase in the body when it is exposed to toxins, such as cigarette smoke, alcohol, pollution, drugs, and pesticides. The stress response also produces hormones that cause free radicals to skyrocket, so stress is a major contributor to free-radical production. Extreme exertion is also a contributor.

Diseases Caused by Free Radicals

Free radicals and other reactive oxygen species have been linked with a wide range of diseases. Free radical reactions cause damage to the tissues, veins, arteries, liver, and kidneys. They attack the DNA, leading to mutation and cancer. They destroy the enzymes and proteins, hobbling the cell's normal metabolic activities. They distort the cell membranes, leading to hardening of the arteries, heart attacks, and strokes.

Besides cancer, arteriosclerosis, heart disease, and stroke, free radicals are also linked with emphysema, diabetes, rheumatoid arthritis, osteoporosis, ulcers, skin diseases, myocardial infarction, apoplexy, cataracts, senility, and aging. According to researchers, disease results from free-radical damage.

How to Stop Free Radicals

Since some people live long and healthy lives without suffering from disease or premature aging, it is clear that the body itself has ways to combat free radicals as part of the body's self-repair healing system. Maharishi Amrit Kalash and all of the Maharishi Ayurveda Herbal Supplements aim to restore balance and enliven the body's inherent healing mechanisms.

The first of the body's self-repair systems resides within the cell itself. While metabolizing food, the cell produces enzymes (such as superoxide dismutase) that dismantle free radicals. These enzymes are produced by the cell to destroy free radicals. They maintain balance in the body as long as the cell's waste removal systems and other systems are functioning well.

The second system involves nutrients the body ingests through food. Vitamins C and E, beta-carotene, and bioflavanoids obtained from food are thought to help the body fight free radicals, although to a much lesser degree. The third system is the DNA's self-repair system, which involves replacing molecules that have been damaged by free radicals.

The Link between Toxins (Ama) and Free Radicals

If children eat foods that are high in pesticides, preservatives, indigestible fats, and other toxins, the digestive system becomes overloaded and ama gets produced. When the liver, the cells, and other detoxifying systems become overloaded with ama—and the body's waste-removal system becomes increasingly sluggish—free radicals are produced in greater number and cannot be removed from the body as easily.

In addition, when ama clogs the cell's waste-removal channels, it also clogs the channels that deliver nutrients to the cells. The cell becomes weaker, and cannot produce the enzymes needed to scavenge free radicals in a large enough quantity to stanch the tide of newly produced free radicals. Also, as waste materials build, the body's defense mechanisms cannot operate properly, and free radicals attack the weakest area of the body.

There is also a link between high cholesterol levels and free radicals. Free radicals often latch onto lipids (fatty substances) and oxidize them, forming lipid peroxides like those found in rancid oils. If a person's lipid levels are up, then lipid peroxide levels (cholesterol) will most likely also be up. A high cholesterol level offers a greater opportunity for free-radical reactions.

How Maharishi Amrit Kalash Combats Free Radicals

Maharishi Amrit Kalash helps purify the channels of the body, clearing the way so that the body's waste-removal, nutrient-delivery, and self-repair systems can work properly.

It also has a remarkable ability to emulate the body's natural antioxidant, the enzyme superoxide dismutase, in scavenging free radicals in the cells. Unlike other antioxidant vitamins and drugs on the market today, Maharishi Amrit Kalash contains a full range of free-radical scavengers, making it the only full-spectrum antioxidant available. This means that it can combat the wide variety of free radicals produced by different cells, whereas vitamins A and C can only combat one or two. Also, synthetic vitamins often are not absorbed by the body and can actually increase free-radical production.

Scientists feel that the time-tested formula, which blends whole herbs together and creates a synergistic effect, is another factor in the success of Maharishi Amrit Kalash in scavenging free radicals. The ancient methods of preparation also enhance its absorption. Because the formula is produced with low heat over a period of days, the long chains of antioxidants get broken down into smaller, more easily assimilated short-chain molecules. Ghee, a soluble lipid, is mixed with the herbs, which makes the molecules lipid-soluble and thus more easily digested.

Research on Maharishi Amrit Kalash

More than forty studies have been done on Maharishi Amrit Kalash worldwide. This unique formulation has been found to increase immunity in humans, as measured by fewer allergic reactions, and in rats in the laboratory, as measured by increased lymphocytes, an indication of increased immunity.

Some families find that when the children take Maharishi Amrit Kalash regularly, they rarely come down with a cold. Research has shown that Maharishi Amrit Kalash is also highly effective in fighting heart disease, arteriosclerosis, high cholesterol levels, and aging. It additionally has been shown to reduce chemical toxicity, for instance following chemotherapy.

Rasayanas for Increased Intelligence, Balanced Emotions

Rasayanas are traditionally known to balance the mind and emotions, creating contentment, happiness, mental clarity, and balance. Research has shown that there is a physiological basis for the increased well-being and decreased depression that Maharishi Amrit Kalash produces.

Other rasayanas are especially helpful for memory and the mind. Intelligence Plus™ (formerly called Study Power) is especially formulated to nourish the mind, memory, and brain during the student years. This nutritious food supplement helps make it easier to function optimally in school.

Researcher Sanford Nidich and others at Maharishi University of Management in Fairfield, Iowa found that when students took Intelligence Plus, their IQs increased by ten points on a test of nonverbal intelligence. Another study by Dr. Hari Sharma, a retired professor of pathology and Director of Cancer Prevention and Natural Products Research at the Ohio State University's College of Medicine, showed that Intelligence Plus improved long-term memory, both because of its ability to scavenge free radicals, and because it increased a chemical in the brain associated with learning.

A Mother's Story

One mother found that a Maharishi Ayurveda rasayana for children, recommended by a physician trained in Maharishi Ayurveda, had a timely and dramatic effect on her son's emotions. This mental tonic, recommended by a physician, helps to build the dhatus and enhances the vitality in the brain. Normally, it must be used for six to seven months to have a good effect, and should be supplemented by a balanced, nutritious diet.

"My normally sweet-tempered, well-behaved two-year-old was going through a period of severe temper tantrums," says his mother. "He would dramatically fling himself on the floor over the smallest of disappointments, thrash about, cry loudly, and even, at times, bang his head on the wall. He wouldn't let us near him when he was in the midst of one of these fits. The crying would go on for hours."

Beside herself with anxiety and fatigue, the mother was worried that something serious might be wrong with her son. She consulted a physician trained in Maharishi Ayurveda, and he recommended the Children's Rasayana (MA 674) to soothe the nervous system and balance the doshas.

"The next day I gave him the Children's Rasayana syrup in the morning, and that day he didn't have a single tantrum. His tantrums have disappeared completely. The same formula also helped my infant son with his digestion. The children like the taste so it's easy to get them to take it."

You have seen in this chapter how Maharishi Ayurveda herbal formulations are both simple and complex. They are simple, because they do not involve extracting the active ingredient, but include instead the whole plant as nature created it. Yet they are highly sophisticated and complex, involving specific combinations of herbs that are prepared in a precise, time-honored way.

Remember that these are food supplements and they work by restoring the body's inner intelligence, not by suppressing symptoms. It is important to follow a healthy daily routine and a toxin-free diet to produce best results.

These herbal formulations have significant implications for children's health. Because they contain the whole plant and not the isolated active ingredient, they do not create harmful side effects. They have been used for thousands of years. Thus they are probably among the safest herbal formulations you could give your child. Yet they are highly effective and potent in their results.

In my practice, I have seen that they can turn around many chronic conditions that have not been helped by Western drugs. Most important of all, they help enhance immunity and break the cycle of sickness. They heal children physically, emotionally, and spiritually.

PART 4
Behaviors That Create Health

CHAPTER ELEVEN
Sleep and the Bedtime Routine

Amber, a nine-year-old girl, was complaining of headaches, fatigue, pressure in the head, and trouble focusing in school. Pulse diagnosis indicated that she had an imbalance in the sub-doshas of Vata concerned with mental activity and sensory overload, and was generally weak and lacking in energy.

After inquiring about Amber's daily routine, the physician recommended that she go to bed between 8:30 and 9:00 p.m. instead of 10:30 p.m., that she do a daily Ayurvedic oil massage (abhyanga) with ghee and coconut oil on the head before bed, and that she make some adjustments in her diet, which was too heavy for Amber's digestion.

He also recommended that Amber spend the last hours of the evening in quiet activities, rather than watching stimulating, violent television shows or playing computer games, as she was accustomed. He explained to her that sleep comes when the mind is prepared for sleep. What she needed was a transition phase when the mind, intellect, and senses are able to withdraw from dynamic activity and allow sleep to take over. The physician recommended Slumber Time® Tea before bed, along with Mind Plus® herbal syrup, to calm her mind and prepare for sleep.

Once Amber understood how to prepare for a good night's sleep, she started sleeping better at night, and within two weeks the imbalance in her pulse and the symptoms disappeared. She realized that by resting deeply in the night and by keeping a proper routine, she could wake up with enthusiasm, energy, and the ability to focus. Once she had the experience of sleeping soundly, she was motivated to continue a good routine.

Amber's story highlights the importance of providing the right balance of rest and activity in a child's routine. In this chapter you'll learn how to arrange the daily schedule so that your child can gain the deep rest needed to have a dynamic day ahead. For you as a parent, the information in this chapter will help eliminate your own fatigue. For your child, establishing a daily schedule that is aligned with nature's rhythms will help him or her establish health habits that will create energy and health for a lifetime.

Nature Has a Natural Rhythm

If you look around in nature, you see that both rest and activity are equally important. The sun sets at night, giving all living creatures a chance to rest after the day's activity. Even when you walk, one foot is resting while the other moves ahead.

The Ayurvedic daily routine makes use of these natural cycles to create the optimum schedule. If you rest when nature is resting, your sleep will be deeper. If you are active when nature is active, you will be more dynamic and successful.

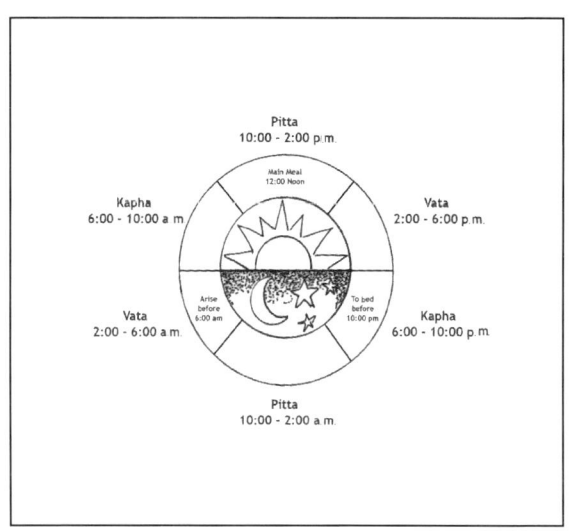

The most powerful influence on our daily rhythms is the sun as it rises, moves across the sky, and sets. In scientific terms the twenty-four-hour cycle of the sun as it rotates on its axis is called the circadian rhythm. Circadian rhythms help determine the daily cycles of sleep and wakefulness, body temperature, metabolic rate, and hormone release. The science of chronobiology has discovered that the human body has a wide spectrum of reactions to medications, for instance, depending on the time of day they are administered. Some medications for asthma only have the optimal therapeutic effect and reduced side effects if administered in the morning. Asthma is twice as likely to occur at night, while other diseases, such as stroke and heart attack, usually occur early in the morning. Thus the timing of a treatment could produce different results depending on the time of day.

In Maharishi Ayurveda, these fluctuations in energy caused by the sun's cycles are linked to the daily cycle of the three doshas, Vata, Pitta, and Kapha. There are actually two twelve-hour cycles of Vata, Pitta, and Kapha.

Different qualities of the doshas predominate in nature at these times. The morning Vata cycle, for instance, starts at 2:00 a.m. and ends at 6:00 a.m. This is the time of day when the air is suffused with energy and lightness. The morning Pitta cycle starts at 10:00 and reaches its peak at noon, when the sun is highest in the sky and is creating the maximum amount of heat. The evening Kapha cycle (6:00 to 10:00 p.m.) is the time of day when the birds come home to roost, and the day's active mode is left behind for the quieter, slower, evening rest. Understanding these cycles gives you clues as to the best times to eat, to sleep, and to be awake.

Children Grow in Their Sleep

Maharishi Ayurveda recognizes sleep as one of the pillars of health. It is during sleep that the body purifies and cleanses itself; the body's self-repair mechanisms depend on sleep. Sleep creates ojas and a strong immune system. It's no coincidence, after all, that pediatricians prescribe plenty of rest for any illness. The body releases stress in sleep. And for children, sleep is also the time when growth takes place.

Children are not "small adults" when it comes to sleep. They have very different physiological needs, due to the fact that they are growing at a rapid rate. Babies sleep as much during the day as at night until their third month, when night sleep starts to take over. Newborns sleep a minimum of sixteen hours, and by one year they will still be sleeping twelve hours, but not in one continuous block of sleep. It can take up until age five or six for children to switch completely to nocturnal sleep. That's why throughout early childhood, napping is essential. The development of nocturnal sleep patterns parallels the development of motor skills.

Infants and toddlers sleep more lightly and experience more wakefulness during the night. A higher proportion of their sleep is the restless, light REM (rapid-eye-movement) sleep with dreaming, and in newborns it's a different type of REM sleep than an adult experiences. Babies awaken easily from that kind of sleep, as any weary parent of a baby knows.

Eight-to-ten-year-olds, on the other hand, sleep very deeply, and it can actually be difficult to wake them up, especially in the first part of the night. They are experiencing more deep sleep, known as NREM (non rapid-eye-movement) sleep.

This type of deep sleep is essential for children to grow properly. In fact, research shows that children do much of their growing during the deepest NREM sleep. Somatotrophic hormone, a growth hormone, is released by the pituitary gland during the first two cycles of NREM sleep, meaning in the first part of the night. If for some reason NREM sleep is interrupted, less growth hormone gets released.

Children need much more sleep than adults. The amount of night rest and napping your child needs varies according to his age, his temperament, and his constitution. Some children are great sleepers from day one, while others wake up during the night. Some need more sleep, and others need less.

Typically newborns sleep about sixteen hours daily in spurts of two to four hours. For preschool children, going to bed before 7:30 p.m. is advisable, because they usually need as much as twelve hours of sleep a night, plus naps during the day. An average twelve-year-old sleeps for ten hours. The typical adolescent today sleeps only six hours a night, but needs much more, nearly as much as babies. Adults require an average of eight hours a night.

The Key to the Daily Routine: Early Bedtime

As a parent, you may not know that there are certain key times for sleep to take place. When your child goes to bed early in the Kapha time of the evening (well before 10:00 p.m.), he will enjoy the deep, heavy quality of sleep associated with Kapha dosha. Sleeping in the early part of the night actually creates a more restful sleep.

As mentioned earlier, NREM sleep takes place during the first part of the night, about twenty minutes after falling asleep, and lasts about an hour. If NREM sleep is consistently interrupted, it can result in sleep disorders or growth and endocrine imbalances. By timing sleep so the NREM sleep takes place during the heavier Kapha period of the day, the deepest part of sleep can be undisturbed and more restful, nourishing the growth of children.

If your child stays awake until 10:00 p.m. or later, this is the Pitta stage of the night. This is the body's natural time for purifying the digestion and for self-repair. If your child falls asleep during this period, his sleep will be more active and restless, like Pitta dosha itself. If he's awake he also might feel hungry and need a snack, which disrupts the self-cleansing mechanisms of the body.

This is also true of adults who regularly go to bed after ten o'clock at night. Try going to bed before ten for a week, and see if you don't feel much more rested. You'll have less chance of feeling restless and waking up in the night. Many people who suffer from insomnia find that if they go to bed during the Kapha part of the night, they fall asleep much more easily. You also might find, as many adults do, that you need fewer hours of sleep to feel rested. By sleeping earlier in the evening, sleep is more restful and comes more easily. Putting your children to bed earlier gives you some necessary downtime, so you can also get to bed before ten.

Why Getting Up Early Is Important

Another reason for getting to bed early is that it's not good for health to sleep late in the morning. After resting the whole night, rising early in the morning brings lightness to the body, freshness to the senses, and clarity to the mind.

Although sleeping past 6:00 a.m. is not recommended for adults because it clogs the microchannels of the body and creates dullness in the mind, preschool children may need to sleep later in order to get enough rest. Usually by the time the child is going to school, he will be ready to start rising at 6:00 a.m. And it is, of course, a good idea for children five years of age and younger to take naps. Sleeping during the day is also important when children are ill, or are tired from traveling, as then the body needs to rest and repair itself. During the summer, when the hot weather keeps the srotas open, the whole family can nap during the day without feeling sluggish.

Set a Bedtime and Rising Time and Stick to It
Putting your child to bed at the same time every night is important. In fact, it's ideal to eat at the same time every day, to go to bed at the same time, and to wake up at the same time. Children thrive on consistency and routine, especially if they have any Vata imbalance. Keeping a consistent routine can cure many sleep disorders. An irregular routine creates imbalances in the doshas and disrupts the body's natural rhythms.

Studies on adults have shown that irregularity in sleep-wakefulness patterns leads to a negative sense of well-being, irregular moods, and the inability to fall asleep at the right time. This is also true of children, although they won't be able to tell you so. They might be hyperactive, feel fatigued, have learning problems, or feel uninterested in school. Sleep is the basis for alertness and attention. For babies, interrupted sleep leads to emotional ups and downs, irritability, colic, falling sound asleep at the wrong time, and waking up in the night. Well-rested children are more pleasant, flexible, happy, and adaptable.

Maintaining an early bedtime at the same time every evening is the key to helping your child stabilize his developing biological rhythms. It is just as important to maintain a regular wake-up time in the morning.

Parents can start gently nudging their children into a routine after the first three months, so that by age one the waking, sleeping, napping, and eating patterns are consistent each day. How much sleep or naptime your child needs will differ with each child and will change as he grows. But the point is to find the right amount and make it a habit.

If you keep a consistent routine, and your child becomes accustomed to falling asleep at 8:00 p.m., he will start to feel drowsy and his eyelids will start drooping at 7:30, making your job a lot easier. This is also true about meals. By eating at the same time every day, the enzymes of the body prepare to digest at that time, making digestion run more smoothly and easily.

Techniques for Getting Your Child to Bed at Night

It is known in Maharishi Ayurveda that if the brain is too active, the body cannot sleep. That is why it's a good idea to avoid exposing your child to too much stimulation at night, such as television. If your child is having a hard time falling asleep, try eliminating TV in the evening, or at least limit it to a half hour well before bedtime.

Soothing nighttime activities include listening to music, singing songs, or playing games. The evening hours before bed can be a time when the family engages in quiet activities and hobbies together.

It's ideal if the child's bedroom can be separate from the playroom, so when your child enters the bedroom, he's primed for sleep. It's important to make a ritual of bedtime, helping your child get ready for bed and crawl under the covers rather than falling asleep in front of the TV. Even babies will feel disoriented if they wake up in a different environment from the one they fell asleep in. Try to keep the bedroom quiet and dark when your child falls asleep, just as it will be when he wakes up in the night. If everything is where it was when he fell asleep, he'll be less inclined to feel disoriented and more inclined to fall back asleep again.

Bedtime should be pleasant, something to look forward to. It helps if you have the same routine every night, one you and your child have agreed upon, so the child knows that he or she can't beg you into another story and thus stay up later. You'll need adequate time to get your child to bed, from ten to thirty minutes, depending on the child.

School-age children also need personal attention before bed. Engage in conversation that fits with your child's age and needs. You could talk about pleasant events of the day, read a favorite book out loud, or listen to music together.

An eleven- or twelve-year-old may be able to get ready for bed by himself, but it's still important for the parent to remind him when it's time for bed. It's also a good idea to stop by his room to say goodnight, to give your child a chance to share his thoughts and feelings with you.

Parents the world over enjoy telling stories or singing a lullaby to their children before bed. Bedtime is also a time when many parents express their feelings of love for their children. Even older children will allow a hug and a kiss then. This is important and healthy, because physical affection settles the heart and balances the doshas, creating a sweet and happy feeling as your child slips into sleep.

The impressions from your child's last waking moments will be carried into sleep, so you'll want the stories to be uplifting, about heroes and heroines or good deeds. The habit of many families to say prayers with their children before bed helps the child remember the good things that happened during the day and to look forward to the next day with a happy feeling.

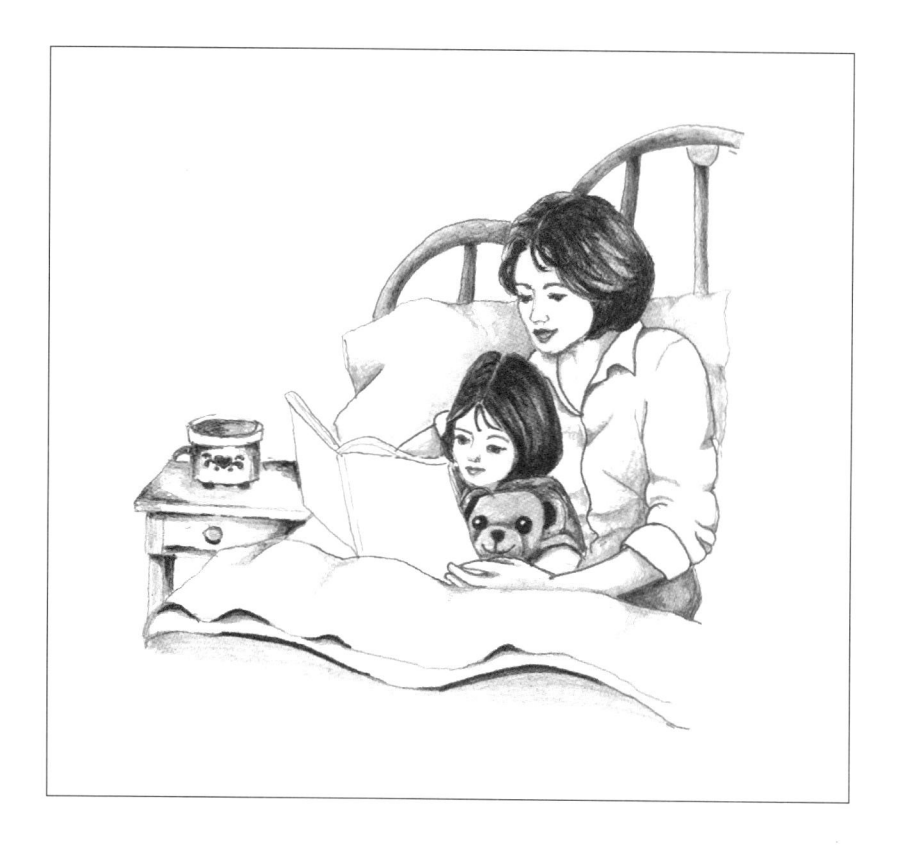

You can also give your child a small amount of warm milk with cardamom before bed. Remember to boil the milk first to make it more digestible. Milk helps to balance Vata and Pitta doshas, both of which are responsible for sleep disorders. If your child tends to wake up frequently in the night and sleeps restlessly, you can add some Rose Petal Preserve to the milk to balance Pitta dosha. For Kapha types, the milk might be a little heavy, so you can add some water to dilute it or raw honey to sweeten it after the milk cools.

For Children Who Can't Fall Asleep at Night

The interesting thing about sleep is that sometimes the less you sleep, the harder it becomes to fall asleep and stay asleep. A child can actually become too tired to sleep. Sometimes older children who are more prone to Vata disorders, including insomnia, get into a vicious cycle of not sleeping enough, which leads to more disturbed sleep patterns. Yet sleep is one of the most important ways to balance Vata dosha. Children who are high-strung and active need more sleep than others to stay emotionally balanced and physically healthy.

Three Types of Sleep Disorders and Solutions

1. Your child has trouble falling asleep easily. His mind is restless and "wound up" before bed.

Possible Solutions
- Balance Vata dosha. Be sure your child's diet is Vata-pacifying. Even small amounts of caffeine or chocolate could keep a child awake, especially if eaten in the evening. Eating too many light or dry foods, such as crackers or cold cereal, can also tip the balance of the body.
- Cut out TV at night. Watching TV excessively is overshadowing to the senses and can create Vata disorders. At night it's better to let the senses be soothed and settled.
- Give your child a nightly abhyanga (see next chapter for directions). For a child who is insomnia-prone and has a Vata imbalance, a soothing, light oil massage right before bed can help remove stress, settle the mind, and soothe him into sleep. Giving special attention to the head and feet can help balance Vata dosha. You don't have to give him a bath afterwards; just use a light amount of oil so it won't stain the bed sheets.
- Try using Slumber Time™ Therapeutic Aroma Oil in your child's bedroom at night. This is a combination of oils specifically designed to facilitate deeper sleep.

- Give your child warm milk with ghee before bed to calm Vata dosha.
- For younger children, make sure they have a nap in the afternoon to help balance Vata dosha.
- Try making bedtime earlier in the evening, before 8:00 p.m., when the heavier qualities of Kapha are more predominant.

2. Your child falls asleep fine, but wakes up with lots of energy in the night, between 2:00 and 4:00 a.m. He has frequent nightmares and sleeps restlessly, tossing and turning and waking up frequently.

Possible Solutions
- Check to see if his diet or routine is Pitta aggravating. Are there too many spicy, sour, or salty foods? Caffeine and chocolate aggravate Pitta dosha and should be avoided. Skipping meals, playing too hard in the hot sun, and confrontational situations can aggravate Pitta.
- Be sure your child goes to bed well before the Pitta time of night, which starts at 10:00 p.m.
- Give him cooled milk (i.e., let it cool after boiling) with a teaspoon of Rose Petal Preserve before bed.
- A massage before bed can also help prevent restless sleep.
- Make sure he's getting the right balance of exercise during the day.

3. Your child is tired even though he sleeps more than fourteen hours a night.

Possible Solutions
- Consult your child's pediatrician to make sure that there is no physiological reason for his fatigue, such as allergy or a hidden disease. A physician trained in Maharishi Ayurveda can determine if accumulated toxins (ama) are causing the feeling of fatigue.
- Be sure the diet is not too heavy and difficult to digest. Add some mild spices to his diet, such as fresh ginger, cumin, corian-

der, and turmeric, Stimulating (Kapha) Spice Mix, and Kapha Tea.
- Make sure that he has time to digest dinner (two to three hours) before bedtime.
- Be sure he's getting enough exercise. Sometimes fatigue is caused by too much inactivity. Limit the TV and computer games and get your child outside playing in the fresh air and sunshine.
- Give your child a morning abhyanga to help remove impurities, creating a fresher wake-up feeling. Older children can learn to massage themselves.
- Try to shift the sleeping hours so that your child is not sleeping in the late morning. Teenagers need a lot of sleep, for instance, but they tend to stay up late and sleep all morning, which clogs the microchannels of the body and aggravates the doshas, especially Kapha. For younger children, move their bedtime up to 7:30, so they can wake up earlier.

By giving your child a good night's rest, you give him the best possible foundation for a dynamic day. In the next chapter, you'll learn the Ayurvedic principles for the daytime portion of the daily routine.

CHAPTER TWELVE
Ayurvedic Massage and the Wake-Up Routine

When most adults look back on their growing up years, they recall that time passed very slowly, with hours of free play. Life was lived at a more leisurely pace, and this is still the case in many countries.

In America, the fast pace of life has reached down to the childhood years. This is especially true when parents, eager for their children to excel, urge them to participate in many types of lessons or extracurricular activities after school. Many children live very structured lives, rushing to lessons or sports events, then facing many hours of homework. As one little girl said, "All the time it's hurry up, hurry up."

Yet the Ayurvedic daily routine does not involve rushing. Rushing destroys ojas and aggravates Vata dosha. Even if there are many things to do in a day, it is up to the parents to structure a schedule that does not create stress in their children.

For this, it is important to know your child. Some children can handle more structure than others. A child who has more Vata may need to rest after school, because his more delicate nervous system may be fatigued and overwhelmed with all the stimulation of the day. Helping him to recognize how to rest and recharge his batteries by taking some time out, or by doing some quieter activities such as reading in his room, will help him structure a happier and healthier life.

If a child is naturally competitive and has a predominance of Pitta dosha, it may be a good idea to direct his or her need for competition into rewarding activities. On the other hand, if a child is already a perfectionist, it's vital that he not feel too much external pressure from his parents and teachers. He already has enough internal pressure, and needs to learn how to take time out when he starts feeling too intense, angry, or frustrated.

For a Kapha child, who may be content to just take it easy, structure may be important to motivate him to use his talents and to keep active.

If your child is showing signs of stress (for instance, if he is often fatigued, feels overwhelmed easily, complains about all that he has to do, does not seem to be enjoying his activities, and exhibits physical symptoms of stress such as nail-biting, wetting the bed, or severe sleep disorders), it could be a sign that he needs his parents and other adults

---

The Daily Routine for Children

Morning
Wake up early
Evacuate bowels and bladder
Ayurvedic oil massage (abhyanga)
Brush teeth, scrape tongue, rinse mouth
Bath or shower
Yoga Asanas and breathing exercises
Transcendental Meditation or Word of Wisdom program
Breakfast

Daytime
School or play
Eat the largest meal at noon
Walk or play
School or play

Late Afternoon and Evening
Yoga Asanas and breathing exercises
Transcendental Meditation or Word of Wisdom program
Light dinner before 6:00 p.m.
Light relaxing activities (games, socializing, music, singing, stories)
Bedtime before 8:30 p.m., depending on age of child and constitution

in his life to help him find a better balance between rest and activity. What Maharishi Ayurveda suggests is to adjust the daily routine to be more in tune with nature's rhythms.

The Morning Routine

At about age six or seven, you can teach your child to rise early in the morning, before 6:00 a.m. As you learned in the last chapter, rising in the Vata time of the day will not only create a freshness and vitality that will last the whole day, but it will also allow time for the morning routine, which includes Ayurvedic oil massage (abhyanga), bathing, dental hygiene, Yoga Asanas (yoga poses), and practicing the Transcendental Meditation technique. For the child, all of these are designed to prepare the mind, body, and emotions for a busy, productive day of learning and fun.

Ayurvedic Oil Massage (Abhyanga)
A very enjoyable part of the Ayurvedic daily routine is the morning oil massage, or abhyanga. Abhyanga is a gentle way to wake up, clearing the cobwebs from the mind and preparing your child for the day ahead. It energizes the body, removes fatigue, and promotes overall health. It helps balance the doshas and releases stress. Because the skin is the seat of Vata dosha, it has a special effect in soothing Vata, which is the "king" dosha. When out of balance, Vata leads the other doshas in creating disease. Abhyanga creates a kind of protection, or special armor, for meeting the world each day. It improves immunity by flushing out toxins and rejuvenating the internal organs.

Abhyanga is good for the whole family, from infants to adults. It works better than a cup of coffee in getting Mom and Dad going for the day and is a thousand times healthier.

Infant Massage
Traditionally, daily abhyanga is started several days after birth, and is a delightful way for parents to bond with their new baby while improving his immunity, flexibility, muscular strength, circulation, coordination, sleep, and digestion. Infant abhyanga helps remove impurities, brings nourishing blood and oxygen to all cells of the body, alleviates gas,

relaxes the muscles and nervous system, tones the baby's muscles, helps keep the baby happy and settled, and enhances immunity. It allows the infant to release the tension and stress accumulated while cramped in the womb for nine months.

Some stunning research on pre-term babies who were massaged showed that these children experienced faster neurological development, greater weight gain, improved mind-body integration, and better sleep. They were less irritable and more responsive, and they developed better interactions with their parents.

You can start giving your child an abhyanga after the umbilical cord falls off. To learn how to give infant massage, it's best to consult a Maharishi Ayurveda health expert.

With the baby massage, you must be especially careful that the room is warm. The bathroom is a good place to do baby massage. You can spread towels on the floor to create a soft, clean place to lay the baby, and be sure to have extra towels on hand. Talk to your baby throughout the abhyanga, to reassure him and to keep him relaxed. It's a special time between parent and child and is very enjoyable. Older infants may sit up or roll over. That's fine. You can incorporate those moves into the massage.

Preschool Children

Even though your child is no longer an infant, you can continue to massage your child throughout the preschool years, using the guidelines given below. Massaging your child has many psycho-emotional benefits. Massage strengthens the tender bond of love between parent and child. It is a way to express your love and affection through touch.

Children generally enjoy abhyanga and look forward to the soothing feeling it creates. As you massage your child, you are giving so much love. You can also explain the health benefits of abhyanga to your child, so he or she understands its purpose. The main thing is to enjoy the abhyanga as a happy time. No need to feel worried if the abhyanga is not done perfectly every time.

You can massage your preschool child before his or her morning bath. But remember that your child will probably slip around a bit. Don't expect your child to sit still—it may be a rather dynamic process.

Plan for this by spreading a plastic tarp on the bathroom floor, or else wipe up the oil afterwards with a damp sponge.

School-Age Children

As they grow older, your children will want to start massaging themselves, and that is a good time to teach them to give themselves an abhyanga.

Use the guidelines below to teach your child abhyanga. By learning to massage themselves, children learn a habit that will help balance all three doshas, create increased immunity, promote better sleep, eliminate fatigue, increase flexibility, purify the body, and create radiant skin for their whole lives.

How to Do Ayurvedic Oil Massage

The procedure is basically the same for all age groups beyond infancy, with a few exceptions. Massage should not be done when the child has a chest cold, because the massage can mobilize toxins (ama) and spread the disease.

Cure the Oil

The first step is to make sure the oil is cured, or purified. Sesame oil is considered the best oil for abhyanga, but in certain cases, olive oil is used for Kapha constitutions and coconut oil is recommended for those with Pitta constitutions.

Buy cold-pressed, unheated sesame oil, preferably organic. The quality of the oil is important, because during abhyanga, oil penetrates the skin and even the cell membranes. You want to be sure the oil is of high quality. Maharishi Ayurveda Vata, Pitta, and Kapha massage oils are also recommended. These do not need to be cured.

To cure the oil, place up to one quart in a stainless steel or glass saucepan and heat it to the boiling point of water, which is about 212° F. You can use a candy thermometer to judge the heat. This takes only about five minutes. Do not leave the oil unattended, even for a moment. If you were to forget it, or it boiled over, it could burst into flames.

Place the covered saucepan in a safe place to cool, far from the reach of small children. Once cooled, you can store it in glass or plastic jars. A quart of oil will last several weeks or more.

Store it in a bottle, and before each massage, warm up the oil to body temperature by placing the bottle under the hot-water tap. You can also use a baby bottle warmer.

Apply the Oil

Traditionally, Ayurvedic oil massage uses the palm of the hand instead of the fingertips. It is not a deep, penetrating massage, but a light-to-moderate stroking of the body. Use long strokes on the long bones of the body (such as the legs and forearms) and circular strokes on the joints. Go easy on the stomach (especially pregnant women).

Apply a light covering of oil to each part of the body before massaging it. The massage proceeds from the head to the feet in a sequence of strokes.

Massage the head, ears, and face first. Using a circular motion, massage the top, sides, and back of the head with both hands. Gently massage the outer ears.

Circle the temple and cheeks. Stroke across the forehead. Stroke across the upper lip and chin.

Next massage the front and back of the neck, using horizontal strokes back and forth. Be gentle over the windpipe.

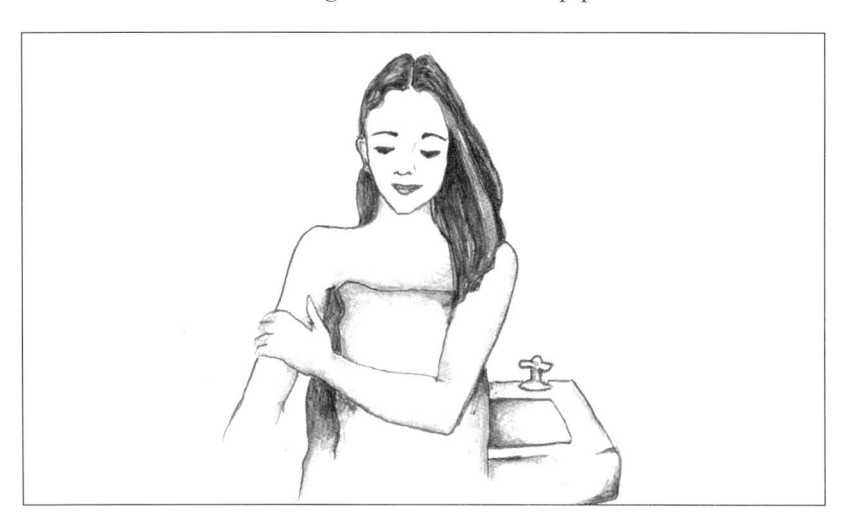

Massage each arm. Circle the shoulder, use long strokes back and forth on the upper arm, circle the elbow, and use long strokes back and forth on the lower arm. Circle the wrist. Massage the palm and the back of the hand, and then gently pull each finger.

For the chest and abdomen, make circles on the chest with both hands, using gentle, circular motions over the heart. Be especially gentle on the abdomen, using a clockwise motion (to follow the natural direction of the elimination system).

On the back, use long strokes to massage up and down the spine and back (as far as you can reach).

Legs are similar to arms. Massage each leg separately, and use long strokes on the upper leg, circular strokes on the knee, and long strokes on the calf. Circle the ankles.

The feet are last, but you'll want to spend more time here. Massage back and forth on the Achilles' tendon, heel, and top of the foot. Use the palm of the hand to stroke the sole of the foot lengthwise. Gently pull the toes.

Dental Hygiene

The Ayurvedic texts give a great deal of attention to dental hygiene for children. Just as we do in modern times, they recommended that children clean their mouths in the morning after waking (as well as at night before bed).

Massaging the Gums

After the Ayurvedic oil massage, and while the oil is still on the body, your school-age child can massage his gums with a little sesame oil. Pour a few drops of oil into his open palm, ask him to dip his forefinger in the oil, and use the oiled finger to massage the gums. This only takes a few minutes and is very healthy for the gums. Sesame oil has been found to strengthen the gums and prevent plaque buildup on the teeth.

Scraping the Tongue

One thing children don't mind doing is scraping their tongues. When you teach your child to use a toothbrush, you can also teach your child to use a tongue scraper, a blunted strip of stainless steel or silver that you gently drag down the tongue to remove the whitish coating that often appears on the tongue in the morning. This whitish coating is ama, and by removing it from the tongue, your child can actually help cleanse his digestive system. Scraping the tongue freshens the mouth and sharpens the sense of taste, which also aids digestion.

Lubricating the Nasal Passages (Nasya)

Sniffing a little sesame oil in the morning is an Ayurvedic method for relieving dryness in the nasal passages and preventing colds and sinus infections. Place a drop of cured sesame oil in the palm of your child's hand. Teach him to dip his little finger in the oil and insert it in the nose and sniff. Repeat for the other nostril. This can be done starting at age four or five.

Bathing and Exercise

After the Ayurvedic oil massage (abhyanga) and brushing the teeth, the child can take a warm bath. This is important not only for washing off the oil, but also for allowing the impurities that have been loosened by the abhyanga to flow out of the tissues and into the digestive tract.

If a warm bath is not possible, at least give your child a warm shower. Encourage your child to dress in fresh, clean clothing after bathing.

The best time to exercise is during the Kapha period in the morning, between 6:00 and 10:00 a.m. Starting at age ten, when they learn the Transcendental Meditation technique, children can also begin doing Yoga Asanas (yoga poses) each morning. Yoga Asanas are gentle, simple exercises that tone all the muscles and purify the organs of the body. They help settle the mind for meditation. Traditionally, Yoga Asanas are done after the morning bath. These are described in the following chapter.

Children's Meditation

The children's meditation is a very important time of the day. If the mother and father meditate, the children will want to do it too. It has many benefits for mental and physical health. As described earlier, children from age four can learn a more active version of meditation, while children aged ten and up can learn the same restful technique as adults, although they do it for a shorter period of time.

Sometimes children forget to meditate and need a little reminder. It's better not to make a big deal about it, but you can set up the schedule to make it easy for them to do it every day. It also helps if you all do it together. One mother with three daughters would start the meditation all together. Her twelve-year-old daughter sat to meditate with her, while her two younger daughters, nine and four, practiced their Word of Wisdom technique while walking about the room. Each daughter let herself out of the room when she was done, leaving Mom to finish her longer meditation alone. Meditating with Mom made it fun and easy to fit into the routine.

You can also help your child feel motivated to meditate by noticing the good effects. Better grades in school, better relationships with their family and friends, getting sick less often, and a happier feeling are some of the benefits children appreciate.

Optimum Time for Meals

Even though breakfast is certainly an important meal for children and should never be skipped, it's best to serve a lighter quantity and quality of food at breakfast and supper, because both of these meals occur during the Kapha cycle, when the digestive fire is much weaker. Overloading it at these times results in the production of ama.

In the Ayurvedic daily routine, the main meal is eaten at noon, because this is the Pitta period, when the sun is at its peak in the sky and the body's own internal sun, or digestive fire, is also at its height. This is why all traditional cultures eat more heavily at noon, when a strong digestion allows heavier foods to be digested and assimilated more easily.

Homework and the Active Time of the Day

For children, the active part of the day is usually taken up in school, exercise, and play. These occur during the Pitta and Vata times of the day, when children naturally feel energetic.

It's also important to consider the time of day for doing homework. Children are often too tired to do their homework right after school, and need a break to relax and get some exercise. Right after lunch or dinner might not be a good time either, as the food is digesting then and could cause some drowsiness. Children with a predominance of Vata dosha might find it hard to fall asleep at night if they study too hard close to bedtime. It's also better for them not to wait until the last minute, when they'll feel some pressure.

During the week, the best time for all children might be in the early evening before dinner. On the weekends they could do it in the middle of the afternoon, after lunch has digested.

Maharishi Gandharva Veda[SM] **Music**

One of the most delightful ways to attune your child to the daily cycles of Vata, Pitta, and Kapha is to play Maharishi Gandharva Veda music. This music is from the Vedic civilization in India, and it expresses the varying frequencies of nature at different times of the day, from morning to night to morning again.

There are eight discrete time periods during the day, and each raga (musical composition) is played only at a particular time because its rhythms and melodies match nature's frequencies during that period. By listening to Maharishi Gandharva Veda music, you can attune yourself to the subtle frequencies of nature that are being expressed at that moment. In this way, you can dissolve stress, disharmony, and fatigue.

The child doesn't have to listen to the music in order to enjoy more peace, harmony, and bliss. Families that play Maharishi Gandharva Veda music quietly in a closet or unused room of the home report that family harmony increases, and that children are more contented and peaceful. The vibrations from the music permeate the home and create the effect even without being heard.

Maharishi Gandharva Veda music is also soothing to play in the bedroom while your child is falling asleep. However, it's better not to play any music in the same room while children are studying or eating, as this will make it difficult for them to focus.

Respect Natural Urges

It's important to teach your children not to suppress their natural urges throughout the day. They should be taught to use the bathroom when they need to. Other urges that should not be repressed are: flatulence, vomiting, sneezing, belching, yawning, hunger, thirst, tears, sleep, and breathing deep breaths when exercising.

Suppressing these natural urges can cause Vata dosha to become imbalanced, since it is Vata that wants to move. Suppressing the urge to go to the bathroom, for instance, can eventually cause constipation (a Vata disorder) or urinary problems. The Ayurvedic texts also explain that these urges should not be forced to occur, as that can also create imbalances.

The Seasonal Routine

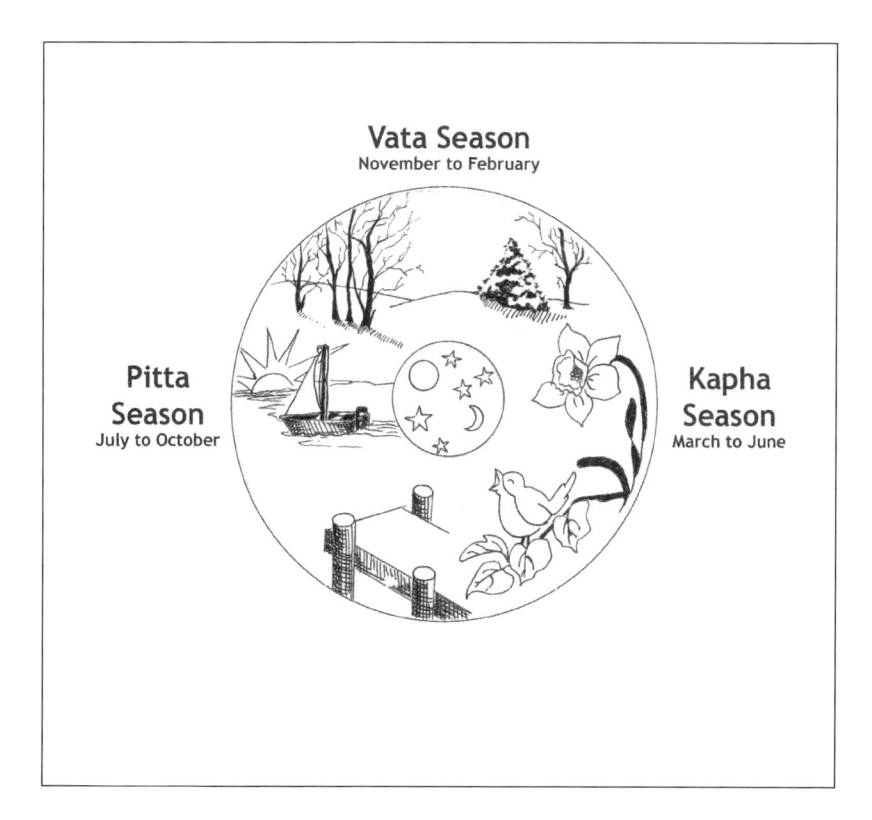

Just as the daily routine responds to the cycle of energy as the sun moves across the sky each day, so the seasonal routine responds to the cycle of the seasons. It's important to culture the awareness of seasons at a young age, so the child can recognize early that he is part of the natural rhythms of nature.

You have already learned how to vary the diet according to the seasons in Chapter Six. There are many behaviors that can be adjusted according to the seasons as well.

Vata Season (November to February)

During the cold and windy Vata season, every mother knows that her children need to protect their heads and necks with hats and scarves. It's also important for children to sleep more during these months. There are fewer hours of sunlight and more hours of darkness, and the body naturally needs more rest during these dark days of decreased daylight in the Northern Hemisphere. Sleep also balances Vata dosha. A regular routine is especially important during Vata season, because the active, fluctuating nature of Vata dosha tends to cause irregularity in the digestion and other systems. Colds and flu circulate during this time, so it's important to increase the digestive fire and the immunity.

Eating more heavy and solid foods is normal during these months, when hearty winter meals help provide extra fuel for the digestive fire and fortify the body against the cold. Serve more sweet, sour, and salty tastes to balance Vata dosha.

Pitta Season (July to October)

During the hot summer, Pitta season, it's important to avoid getting overheated and overly competitive. Keep your child out of the sun at noon, when the sun is at its strongest, especially if your child is prone to Pitta disorders. Help him or her find summer recreation that is cooling, such as swimming.

Supply hats and sunscreen to protect your child's skin during summer. Provide plenty of liquids at home and on family outings. Children can drink cool drinks but should avoid ice-cold beverages, as the icy temperature of the liquid squelches the digestive agni and can cause digestive problems.

It's a good idea to provide a more relaxed, easygoing schedule during the summer months. Rushing around is never a good idea, but in the hot months it will only aggravate Pitta. It's OK for the whole family to take naps during Pitta season, as the heat keeps the srotas open and flowing. Everyone needs to slow down in the heat.

Serve more bitter, astringent, and sweet tastes to cool Pitta dosha.

Kapha Season (March to June)

In the wet and cool Kapha season, it's important for children to eat warm meals that are nourishing yet light. Colds and flu are also common during Kapha season. (It's interesting that the word "cold" describes both Vata and Kapha doshas.) Older children should avoid napping during the day (which creates the duller, heavier qualities of Kapha) by going to bed earlier and getting more sleep while the sun is down, and then waking up early with the rising sun. Exercise is especially important in this season, as it helps stimulate the digestion and helps purify toxins. But warn your children to stay warm and dry.

Serve more warm, light foods and soups, and more bitter, astringent, and pungent tastes.

Ways to Prevent Imbalances throughout the Seasons

Common Imbalances during Vata Season and for a Vata-Predominant Child in Any Season

- Excitability
- Fluctuations in energy, fatigue
- Irregular digestion—hungry one meal but hardly eats the next
- Nervousness, more fears than other children
- Difficulty falling asleep

Ways to Create Balance

- Make sure your child goes to bed early, as sleep is stabilizing. Warm milk with ghee before bed can help with sleep.
- Give your child daily abhyanga in the morning and, if insomnia is a problem, before bed.
- Limit TV and computer games, as these aggravate Vata dosha.
- Stick to regular mealtimes; stay on a regular routine.
- Be careful that your child doesn't overexert in sports and gets plenty of rest.

- Serve warm, cooked foods that are unctuous and sturdy. Include more sweet, sour, and salty tastes.

Common Imbalances during Pitta Season and for a Pitta-Predominant Child in Any Season

- Anger, irritability, or impatience
- Sensitivity
- Perfectionism
- Competitiveness
- Easily overheated
- Prone to rashes

Ways to Create Balance

- Make sure your child takes frequent play breaks and time out from a structured schedule.
- Reduce pressure of competition, of doing things perfectly.
- Give your child milk with Rose Petal Preserve before bed.
- Teach your child to avoid getting overheated, to stay out of the sun at midday, to wear a hat for protection from the sun, and to play sports that are more cooling.

Common Imbalances during Kapha Season and for a Kapha-Predominant Child in Any Season

- Slow learner
- Lethargic
- Overweight
- Prone to colds and flu
- Lacking in motivation

Ways to Create Balance

- Be patient and allow him to complete tasks at his own pace, because he does things thoroughly and well if given a chance.
- Provide lots of opportunity for activity and sports.
- Teach him to eat foods that are lighter, less oily, more stimulating (pungent, bitter, and astringent tastes).

- For older children, teach them to avoid sleeping during the day.
- Provide a stimulating environment with lots of new experiences.

Helping Your Child Make the Right Choices

In recent years, researchers have recognized lifestyle as a critical component of health for children. A child's habits today create the man or woman of tomorrow. Studies show that many unhealthy behaviors often start before adolescence, including poor dietary habits, lack of exercise, and use of harmful substances.

It's important to teach your child that he has a choice. He can choose health or sickness. If he feels dull and fatigued, help him to see that it is from eating something unsuitable or from going to bed late. We all make choices, every day. The more your child sees the connection between the choices he has made and the way he feels, the more he will respond to his body's needs.

You can point out to your child that if he is doing what his friends are doing, but it's not right behavior, then he must make a choice. It's important to explain to a child how peer pressure affects him.

As a parent, you first make the choice for healthy living yourself, and then you help your child to make that choice. This is how to develop independent, responsible children who live life in tune with natural law. If you want to act in tune with nature, to have maximum success, to bring good relations to your family, then it is important to take your time. Nothing should be done in a rush. Every action is for perfection, for fulfillment. But this will only be possible if you are living in concert with the daily rhythms of nature, going about your daily life without strain or undue effort. If you follow the natural rhythms of the daily routine outlined in this chapter, you will find yourself and your family living a life that is more simple, more fulfilling, and more healthy.

CHAPTER THIRTEEN
Improving Health with Ayurvedic Exercise

Exercise is something the whole family can do together. Besides its obvious health benefits, it cultivates much more communication and bonding than sitting in front of the TV. Riding bicycles together, playing baseball, or shooting hoops can be easily incorporated into a family's lifestyle without much expense.

It's not only healthy, it's fun. And that is important for children, to learn that exercise is an entertaining and comfortable event. Children who have fun while exercising will be more likely to exercise as adults, thus setting the pattern for lifelong health.

The Value of Exercise

According to the Ayurvedic texts, exercise is an important part of the daily routine. It improves immunity, removes toxins from the body, and increases strength. It creates stability, lightness in the body, ability to work, resistance to discomfort, and improved power of digestion. It balances the doshas (especially Kapha); makes the body light and glossy, firm and compact; banishes fatigue and weariness; makes the body stout and strong; helps the symmetrical growth of the limbs and muscles; leads to a disease-free existence; is the best means to reduce overweight; improves complexion; and prevents laziness.

Modern research reports many positive benefits for children who exercise. Young children who are physically active and feel successful at movement activities tend to develop greater self-esteem and a greater sense of accomplishment. Physical activity also helps children develop more stamina and resistance to fatigue. They are also more alert in school. Exercise helps develop healthy muscles, bones, and tissues. Research shows that children who engage in daily physical activity enjoy improved muscular strength, flexibility, cardiovascular endurance, and strong bodies.

American Children Sit Too Much

Childhood in America is not as active as it used to be. Long summer days spent swimming, biking, and playing outdoor games are no longer the norm. Whether due to the allure of TV and computer games, the problem of unsafe neighborhoods, or the tendency to spend more time in structured lessons and daycare, today's children spend much less time outdoors in vigorous free play. Just being a kid does not ensure that your child is getting enough exercise.

Some studies show that 50 percent of American children are not getting enough physical activity. An even more shocking statistic shows that children at the tender ages of two to five spend an average of twenty-five hours a week watching television. This frightening scenario does not take into account other sedentary hours spent playing computer games.

Unfortunately, this trend is taking an enormous toll on children's health. The number of overweight children has doubled in the last decade. The U.S. Department of Agriculture's Children's Nutrition Research Center has conducted surveys over a twenty-year period, finding that today's children are exhibiting a dramatically higher level of obesity than in earlier years. One in three girls and one in four boys have body-fat levels at the obesity level.

It is well known that obese children tend to become obese adults, and that children with high blood pressure are likely to have high blood pressure as adults. Thus, correcting the imbalance in childhood is the best way to protect against disease in later life.

The surgeon general has suggested that children under eighteen need one hour of physical activity per day (note that this can consist of shorter periods of exercise that add up to one hour). In a poll that questioned children about their own habits, only three-fifths said they played outdoors with friends daily, and only 55 percent said they walked every day.

Other surveys show that fewer than one in four children receive even half an hour of any kind of physical activity every day, and only one in four gets twenty minutes of "huff and puff" activity each day. "Huff and puff" means the vigorous activity that increases the capacity of the heart and builds muscle strength and endurance, healthy bones, muscles, and joints.

It's Up to Parents to Set the Pace

Children who eat healthy foods and spend time in daily exercise learn these health habits from their parents. It's up to you to turn off the TV and computer games and to structure time for outdoor, active play for your children. Most of all, you need to set an example by getting regular exercise yourself. If parents make exercise a priority, children will too. Just growing up in a home where healthy foods, daily exercise, and daily meditation are the norms will be the best insurance that children will be healthy throughout life.

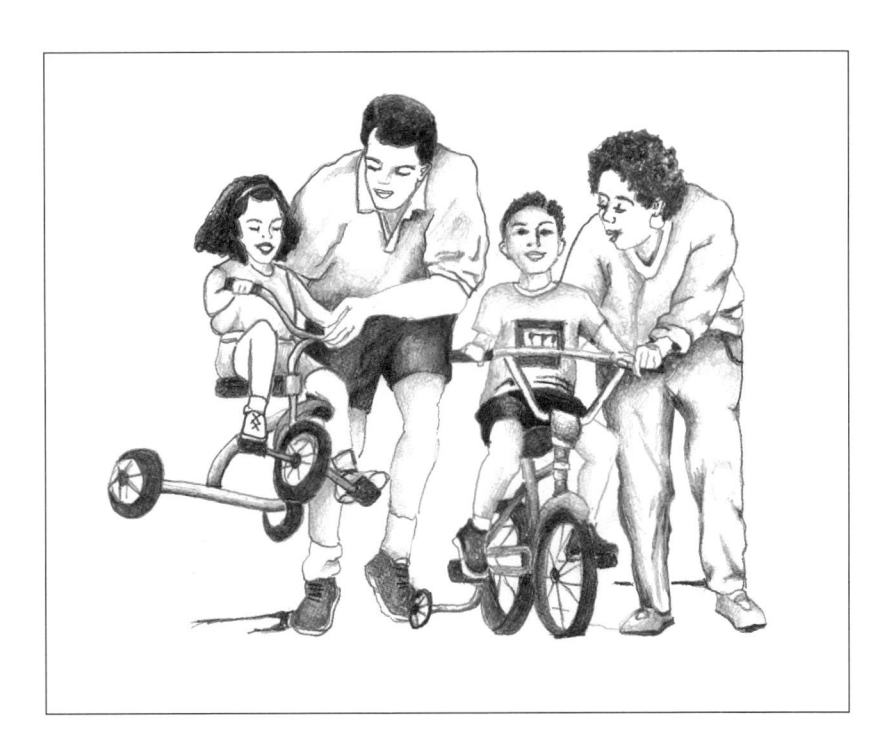

It's also important to cultivate a healthy, relaxed attitude toward sports. Many children suffer their greatest emotional traumas on the playing field. This can be minimized if the child has grown up with daily physical activity and has learned to love it. He or she will feel more confident, competent, and coordinated. Studies show that children who have a higher level of overall fitness (just by playing vigorously every day) have greater success in other physical activities. Children who exercise are more likely to participate in a wide variety of sports, dancing, and games.

Free Play for Preschool Children

It is the nature of young children to be active. Healthy children like to run around and play. How many times have you thought, "If only I had that kind of energy"?

When they play outside, children get not only exercise, but also sunshine and fresh air. Vitamin D from sunshine aids in the absorption of calcium, and everyone needs at least 15 minutes of direct sunshine on the hands and face daily to get their minimum daily dose. In Maharishi Ayurveda, the early morning sun is considered beneficial for health, which is why a walk at sunrise is recommended for adults. But children can also benefit from moderate exposure to the sun early in the morning or later in the afternoon.

Children need a minimum of 20 minutes of fresh air every day. The cells need oxygen to form tissues, and many buildings today do not supply a healthy source of oxygen. Getting your child outside and running around is the best way to keep his cells supplied with fresh oxygen.

Free play is important for preschoolers, to give them time to act out their imaginings. However, just because your child is outdoors doesn't mean that he's getting exercise. One group of researchers found when five-year-olds were given time for free play in the schoolyard, only 10 percent actually rode tricycles or played tag. The rest of the children sat, stood, or socialized.

You may want to introduce a game to get your child moving, such as bouncing a ball, rolling a ball, or playing tag. This can be a fun time for you and your child, a time that he will associate with good feelings and that will make him receptive to other physical activities throughout childhood. It's a good idea to get him to "huff and puff" for short periods, the length of time depending on the child's endurance and constitution. Children who are sturdy and Kapha-like can benefit most from longer stretches of vigorous exercise, while Pitta children should be careful not to get overheated, and Vata children should not become fatigued.

As children get older, it's healthy for them to continue to enjoy running, biking, and swimming in an unstructured environment. In addition, some children may want to play structured sports at school, depending on their desires and disposition.

Choosing the Right Exercise for Your School-Age Child

Exercise for children should be fun. If your child is reluctant to participate in any sports or physical activity, it may be that he has had a bad experience trying to succeed at a sport that he is not suited for. You can help him find the right type, amount, and intensity of exercise to suit his mind-body makeup.

Children have their own natural rhythm, and that is nature's rhythm. This refers, first of all, to the rate that children develop particular motor skills. Children do not grow at the same time or rate. Some children develop motor skills or athletic abilities more slowly than others, which may make them appear clumsy at a certain age. But if given encouragement, support, and a supportive environment, a currently uncoordinated child could become an excellent athlete a year later. If the parent or teacher says, "he's not athletic," the child will absorb that self-image, even though it is wrong.

Every child can be an athlete, and every child can enjoy physical activity—if it is suited to his constitution and inner nature. The child's temperament has a bearing on what types of sports he enjoys playing and excels at, and thus must be respected by the parents.

Children are naturally drawn to the types of activities that suit them best. A thin, small-boned Vata child will be less likely to want to go out for football than a hefty, strong-muscled Kapha type. It's not a good idea to force children to take up sports they are not naturally drawn to. Instead, help your child find the type of exercise that makes him feel balanced, competent, and energized.

For Vata Body Build

Vata children may like a more slow and easy-paced exercise, and should never be encouraged to exert to the point of exhaustion. You may need to encourage the Vata child to pay more attention to his body signals, and to rest before he is tired. Walking, Yoga Asanas, light dance, and water aerobics are examples of preferred exercises for Vata children. Vata body builds tend to get overstimulated, so exercise should be relaxing rather than vigorous. Vata-built children may sustain short bursts of energy, as when running sprints. They may need to rest afterwards, lacking the stamina to keep running long distances.

For Pitta Body Build

Pitta children should be encouraged to avoid playing under the noon-day sun, and to engage in cooling sports such as swimming, skiing, and ice-skating. Sports such as tennis and track and field are also a healthy way to channel their competitive natures. They like to win and enjoy individual competitions.

For Kapha Body Build

Kapha children may require gentle prodding to exercise; yet they need vigorous exercise every day to stay balanced. For them, team sports are a good idea because the structure forces them to exercise regularly. They excel in sports that require stamina and physical endurance, such as cycling, aerobics, running, football, and soccer. They also excel at sports that require a high degree of mind-body coordination, such as baseball and golf.

Exercise Ideas for Different Constitutions

Vata: walking, Yoga Asanas, light dance, ballet, water aerobics, swimming, golf, baseball, bicycling, archery

Pitta: swimming, skiing, ice-skating, soccer, tennis, track and field, touch football, water skiing, martial arts, cycling, kayaking, rowing, hiking in shady forests

> **Kapha**: team sports, Yoga Asanas, track and running sports, soccer, gymnastics, basketball, baseball, calisthenics, fencing, roller-skating, rowing, martial arts, tennis, volleyball, hiking in hilly terrain, spinning

A New Model for Exercise

The Ayurvedic model for exercise is ideal for children, because it does not involve straining. The "no strain, no gain" type of conditioning that often results in injuries has no place in Maharishi Ayurveda.

Rather, exercise should always be comfortable and enjoyable. The whole point is to stop before the point of fatigue, pain, or overstimulation. The child is taught to be more in tune with his body, and to listen to signals of discomfort before they balloon into pain or exhaustion.

Also, exercise should be tailored to the individual child. A coach should not say, "Everyone run two miles today." Better to say, "Everyone run for 15 minutes." Some children would do a half-mile in that time, others would do more, depending on the child's capabilities and body type—and how he or she is feeling that particular day.

Children excel when they are enjoying. They should be encouraged to play within a range that makes them feel confident and masterful.

Children at Maharishi School of the Age of Enlightenment in Fairfield, Iowa, who are taught these techniques of exercise and practice the Transcendental Meditation technique, have noticed many positive results in their tennis matches, basketball games, and daily physical education classes. The students feel that these principles help increase their coordination, mental concentration, and stamina. These children consistently perform well in competitions at local and state levels.

Here are some of the basic ideas behind Ayurvedic exercise. You can follow these principles yourself while you exercise or practice sports with your child.

Exercise every day. It's best to make a habit of getting exercise each day. For adults the minimum is half an hour, for children it should be more, but some of it should be in the form of unstructured play. Children who enjoy physical activity can spend much more time being active each day—as long as they are not feeling fatigued and are enjoying it.

Research shows that for children, it is regular physical activity that helps enhance overall health and reduces risk factors for chronic disease. The correct type, intensity, and amount of regular exercise help reduce LDL (bad) cholesterol while raising HDL (good) cholesterol. Moderate exercise may increase the cell systems that are important in immunity, and also helps reduce stress.

Make sure the exercise is suitable for your body type, and that the intensity and duration of the sport is adjusted to suit your needs. You've learned the types of sports that are suitable for different body types. It's also important to adjust the intensity of your child's activity. A Kapha child can sustain longer periods of intense physical effort. It would be unreasonable and even damaging to expect a thinner-build Vata child to have the same kind of stamina. Vata types should maintain low intensity for a shorter period of time. Pitta children are somewhere in the middle, needing moderate intensity for a moderate length of time.

Stay in your comfort zone at all times. According to Ayurvedic texts, exercise is healthy as long as it only requires 50 percent of capacity. In other words, children as well as adults should stay well within their comfort zones while exercising. Perhaps your child could push his body and run for three miles, but at that point he'd feel exhausted and would probably have to rest the next day to avoid injury. Better to stop at one-and-a-half miles.

In the Ayurvedic model of exercise, the child doesn't gain by straining. It's not healthy to push beyond his capacity one day and have to rest to recover his strength the next. Rather, it's best to exercise easily each day, and in that way he will naturally and painlessly increase his capacity and stamina.

By the time a child's body cries out in pain, it has already been damaged. Then the body has to repair the damage, rather than building up strength. Shaky knees, heavy breathing, and a pounding heart are all signs of overexertion, and have been correlated with the buildup of free radicals in the body. So encourage your child to keep a moderate pace while exercising, and that means not too much and not too little.

Injuries are caused by straining to reach an external goal. The goal here is to stay in tune with your body, listen to its signals, and to stop when there is any discomfort.

Breathe through your nose when exercising. This enlivens the sinuses, warms cold air before it hits the lungs and thus protects the bronchial passages. It also provides a natural way for your child to monitor himself if he is overexerting. If he can no longer breathe through the nose, but must start gulping air through the mouth, it's time to slow down or stop until he can breathe comfortably through the nose again. This is something that you can teach your child at an early age.

Keep your attention on your body. Just as digestion performs better when you pay attention to the food, exercise is safer and more effective if you let your mind easily be on your body while you do it. This improves mind-body coordination, and helps avoid injuries that can happen if your child is not paying attention to his body's signals. For this reason, it's not a good idea to exercise while listening to music.

Don't do vigorous exercise right before bed. This is especially important for children with a Vata imbalance, who may get so keyed up that they can't sleep. If for some reason this happens, a soothing massage can help calm deranged Vata.

Don't exercise on a full stomach. Ask your child to allow at least one hour or more after a full meal before swimming, playing in a soccer match, or engaging in other vigorous sports (adults should allow two hours). This will give the digestive process a chance to take place smoothly and completely. Light walking or biking is fine after a meal.

Yoga Asanas and Salute to the Sun (*Surya Namaskara*)

There are two types of exercise that are balancing to all three doshas. They create neuromuscular integration and mental stability, and they cleanse the body of toxins. They also increase circulation, mind-body coordination, enliven the flow of consciousness, reduce stress, eliminate fatigue, increase stamina, and improve oxygen flow to the brain and other organs. They have equally impressive benefits for the mind, reducing mental stress, improving concentration and mental alertness, increasing inner calm, and creating bliss.

Yoga Asanas: Children usually begin learning Yoga Asanas at age ten, when they start to practice the Transcendental Meditation technique. Yoga Asanas are best learned with personal instruction at a Transcendental Meditation center.

Benefits of Yoga Asanas and Salute to the Sun (Surya Namaskara)

For the Body
Enliven and rejuvenate different organs, glands, and systems
Increase circulation
Increase coordination
Improve mind-body coordination
Enliven the flow of consciousness
Reduce physical stress
Eliminate fatigue
Increase stamina
Improve flexibility
Purify the body
Create neuromuscular integration
Increase oxygen flow to the brain and cells

For the Mind
Develop inner calmness
Increase bliss
Enhance mental stability
Improve concentration
Increase mental alertness

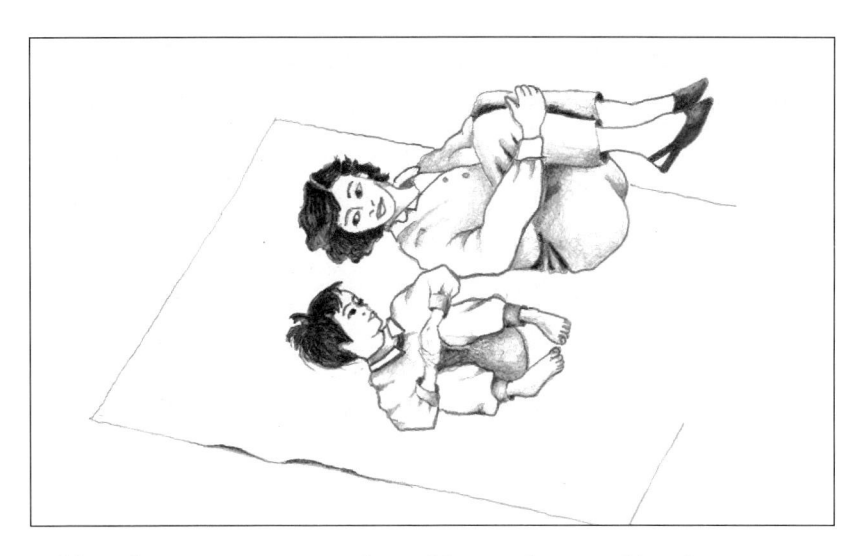

Yoga Asanas are very simple, mild, stretching and bending exercises that produce profound effects. They enhance the flow of consciousness in the body and rejuvenate each organ. They also help the child develop inner stability, inner happiness, and better concentration.

With names such as "lion" and "cobra," Yoga Asanas appeal to children because the positions resemble the animal that they are named after. The positions are simple, yet enliven key vital points in the body. Children can begin selected Yoga Asanas for specific disorders as early as age eight, as recommended by a physician trained in Maharishi Ayurveda.

One reason Yoga Asanas have such a profound effect on the entire body is that they help keep the spine flexible and straight. As is well known, the spine is the center of the nervous system. All the sensory and motor nerves, which control the organs of the body, run through the spine. The spinal cord is also connected to the brain. Thus Yoga Asanas, by keeping the spine supple and clear of toxins and obstructions, help the functioning of the senses, motor reflexes, organs, and brain.

Starting at age ten, children can practice Yoga Asanas for a few minutes in the morning and a few minutes in the evening, right before practicing the Transcendental Meditation technique. It's important that they do not strain in any way, but just bend as far as the body wants to bend. Children are naturally flexible, so it is not usually difficult for them to do Yoga Asanas. By starting Yoga Asanas in childhood, they can maintain that flexibility throughout life.

One asana that children (and adults, too) should never perform is the headstand. This pose creates far too much pressure on the neck and head, and could result in injuries.

Salute to the Sun (Surya Namaskara): Traditionally, these exercises are done in the early morning as the sun is rising, and are a way of acknowledging our earth's benefic source of energy. If practiced regularly, they improve stamina, neuromuscular integration, and inner calm. Children can start doing these gentle exercises even in first grade, and can increase the number of repetitions as they grow older.

Special Breathing Exercises (Pranayama): This simple coordinated breathing exercise enlivens the neurorespiratory system right before the practice of the Transcendental Meditation technique. Pranayama enhances mind-body coordination, creates inner calm, purifies the senses, coordinates the breathing, and settles the mind for meditation.

Pranayama produces balanced, relaxed breathing and revitalizing energy throughout the mind and body. It purifies and refines the life breath, or prana. Pranayama infuses the cells with oxygen, clears the channels that remove waste and carry nutrients to the cells, and removes fatigue. It strengthens the lungs, nasal passages, and throat, helps prevent coughs and colds, and in some cases has been effective in treating asthma. To learn how to do Salute to the Sun and pranayama, consult a physician trained in Maharishi Ayurveda. You can also learn from a teacher of the Transcendental Meditation technique.

Special Nutrition for Young Athletes

Children may need instant nutrition after competing or playing hard. Here are some satisfying energy-boosters that contain no harmful additives or preservatives.

***1. Drink Almond Energy*™ *with Raja's Cup*®** for energy pickup and eliminating free radicals. Mix one cup brewed Raja's Cup with four teaspoons of Almond Energy and one cup water. Recommended for children with strong digestion.

2. Eat a summer fruit to nourish the plasma (rasa dhatu), the raw material for all bodily tissues. You can also make fresh fruit juice with an electric juicer and serve it to your child.

3. Drink sweet lassi (see recipe in Chapter Seven).

4. Drink plenty of water. If children are exercising or participating in competitive sports, it's very important that they drink enough fluids. Children who play sports cannot drink too much. They can hydrate with several glasses of water a half-hour before the competition, and every 20 minutes during play. This is especially important if the sun is hot.

Have you ever noticed that your child sleeps deeper when he exercises more? And when sleep is deeper, children are more dynamic during the day. The two affect each other; both rest and activity need to be balanced to produce health. Children today, with so many hours spent in front of the computer and TV, need to exercise in their daily routine more than ever before. If you are concerned that your child is not active enough, now is a good time to make changes. Find an activity your child enjoys and help him structure his schedule to fit it in every day.

Remember, exercise must be fun if you expect your child to do it willingly. A Gallup poll showed that children understand the value of regular physical activity. They agree that it is important for good health. Yet those who were physically active said they did it because it was fun and they enjoyed it. Few children said better health was the reason that they exercised every day.

The techniques from Maharishi Ayurveda that you have learned in this chapter can make exercise fun for every child, no matter what the level of athletic abilities or skills.

CHAPTER FOURTEEN
Emotions, Behavior, and a Nourishing Family Environment

Of all the suggestions for improving your child's health mentioned in this book, probably the most effective one is to give your child a healthy dose of love and affection every day. It's also the least expensive—giving a hug or a kind word costs you nothing. Yet cultivating a positive home environment, and positive emotions, is a powerful way to contribute to your child's health.

As a parent, you are responsible for creating a safe and nourishing home environment for all the children in the family.

The Role of Positive Emotions in Creating Health

Joy is experienced in the first months of life, as is anger, pleasure, distress, surprise, and disgust. By the first year, most children have experienced the full range of the emotional spectrum, including fear and sadness.

It is well-known that positive emotions boost the immune system and protect against infectious disease. Psychological stress can make people more susceptible to infections such as colds. It also affects the duration and outcome of cancer, autoimmune disorders, allergies, and infectious diseases. Recent research shows that acute and chronic stress, for instance, can trigger asthma attacks in children who already have a breathing disorder.

The endocrine system also responds to emotions and stress. Positive social interactions and loving relationships are known to modulate the endocrine system and the autonomic nervous system, creating many health benefits.

The Role of Behavioral Rasayanas

It is important that you teach your child that his behavior will either make him more healthy or less healthy. The best way to teach, of course, is by example. If your child sees you behaving in a way that is harmonious, he will naturally copy those habits. When he does make a mistake, and behaves in a way that brings him discomfort or ill health, you can ask him how that behavior made him feel. That way he very naturally becomes aware of how his behavior affects his life.

In Maharishi Ayurveda, behavior in tune with natural law is considered to be a powerful medicine. You'll remember from Chapter Ten that rasayanas are herbal compounds that create ojas in the body and nourish rasa dhatu (blood plasma), the essence of food. Yet according to the Ayurvedic texts, certain healthy behaviors, called achara rasayana, or behavioral rasayana, also nourish the body and create ojas. These positive behaviors include truthfulness, nonviolence, calmness, sweet speech, meditation, cleanliness, charitableness, freedom from anger, and respect for teachers and elders.

These simple behaviors help cultivate a feeling of security and happiness in the child. If the child grows up in an environment where his parents speak well of others, for instance, he will feel more trusting and positive toward his friends and acquaintances. If his parents are both truthful and not prone to anger, he will find it easier to speak the truth (especially when he has done something wrong).

Qualities of a Person who Practices Behavioral Rasayana
(*Achara Rasayana*)

Truthful, free from anger, nonviolent, not exerting to the point of exhaustion, calm, sweet-spoken, stable and steady, practicing meditation, engaged in cleanliness, persevering, observing charity, practicing religion, devoted to love and compassion, balanced in sleep and wakefulness, using ghee regularly, behaving with propriety according to the time and place, unconceited, well-behaved, simple, in control of the senses, keeping the company of elders, holding a positive outlook, self-controlled, nonindulgent in alcohol, and respectful toward teachers, preceptors, and elders.

EMOTIONS, BEHAVIOR, AND A NOURISHING FAMILY ENVIRONMENT

It is said in the Ayurvedic texts that a person who displays these qualities gains the same health benefits as if he continually uses an herbal rasayana.

You can see that behavioral rasayanas include many of the behaviors that we included in the last chapters on the daily routine. Practicing the Transcendental Meditation technique each morning, having balanced sleep and wakefulness, and not overexerting while exercising all refer to the daily routine.

One mother of two explains, "Following the behavioral rasayanas are a natural part of our home life. For instance, I try to teach my children from a young age to keep their voices warm and gentle with each other. I've always felt that if I'm sharp, it just creates sharpness in them. What we give out comes back to us. With my twelve-year-old son, if I'm ever sharp, it disconnects us. Then I can't work with him anymore. Ever since he was little, I realized that a sharp 'no' never needed to be said. Instead I've found that it works better to speak sweetly, always pointing out the good and then bringing out the small point that needs to be worked on. If I treat him with kindness he goes out to the world with that kindness in his heart.

"Also, I've always taught my children to be respectful to adults, to say 'thank you' if another mother fixes a meal or gives them a lift home from school. They've learned how to look directly at the adult who is addressing them, to acknowledge what the adult said and to give a pleasant remark back. At one point there was an elderly woman living in our apartment building, and I asked the children to help me bring her food, so my children could learn to take care of their elders."

The Role of the Transcendental Meditation Technique in Developing Positive Behavior

Of course, it's not possible to just decide to be a perfect person and have it happen. A child can only be what he is. He can't pretend all day to be helpful and nice to others. It has to come from the inside. Even if it were possible for him to keep up such forced behavior, it would not be healthy. It would create a strain in the mind and body.

If there is stress in the nervous system, it might be difficult for a child to behave well. That is why practicing the Transcendental Meditation technique every morning and evening is the most important behavioral rasayana. By dissolving mental and physical stress, it allows positive qualities to grow in the child, such as creativity, more quietness within, more tolerance, more openness, more inner peace, and more spiritual qualities. These inner qualities grow and become so stable that even when confronted with chaotic or challenging situations in their environment, children can retain their stable sense of right and wrong. It will help them to spontaneously think more clearly and to remain calm, rested, and happy.

A mother vividly remembers the day her son learned his Word of Wisdom technique, because it created an unexpected change in his behavior. "My four-year-old son and I loved each other boundlessly, yet he never knew how to say, 'I love you.' When I would say to him, 'I love you,' he'd only say, 'OK.' The day he learned to meditate, he said, 'I love you, Mommy,' and he kept saying it all day long, until finally he said,

Percentage of Prosocial Responses for Students at Maharishi School, Just Community Schools (JCS 1 and JCS 2), and Other Private and Public Schools

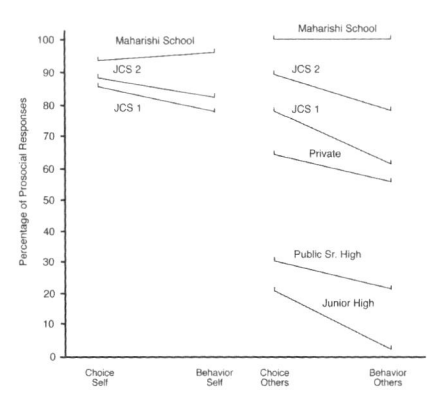

This graph illustrates the total percentage of prosocial responses for Maharishi School, two Just Community Schools, and Maharishi School students' perceptions of the schools they previously attended. Prosocial responses were found to be highest for Maharishi School.

Reference: R.J. Nidich and S.I. Nidich, "An Empirical Study of the Moral Atmosphere of Maharishi International University High School (Maharishi School of the Age of Enlightenment)," presented to the American Educational Research Association (Chicago, Ill.), April 1985.

'Mommy, I'm so tired of saying I love you, but Mommy, I love you so much.' It was a total transformation."

Later, at age ten, her son learned the Transcendental Meditation technique and began practicing it twice a day. "I can see that he feels more relaxed and easier inside afterwards," says his mother. "I asked him, 'What do you feel when you meditate?' and he said he feels happier, and life feels happier."

One research study showed that children who practice the Transcendental Meditation technique actually think more in the direction of right behavior. They exhibit higher moral reasoning.

The Importance of *Transcendental Meditation* Practice for Parents
The need to dissolve stress in daily life also applies to parents. Parents the world over are facing more stress and challenges even though they are certainly trying their best to be good role models for their children. Pressures of making a living and raising a family in today's world can be daunting. Lack of sleep, lack of time, and lack of resources can put unreasonable strain on parents.

In the past, and in many traditional cultures even today, the grandparents and extended family participated fully in raising the children. Parents today are often left without any help. Also, even just a hundred years ago, when most families farmed, both parents worked at home, and childcare was easily integrated into the parents' working life. Today not only the fathers, but also the majority of mothers, work outside the home. This leads to many challenges for parents. One recent survey showed that working mothers experience much higher levels of the hormone cortisol, which is associated with mental distress and feelings of a lack of personal control. And today a large percent of households are single-parent homes, with one parent trying to do the work for two.

Yet by following the procedures mentioned in this book, it becomes easier to behave in a more ideal way. If you get enough sleep, for instance, and practice the Transcendental Meditation technique each morning and evening, it becomes easier to not lose your temper with your children. Practicing the Transcendental Meditation technique is probably the most important thing you can do to make your home environment more peaceful, because by releasing stress in meditation, you can feel more relaxed and giving when you're with your children.

Cortisol levels, for instance, are found to decrease greatly during the Transcendental Meditation technique.

The wisdom presented in this book will help you to nurture your child and to develop his full potential. For this it's important to take care of your own happiness and well-being. Giving to your child doesn't have to be a constant struggle; instead you can feel like a gentle river of nurturing, flowing support.

Storytelling and Other Behavioral Models

Reading stories of heroes and heroines can help teach your child about good behavior. In every culture, there are stories that the elders have told the children for generations to teach the important lessons and concepts of the culture. The great stories from your own religious tradition, such as stories from the Bible, teach children concepts of right and wrong. From myths and traditional stories, children learn to respect others and to follow rules of social conduct.

Stories from the Vedic tradition of knowledge, the oldest living tradition on earth, are also inspiring to children. The Ramayana epic, for instance, tells the story of the ideal warrior-prince, Rama, who lost his kingdom and then redeemed it by overcoming the forces of darkness. These stories are exciting to children, because they contain good and bad, warriors and maidens, and kings and queens. The good hero or heroine always wins in the end, giving the child a sense of security that good will triumph in the natural order of things.

The Vedic stories also are helpful because they explain the qualities of pure consciousness to the child, broadening his or her awareness and inspiring a desire to evolve and become great.

Here is a story from the Upanishads, one of the forty aspects of the Veda and Vedic Literature, which illuminates the highest level of human development. The story is set in Vedic times. It illustrates the principles of Vedic knowledge, which predates any organized religion and refers to laws of nature that can be found at the basis of all religions and all cultures. The word *Brahman* in the story is a Vedic term that can be understood as "wholeness." The story teaches the child that he is Brahman; he is the universe. This makes an ideal bedtime story.

Satyakama—The Seeker of Truth

From the Chhandogya Upanishad*

Long ago, in a small hut in the dense forests of India, lived a boy and his mother. The boy's mother named him Satyakama, which means "seeker of truth."

More than anything, Satyakama wanted to live the life of a student, meditating and studying about Brahman (wholeness) in the dwelling of his teacher. To become a student, he had to know his father's family name, because in those times teachers only accepted students from certain families.

So Satyakama went to his mother, Jabala, and said, "Mother, I want to live the life of a student of sacred knowledge." Jabala was pleased with her son's desire to study Brahman.

"Dear Mother, of what family am I?" Satyakama asked.

"My name is Jabala and your name is Satyakama, and I do not know your family name, my precious son," his mother said.

"Then what shall I tell my teacher, dear Mother?" asked Satyakama earnestly.

Jabala led a pure life and knew the power of truth. "Tell him just what I have told you, my beloved son," she said. With his mother's blessings, Satyakama left his boyhood home. He walked through thick forests where the light of the sun never touched the ground. He saw foaming streams splashing on rocks. He passed by lakes as still and glassy as ice.

Soon he came to the home of the great teacher Gautama, who lived in his ashram, his Vedic school, by the edge of the forest. Satyakama bowed to the teacher in respect. "Please, honored Sir," he asked, "will you accept me as your disciple? With your blessings, I wish to become a knower of Brahman."

Gautama thought the boy looked healthy and bright. But to accept him as a student, Gautama needed to know the boy's family background. And so he kindly asked, "Of what family are you, my boy?"

---

* This story is excerpted from the book *All Love Flows to the Self: Eternal Stories from the Upanishads* by Kumuda Reddy, M.D., Thomas Egenes, Ph.D., and Linda Egenes, Samhita Productions: Schenectady, New York, 2000.

"My mother said to tell you that her name is Jabala and my name is Satyakama—and I know nothing more about my family," Satyakama explained without fear. "So I am Satyakama Jabala."

Gautama was pleased that the boy's mother had taught her son to tell the truth. "Only one from the best of families could give this explanation so sincerely," he said. "I will gladly accept you as my student. Bring the firewood inside, my boy."

Satyakama's heart felt warm with happiness. At last he would be able to study the knowledge of Brahman.

The next day, Gautama said, "I will now begin teaching you the knowledge of Brahman, which is called supreme knowledge (Brahma Vidya). The first step is to know your Self." And so Gautama initiated Satyakama in meditation to settle his mind and heart. With a quiet mind, Satyakama experienced his own inner Self, which was like a vast ocean of silence.

After teaching Satyakama to meditate, Gautama did something unexpected. He took Satyakama to the pasture where hundreds of cows were grazing. To Satyakama's surprise, Gautama separated out four hundred thin, weak cows.

"Take these cows to another part of the forest and live, my dear boy," he said. "Tend them carefully. You may return when they have multiplied to a thousand!"

Without any doubts in his heart, the obedient Satyakama drove his four hundred cows to a lush meadow on the other side of the forest.

At first Satyakama felt lonely, since he was all by himself in the forest. But he sang to the cows and they mooed back to him as he slept. Satyakama began to enjoy his life in the forest. His cows ate nourishing green grass and drank pure water from a spring-fed pond. Satyakama watched his cows grow plump and happy.

Satyakama stayed many years with the cows, living a peaceful life in the warm grassy meadows and cool forest. His days began and ended with meditation. As his mind became more and more quiet, he was able to comprehend the profound wisdom his teacher had given him.

He carefully tended the cows, always finding rich pastures for their grazing. As Satyakama grew older, the herd of cows began to multiply. However, he was so contented with his life of meditation and knowledge that he noticed neither the passage of time nor the increasing size of his herd.

Nevertheless, a profound change was taking place in Satyakama. In his peaceful life in the forest, he was coming to know the Self. His mind became serene, his heart filled with love, and his face glowed with light.

Satyakama never felt alone. He became friends with the proud peacocks, the rippling streams, and the swaying trees. He even became friends with the sun and the moon. Every living creature became part of his family. He remembered the saying his mother had taught him, "The world is my family" (*Vasudhaiva kutumbakam*).

At night, as the cows slept, Satyakama gazed at the infinite span of stars, scattered across the sky like a thousand sugar crystals. He felt as if all nature were speaking to him. In the bright morning, the dew bathed his feet. White gardenias greeted him with their sweet scent. Wispy clouds and distant rainbows delighted his imagination. Cool rain splashed his skin.

"All this beauty is a part of Brahman," he thought. "Everything that grows and decays is a part of the great totality." He felt that he, too, was a part of the eternal cycle of life.

One day, the head of the cows, a wise bull, spoke to him. "Satyakama!"

"Yes, honored Sir," answered Satyakama, who respected all living things.

"We are now one thousand cows," said the bull. "Please take us to your teacher's hermitage. And I will teach you the nature of Brahman, which has many aspects."

"Yes, please tell me," said Satyakama.

"Brahman shines from the east and the west," the bull told him, "and from the north and the south. This is because Brahman is everywhere. It is universal. This is one quarter of Brahman." Then the bull said, "The fire, Agni, will teach you more about Brahman."

Satyakama began to drive the cows back to his teacher's ashram. When evening came, he put a rope around a large area to protect the cows. Then Satyakama lit a fire. He sat down on the west side of the fire, facing east. He gazed at the dark sky, filled with his friends, the stars. After some time, the fire, Agni, spoke to him about the nature of Brahman.

"Brahman is the earth and the atmosphere," said Agni. "It is the sky and the ocean. This is because Brahman is endless. It is without beginning or end. This is one quarter of Brahman."

Then Agni added, "A swan will tell you more about Brahman."

The next evening, after traveling with his cows, Satyakama again lit a fire by the side of a river. He sat down, facing east, and saw a great white swan gliding down the river toward him. The swan began to teach Satyakama about the nature of Brahman.

"Brahman is fire," the swan explained, "and Brahman is the sun. Brahman is the moon, and Brahman is lightning. This quarter of Brahman is light. Brahman is the light of life."

Then the swan said, "A bird will tell you more about Brahman."

The next evening, after settling his cows in a safe place beside a hill, Satyakama again lit a fire. He sat down on dry, soft grass, facing east. This time a purple sunbird flew down from the limb of a tree. Like silk woven with gold, its wings caught the brightness of the fire.

The sunbird sang, "Brahman is the breath, and Brahman is the eye. Brahman is the ear and also the mind. This quarter of Brahman is the seat, the resting place. Just as the eye is the seat of what is seen, and the mind is the seat of what is thought, so Brahman is the seat of everything. Everything rests upon Brahman."

Finally Satyakama arrived at his teacher's dwelling. His teacher noticed how Satyakama's face was shining, and he said to him, "I see that you have found Brahman. For it is said that the knower of Brahman has settled senses, a smiling face, freedom from worry, and has found the purpose of life."

But even with these words of praise, Satyakama spoke humbly. "Please, honored Sir, teach me about the nature of Brahman." For Satyakama wanted to learn from his teacher about the true nature of Brahman.

"You have heard that east and west are Brahman, that the earth and sky are Brahman, that the sun and moon are Brahman, and that the eye and ear are Brahman," his teacher replied. "Like waves stirring within the ocean, all these are a part of Brahman. This is because Brahman is everywhere. Brahman is everything. It is endless. It is the light of life. Everything finds its rest in Brahman.

"And Brahman is realized by knowing the Self, your true nature. When you realize that you are everywhere, you are endless, and you are radiant. This is the supreme knowledge, *Brahma Vidya*. Yes, this is the supreme knowledge, Brahma Vidya."

And that is how through meditation and knowledge Satyakama came to know Brahman, and grew up himself to become a great teacher of Brahman.

Behavior and Discipline

Behavior is learned by example, and the mother and father are the primary teachers. The mother is so closely connected with her child that she is in the position to influence him the most.

You can't teach a child with words. Children absorb lessons from your actions and feelings, which is why it is so important to nourish yourself and feel healthy and happy within yourself.

In the Ayurvedic tradition, the child is seen as divine. Discipline is not imposed on the child during the first two years. The child is nurtured, pampered, and loved unconditionally.

After the first two years, gentle discipline begins. Discipline starts when the child needs to learn what is right and what is wrong. The ideal of discipline is to cultivate a child who is not self-centered, but is aware of others.

Sometimes if you tell your child that he is doing wrong, he may not agree in the beginning, but later he will be thankful that you alerted him to the danger. Otherwise, if you don't tell him, he may later say, "Why didn't you tell me?"

In his book *The Science of Being and Art of Living*, Maharishi Mahesh Yogi writes:

> It is a regrettable tendency in parents today that although they believe that whatever they say should be followed by the child, if they see the possibility of the child resenting their advice they keep quiet and do not give it. It is not kindness or love, and it is not right for the parents to take this attitude. The child is young and inexperienced and does not have a broad vision or experience of life. The parents should tell the child freely and with love and kindness that this is wrong and that is right. If he resents it the parents should not insist, because if he disobeys it will naturally result in an experience proving to him that his parents were right. This is the way to cultivate a child's tendency to obey and act according to the wishes and feelings of the parents. The child is informed of right

action by his friends, teachers, and neighbors—by individuals the child loves and obeys. For it is the duty of the parents to see that the child grows in wisdom and goodness.

Children are flowers in the garden of God and must be nourished. They themselves do not know the way that is best for them. It is for the parents to lead them on to a path, which is free from suffering. It is part of a parent's role to punish a child if he does not obey and does wrong. But children should be punished in all love.

The modern tendency to put the fate of children completely in their own hands is highly dangerous. It only leads to uncultured growth in the younger generation.

Nourishing the Five Senses in the Home Environment

The senses are recognized in Maharishi Ayurveda as an important avenue for maintaining emotional and physical balance. The senses are considered to be part of the mind in Ayurvedic medicine, and Western research in recent years has demonstrated the close link between the senses, brain, and emotions. The sense of smell, for instance, is directly wired to the limbic system, the center for emotion in the brain. If you have ever had the experience of smelling a familiar aroma from your childhood, such as bread baking, and then being suddenly transported back to the exact emotions and feelings of that period in the past, then you have experienced the power of the sense of smell.

For infants, taste is their most developed sense, which is why they try to put everything in sight in their mouths. This is how they are gaining information about the world. All throughout the preschool and early school years, concrete sensory experiences develop the brain and its intricate wiring.

Effects of Excessive Use, No Use, and Wrong Use of the Senses

It can't be emphasized enough how important it is to provide positive sensory experiences throughout childhood that will nourish the child's mind and body. The senses can be a source of balance or imbalance. According to Maharishi Ayurveda, sensory stimuli cause disease when they are experienced in excess, when they are absent, and when they are of the wrong type.

To understand how this works, think about the sense of hearing for a moment. It's easy to see how extremely loud noise could damage the ears (and research has shown how preadolescent and adolescent children have actually suffered ear damage by listening to excessively loud music on their MP3 players and at rock concerts).

Children are sensitive to the sounds, sights, tastes, smells, and textures around them. It's especially important to avoid exposing infants to bright lights, stressful noises, or toxic smells.

Yet too little auditory stimuli could be just as damaging. It is early-childhood sensory experiences that directly influence the structure and function of the brain. Without a nourishing sensory environment, the brain cannot develop properly. Genes direct the growth of axons, dendrites, and synapses, but only the synapses that are stimulated by the child's sensory environment become part of the permanent brain wiring. Synapses that are not stimulated wither and die.

Thus everything the child hears, touches, tastes, smells, and sees shapes his brain. Children who are raised in a rich, nourishing sensory environment grow much more complex and intelligent brains, while children who are raised in sensory-deprived environments have impoverished brains and poor health. In fact, it is each child's unique sensory experiences in life that determine which connections survive and which ones atrophy, creating a unique map of each child's sensory environment inside his brain.

And how do harmful auditory stimuli cause disease? Studies show that rock music makes plants wither. Certain types of rap music have incited anger in crowds. A study comparing hard rock music with the primordial sounds (the basic impulses of Veda and the Vedic Literature) known as Sama Veda found that cancer cells grow faster with hard rock, and with Sama Veda they transform into healthier cell structures. Intense music is a stimulus that should be kept away from children.

There can also be unlocalized effects from overuse, under use, or wrong use of any one sense. On the surface you see the eye, or the ear, or the nose, but each of these sensory organs is also connected to different areas of the brain. For instance, if a child reads while lying down and strains the eyes, watches too much television or sits too close to the

TV screen, or plays too many hours on the computer, over time this straining of the eye muscles can result in common headaches, migraine headaches, sinus disease, congestion, disorientation, inability to focus, behavioral problems, psychological imbalances, increased stress, anxiety, depression, or sleep problems. Wrong use of the sense of hearing can even result in Attention Deficit Hyperactivity Disorder (ADHD), a problem that often has its basis in a Vata imbalance.

Creating Balance in the Senses

Maharishi Ayurveda offers therapies for all five senses, which help to balance the three doshas and create overall health for the body, mind, and emotions. These can be used in your home on a daily basis.

Maharishi Gandharva Veda music and the practice of the Transcendental Meditation technique use the sense of sound. Abhyanga uses the sense of touch. Getting enough sunlight and wearing bright, cheerful colors according to individual liking and prakriti of the child enliven the sense of sight. The sense of taste is enlivened through eating all six tastes, eating lovingly cooked, delicious food, and eating various qualities of food (heavy, light, dry, moist) according to the doshas. Aromatherapy and pleasant cooking smells enliven the sense of smell.

Young children can become overwhelmed by too many sensory impressions, especially when they spend many hours at activities or day care outside the home. This is why it's unhealthy to push preschoolers, kindergartners, and first graders to do too much after school. Sometimes they just need unstructured quiet time. The noises and sights of a busy school day might cause an imbalance in Vata and Pitta if the child is not allowed to recover afterwards.

Sometimes a preschooler or kindergartner will want to stay home from school for a day and rejuvenate. This is fine, if you can manage it. It's better not to force young children. After a day at home, your child will likely feel refreshed and will want to see what the other children are doing.

Television or No Television?

One of the most dominant effects on the sight, hearing, and emotions of young children today is television. Today's children watch an average of four hours of television a day. By the time he graduates, the average high school student has spent 15,000 hours watching TV—and only 13,000 hours in the classroom. A research study at Case Western Reserve University viewed the TV habits of more than 2,000 children. They found that those who watched the most TV were most likely to feel depressed, anxious, or angry.

Note this Vedic saying, "What you put your attention on grows stronger in your life." This is a subtle but powerful principle to keep in mind when choosing entertainment for your children. Do you want them to grow in the qualities of love, happiness, sweetness, intelligence, creativity, and nonviolence? Then you must expose them to those qualities in the environment, including the people they spend their time with and the books, stories, movies, computer games, and TV shows they see.

Many parents screen what their children watch, providing wholesome videos on weekends and limiting children to one-half hour of television on weekdays. Surely there are many beautiful videos and TV programs that children can benefit from. Nature programs, history programs, and programs made especially to educate children can be healthy in moderation. I am certainly not advocating that children be restricted from television altogether. I just want to point out the research that shows that excessive viewing is harmful to children. The average child is watching too much TV too soon.

Seven Health Risks from Playing Too Many Computer Games and Watching Too Much TV

1. Excessive exposure to computer games and television can create Vata imbalance in any child, whatever their age. Children are much more sensitive to sensory overload than adults, and most TV tries to heighten sensory stimulation.

Preschool children, who are still developing their sensory abilities, can be especially affected by too many hours in front of a screen. It can take up valuable time when they should be exploring the world around them by using their senses. Older children are missing out on developing valuable social, cognitive, and emotional skills, because they are not interacting with real people and the real environment.

2. Violence on TV can be frightening to your child. One researcher, Joanne Cantor, a professor of communication arts at the University of Wisconsin-Madison, has found that children are far more disturbed by violent television shows than adults realize. From age two to seven, children can be terrified by wild animals, grotesque monsters, and ugly images. Eight-to-twelve-year-olds are more frightened of violence to themselves or their friends. Today's news stories also frighten children—especially when they are about violence against children. Surely, older children need to be informed about the world around them, but in a way that does not damage their emotions.

The combination of sound, music, and images on television creates a much greater impact on the tender imagination of the child. Children's fears can affect their sleep and their confidence when awake. In her research, Cantor found that it is much more common than adults realize for children to be so frightened by a movie or TV show that it actually stops them from enjoying a particular activity.

3. Children who are exposed to media violence in television shows, movies, computer games, and music are more likely to see aggression as a way to deal with problems and can become desensitized to the effects of real-life violence. Four major medical associations—the American Medical Association, the American Academy of Pediatrics, the American Psychological Association, and the American Academy of Child and Adolescent Psychiatry—recently issued a joint warning to parents after reviewing more than 1,000 research studies that linked violent behaviors in children with exposure to violence in the media.

4. Besides cultivating aggressive behavior, many TV programs provide negative role models. In choosing books, movies, and entertainment for children, choose those without too much contrast. Extreme negative emotions that express fear, terror, anger, violence, or hatred are simply not suitable for children. And unfortunately, much of television programming includes just those emotions. They also feature dysfunctional families that do not follow the behavioral rasayanas mentioned earlier in this chapter and do not provide good role models by any measure. It is up to the parents to take charge of the situation and protect their children from the negative effects of unsupervised television.

As one mother says, "I don't allow my twelve-year-old son to watch R-rated movies, but unfortunately some of his friends watch them. One of his friends is having trouble sleeping at night and is sometimes rough in his behavior. He's a very sensitive child, and I can see that watching lots of R-rated movies is making him more aggressive and fearful. I wish his parents could see the connection."

5. Watching too much television can contribute to childhood obesity, according to a recent study by the Stanford Center for Research in Disease Prevention. Children who sit in front of the TV instead of playing outdoors or participating in sports will naturally have more problems avoiding weight gain. They also are more likely to eat in front of the TV, which causes digestive problems and lack of awareness of hunger levels.

Social and emotional development can also be stunted if children watch a screen all day instead of interacting with real people. As an example, in his nonfiction book *Among Schoolchildren*, Pulitzer Prize-winning author Tracy Kidder describes neglected children who watch too much TV late into the night as pale in complexion, lethargic, and zoned out. They have a problem connecting with the world.

6. Many commercials are geared for children, and try to persuade them to eat foods that are unhealthy. The average child will be exposed to 350,000 commercials by the time he graduates from high school, and 55 percent of those will advertise food. More than half of this food will be made with heavy amounts of sugar. This can create conflict if you are trying to feed your children a healthy diet, and they are being indoctrinated to eat unhealthy foods by watching television.

7. Computer games create unnatural strain on the eyes and brain, which is another reason their use should be limited to a few hours a week.

You have seen that the family environment is a powerful influence on children's behavior. In the next chapter, you'll learn how to protect your child from environmental risk factors both inside and outside the home.

PART 5
Using the Near and Far Environment to Enhance Immunity

CHAPTER FIFTEEN

Ten Ways to Protect Your Child from Environmental Risk Factors

Unfortunately, today's children live in a toxic world. Your child can be exposed to unsafe levels of toxins just by eating an apple. Fortunately, there are many things you can do to protect your child against these environmental factors. Here's a program for keeping environmental toxins from harming your child.

1. Buy Organically Grown Food

As much as possible, buy organically grown foods for your children. This is becoming increasingly important as the levels of pesticides, chemicals, toxins, and other harmful substances are increasing in our environment and in our food and water supplies.

High Risks for Children

Since the mid-1900s, most crops in America have been grown using pesticides and chemical fertilizers. These toxins pose a much greater health risk for children than for adults, because a child's mind and body are still developing. It is well-documented that certain pesticides and toxins can have a seriously detrimental effect on the developing brain. A special committee formed by the National Research Council noted that exposure to certain pesticides early in life can lead to a greater risk of chronic diseases in adulthood. Such effects include cancer, neurodevelopmental impairment, and immune dysfunction.

In recent years, research on animals has made scientists suspect that pesticides may cause developmental problems in children, such as impaired ability to learn and remember, autism, hyperactivity, and aggressive behavior. Each of these is dramatically on the rise. Just as one example, autism, a neurological disorder that in 1985 affected one in 2500 children, is now occurring at the rate of one in 500. Researchers cannot rule out pesticides and other neurotoxins that can have lasting effects on the developing brain.

Why Children Are More at Risk Than Adults

Children can more easily ingest higher concentrations of pesticides because they have smaller body weights and consume more calories per unit of body weight than adults. The average American child also tends to devote a larger portion of his diet to certain foods that are high in pesticides, such as apples (including apple sauce and apple juice). A Consumer's Union report found that seven common fruits and vegetables—apples, grapes, peaches, pears, green beans, spinach, and winter squash—actually contained pesticide levels that were hundreds of times greater than those of other foods. Some apples are so toxic that just one bite can deliver an unsafe dose of organophosphate insecticides to a child under five.

According to a report by the Environmental Working Group, which analyzes statistics supplied by the U.S. government, more than a quarter million American children ages one through five ingest a combination of twenty different pesticides every day, and overall more than one million American children under the age of five eat an average of eight pesticides a day. Every day, 610,000 preschool children consume a dose of neurotoxic organophosphate insecticides that is above the amount *considered safe for adults*. These multiple pesticides are known or suspected to cause cancer, hormone interference, and brain and nervous system damage.

Despite the obvious risks for children, toxicity levels have been calculated for adults only. The safe levels for children are not yet established. In its 1993 report, *Pesticides in the Diets of Infants and Children*, the National Research Council recommended that new tolerance levels be established for children, since safe adult levels could be toxic for some children. Yet this has not yet happened, and it will take years to test the hundreds of pesticides on the market and to set tolerance levels for children.

Laws are slow to change. In the meantime, it is up to you to protect your children, for the government will not necessarily do it for you. On a good note, the EPA banned the use of two highly toxic pesticides (methyl parathion and azinphos-methyl) that are used on apples, peaches, wheat, rice, sugar beets, and cotton. In making their decision, EPA officials cited studies that measured the effects of these pesticides on children rather than adults.

The health risks are even greater when children are exposed while in the womb or while of nursing age. There are brief moments, or windows of vulnerability, when exposure of the fetus or newborn to high levels of toxins can alter the development of organ systems. Even chemicals that are relatively benign may combine with other compounds to multiply toxic effects.

DDT Is Still Here

The most harmful fat-soluble toxins, including PCBs, dioxins, and DDT, are actually increasing in the bodies of Americans even though these chemicals have been banned in America for more than two decades. In the 1980s these chemicals were shown by researchers to be declining in the bodies of Americans, and at that rate their presence should be about zero by now. Researchers suspect that there is a sudden increase because these deadly substances are still used in many developing nations, who do not have bans on them.

In recent years, the United States is importing large amounts of fruits and vegetables from Mexico and South America that are grown using highly toxic chemicals that are banned in America. (A government report estimated 7.3 percent of fresh fruits and vegetables that were tested had chemicals in them that are illegal in the U.S.) These chemicals are also borne in water and air, causing some amount of background exposure for almost everyone. Ironically, Mexico purchases many of these chemicals from companies in the U.S., who are banned from selling them in America but are free to sell them in developing countries.

Some of the health risks for these toxins may include forms of cancer, endocrine disruption, reproductive problems, suppression of immunity, neurological problems, cognitive disorders, liver damage, and skin problems. High levels of these toxins found in utero or in nursing children have been linked to decreased cognitive ability and increased behavioral problems. Indeed, during the last twenty years there has been a dramatic rise in cancer rates for children and adults, and the link between breast cancer and toxins in the environment has been suspected by numerous researchers. Cancer is the third leading cause of death in American children today.

This is why I urge my patients, especially children, to eat organically grown food whenever possible. Organic foods are becoming common even in commercial supermarkets. Look for the "Certified Organic" label. If you and other consumers ask for it, your supermarket will start to supply it. The organic foods sector is the fastest growing part of the commercial foods market, with a growth rate of 20 percent, so you will not be alone.

You can also try to purchase locally grown produce at your local farmer's market because small farmers tend not to use as many pesticides and chemical fertilizers as on large commercial farms. Many local farmers use no chemicals at all. When you can meet the farmer face-to-face, you can ask him or her directly how much he is spraying the crops.

Be sure to wash all your produce thoroughly with a vegetable brush and a mild detergent. This removes surface pesticides (and also removes any fertilizer residues from organic produce). Be sure to rinse thoroughly. Peel any fruits or vegetables that have been waxed (such as apples and zucchini), because the wax traps the pesticides. If you have a green thumb, try starting a vegetable garden. The veggies will be fresher and much safer for your child. And an added bonus: children tend to have more positive attitudes toward eating fresh vegetables when they have been involved in growing them from seeds.

2. Avoid Genetically Modified Foods

Another reason to buy organic foods is that there is now a new health risk for children: genetically modified (GMO) foods. In just the past few years, much of the soybeans, corn, and canola oil for sale in the U.S. has been grown using genetically modified seed. Thirty genetically modified foods are currently on the market, and many others are slated for release during the next few years. Since so many commercial products contain soy oil, cornstarch, corn syrup, or other corn by-products, it is estimated that as much as 70 percent of the food on your grocery shelves contains one or more components of genetically engineered foods, without any labeling to identify them to consumers. Since organic foods do not contain GMO ingredients, buying organic is the only way to be sure you are not eating GMO foods.

Unfortunately, these radically modified foods have been approved by the FDA without adequate testing to guarantee their safety. There are many reasons for parents to be concerned. You and your children are, in effect, being used as guinea pigs to test the safety of a new scientific technology.

What Is a Genetically Modified Food?

First of all, let's clarify what a genetically altered food is. Perhaps you have some vague memory of your high school biology class, where you learned how the Austrian monk Gregor Mendel crossed tall and short pea plants and discovered the secret of dominant and recessive genes. This method of crossbreeding plants of the same or closely related species was later used to create hybrid corn and other agricultural advances. Unlike these methods, which use nature's own reproductive methods of cross-pollination, genetic engineering involves cutting, splicing, and recombining genes of two completely different species in the laboratory. Scientists actually take the genes of one organism and inject it into another to create completely new DNA blueprints and new organisms. A cold-water fish gene, for instance, was injected into a tomato to make it more resistant to cold. The genes of viruses, bacteria, insects, and even human genes have been injected into crops.

Genetically Modified Foods Currently on the Market[*]

• *Corn*—Corn and all related foods such as sweet corn, cornstarch, popcorn, cornmeal, corn syrup, high fructose corn syrup, and polenta. Does not include blue corn.

Soy—Soy flour, soy lecithin, soy oil, soy powder, soymilk, tofu.

• *Canola oil*—Fifty percent of the North American canola oil is now genetically modified, and it is found in many health foods and packaged foods in commercial grocery stores.

---

[*] Potatoes—because of research that raised an alarm about possible ill effects from genetically modified potatoes, they were taken off the market.

- *Milk and Dairy Products*—Thirty percent of the nonorganic milk in the U.S. is from cows that have been injected with the genetically modified recombinant bovine growth hormone (rBGH). Scientists in Canada and Europe have banned its use due to concerns over its safety and possible links to high toxicity and cancer. Because rBGH weakens cows and causes them to need more antibiotics, dairy products from cows injected with rBGH contain higher levels of antibiotics. They also contain higher levels of growth hormone factor IGF-1. There may be other differences due to the stress and hormonal cascades created by rBGH in the cow.
- *Yellow Summer Squash and Zucchini*—Several varieties of yellow summer squash and zucchini are genetically modified, including yellow crookneck squash.
- *Cottonseed Oil*—Cotton and cottonseed oil are genetically modified.
- *Hawaiian Papaya*
- *Additives, enzymes, flavorings, and processing agents*—Many of these genetically modified additives are found in thousands of processed foods on the market. A genetically modified version of rennet is used to make cheeses. The diet-sweetener, Aspartame, is genetically engineered. Xanthan gum is often genetically engineered, as are many bacteria and fungi used in the production of enzymes, vitamins, and processing aids.
- *Other Foods Approved for Release but Not Yet Marketed*—Sugar beet, wheat. Genetically engineered tomatoes, including cherry tomatoes, are approved but are not currently being marketed.

Health Risks for Children

What are the health risks of genetically modified foods? There are far too many to discuss here, but here are just a few.

1. Food Allergies. One health risk is increased allergies in the people who eat genetically modified foods. Because genetically modified foods might involve the splicing of a fish and a tomato, people who are allergic to fish may then eat those tomatoes without realizing that they are actually eating fish genes. Researchers have already noted that the introduction of genetically modified soy several years ago is correlated with a 50 percent increase in soy allergies and digestion problems caused by soy during those same years. Researchers at the York Nutritional Laboratory in northern England noted that this time period coincided with the dissemination of genetically modified soy products, and concluded that the findings raise serious questions about the safety of genetically modified soy.

2. Decreased Effectiveness of Antibiotics. Scientists are routinely splicing antibiotic-resistant genes into GMO foods as "markers" to test whether gene modification has been successful. This practice has already raised concerns among scientists, who claim that these may encourage the growth of antibiotic-resistant strains of diseases.

3. New and Higher Levels of Toxins. Biotechnology firms aim to develop plants that kill pests. This means even greater levels of pesticides in your child's food and in the water.

The EPA recognizes this problem of increased toxins in genetically modified foods. They now classify corn and potatoes that have been genetically engineered to kill insects as pesticides rather than vegetables. That is truly astounding—that the corn and potatoes your child may be eating are actually so toxic as to be classified as pesticides.

4. Unknown Hazards to Human Health and the Environment. Scientists simply do not know how these new species will affect the environment. The ecosystem consists of millions of smaller organisms. Even a teaspoon of soil contains 1,000 different types of bacteria. No one knows how genetically engineered foods will change the delicate balance of nature. Already there are signs, though, that the effects could be disastrous. Headlines were made when a research study published in *Nature* magazine showed that the caterpillars of Monarch butterflies were killed when they ate the pollen of corn that had been genetically modified.

Fortunately, consumers are starting to wake up to the potential hazards of GMO foods. A panel of Canadian doctors voted to ban the use of rBGH in Canada, citing research that revealed harmful levels of toxins in the cows injected with the genetically modified growth hormone. They also cited increased lameness and udder infections, which could increase the need for antibiotics, as reasons to ban its use. They felt the toxic effects on the cows could also be experienced by humans, and asked that more testing be done before putting it on the market. Unfortunately, rBGH has been approved by the FDA since 1993, which is why, in the U.S., organic milk is safer to drink.

The point here is that the effects of eating genetically modified foods is unknown. Yet they could be potentially dangerous to health. To ensure your child's safety, buy organic soy, corn, and dairy products.

3. Encourage Your Child to Drink Plenty of Pure Water

Headaches, constipation, and fatigue are sometimes caused by not drinking enough water. Drinking five to eight glasses of water a day is a simple and inexpensive way for your child to boost his or her health.

To be effective, it's important not to drink too much at mealtimes. One glass of water is enough to aid digestion and quench thirst. More than one glass of water could douse the digestive fire and cause impurities (ama) to be produced. It's best to drink larger quantities of water between meals, as it cleanses the stomach and helps the body flush out toxins.

Drinking water is especially important before and during sporting events. Children should be advised to drink several glasses of water a half-hour before the event starts. If the event lasts more than an hour, they should also drink at rest periods throughout the event. Dehydration is especially a risk during the summer months.

It's important that the water be pure and clean. City water that has been treated with chlorine should be purified with a carbon filter. You can buy simple carbon pitcher-filters (which are easy to use because you just fill the pitcher with water and let it drip through the filter) at most discount-variety stores. You can also buy a charcoal filter for your showerhead, which is a good idea because you absorb water through the skin when you bathe.

If you suspect that there may be nitrates or other harmful chemicals in your drinking water (which is highly probable if you live in a farming area), then you may want to purchase a good-quality water purifier that will filter out chemical pesticides and fertilizers. Buying spring water for drinking is also a good idea, but be aware that there are few governmental standards for spring water and no guarantee of the quality. Be sure to read the labels and investigate the legitimacy of the company's claims if you plan to buy it on a regular basis.

4. Avoid Chemically Harsh Household Cleaners and Detergents

Commercial detergents can contain many synthetic ingredients that could irritate your child's skin. Also, breathing strong household cleansers can contribute to allergies, asthma, and other respiratory illnesses.

It's best to use the most gentle, nontoxic detergents and household cleansers. Many different nontoxic brands are available in health food stores, and even discount stores sell nontoxic lines of detergents and cleansers.

You can teach your child the environmental advantages of using household products that are free of harmful chemicals and phosphates. The health of our waterways and the fishes and other creatures that live in them is something that we all need to be concerned about, and by teaching your child at an early age to respect the environment, you will be teaching an important lesson for life.

5. Provide Natural and Comfortable Clothing for Your Children

The skin is the largest organ in the body, and it needs to breathe to be healthy. Children have sensitive skin, and it's best to keep synthetic clothing and bedsheets away from them.

Synthetic clothing, such as polyester and acrylic, can feel more like a plastic bag than breathing, living fiber. It can cause wide-ranging discomforts, from skin rashes to headaches. Cotton, linen, flax, hemp, wool, cashmere, and angora are natural fibers that allow the skin to breathe. Natural fibers are cooler in the summer and warmer in the winter. Organic cotton is much less toxic than commercial cotton. Commercial cotton is a crop that is sprayed many times with highly toxic pesticides, and these have an effect on the skin. Cotton is also genetically engineered.

Clothing should be comfortable and not too tight, especially around the stomach. Tightness there can disturb digestion and cause unhealthy side effects.

6. Avoid Exposing Your Child to Environmental Toxins

In May 2010 the President's Cancer Panel urgently recommended new research on the link between cancer and the nearly 80,000 chemicals that American children and adults are exposed to in the air, water, food, and everyday objects such as bedding, plastic toys, and car seats. The effects of only a few hundred of these chemicals have been researched.

One of the most toxic environmental hazards for children is lead. Exposure to lead has been linked to mental retardation and learning problems in children, and a new study shows that lead exposure is also linked to dental cavities in children and adolescents.

Much effort has been expended to eliminate lead in paints, water pipes, and ceramic dishes in the U.S., yet tests show that nearly 900,000 children under the age of six harbor dangerously high levels of lead in their tissues.

Most of the children at risk for lead poisoning are underprivileged children living in older buildings with lead pipes and walls painted with lead-based paint. Yet any child could be exposed to lead poisoning in older buildings. If you suspect there are lead pipes in a building where your child goes to school, lives or visits regularly, it would be a good idea to have the pipes tested.

7. Avoid Too Much Direct Sunlight on the Skin

The sun is not quite as benign as it used to be. Although it's important for children to be out in the fresh air and sunlight every day, and sunlight helps the body absorb calcium by supplying Vitamin D, fifteen or twenty minutes of direct sunlight on the face and arms is enough. Too much direct sunlight can increase the risk of skin cancer.

As has been widely reported in the media, the ozone layer is thinner now due to pollution, and thus the sun's ultraviolet rays are stronger than before. You'll want to keep your child out of the sun at noon in the

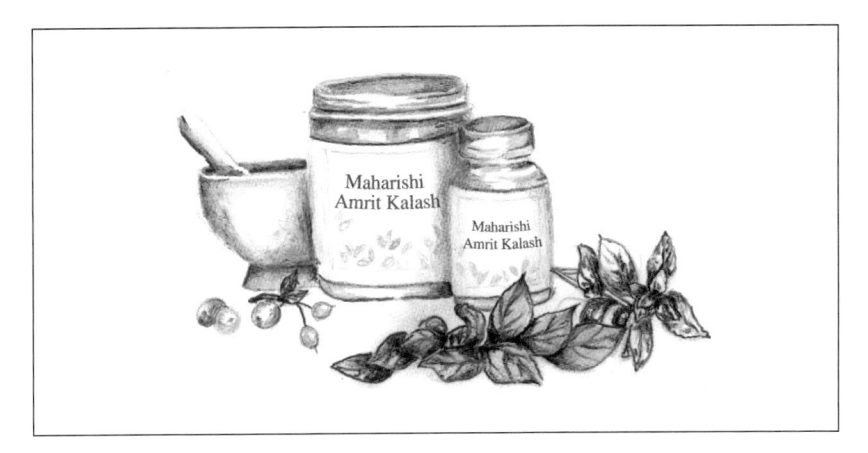

TEN WAYS TO PROTECT YOUR CHILD FROM ENVIRONMENTAL RISK FACTORS

summer, when it's the strongest. Providing hats and light clothing will also protect the skin from the sun.

It's especially important to protect fair-skinned children with Pitta imbalances from excessive sun exposure. Severe sunburn (to the point of blistering) in childhood can lead to skin cancer later in life. It's up to the parents to be on the alert during the summer months, when the sun is hot, the beach is inviting, and it's easy to forget how abrasive and painful a sunburn can be.

8. Give Your Child Maharishi Amrit Kalash

All these harmful environmental influences accelerate the production of free radicals. As you'll remember from Chapter Ten, free radicals are thought to cause many diseases. But try as you might, it's not possible to protect your child from all environmental toxins at any given moment. It could even be harmful to be so restrictive. Children need to feel like they are a part of the world, and need to feel free to experience new foods and new environments without fear.

By giving your child Maharishi Amrit Kalash on a daily basis, you can help diminish the production of free radicals caused by environmental toxins, greatly minimizing their negative effect. Thus even if your child is exposed to more toxins than you would like in our imperfect world, this is something you can add to the diet to protect him or her from negative environmental influences.

9. Purify Toxins with Daily Ayurvedic Oil Massage (Abhyanga)

Daily Ayurvedic oil massage (abhyanga) has a remarkable ability to purify toxins from the cells of the body. This is because the oil penetrates the skin and even the cell membranes, which are composed of lipids (fats). The fresh, uncontaminated oil molecules actually replace the old, tired, toxic lipid molecules, creating a cleansing, purifying effect. As discussed earlier, be sure to use pure, organic sesame oil that has been cured.

10. Use Vedic Architecture to Create Health

To help your child's health, make sure that the buildings he lives in and goes to school in are healthy. You have already learned about the problems of sick-building syndrome, which can arise when children are exposed to poor ventilation, toxic carpets, and toxic building materials.

Maharishi Ayurveda takes the concept of healthy buildings to a much deeper level. In the Vedic science of architecture, also known as Maharishi Sthapatya Veda® design, buildings are designed to be in harmony with nature. The Sanskrit root "stha" means "established," meaning that the buildings themselves contribute to the inhabitants becoming established in pure consciousness.

The buildings are placed on a carefully measured site, called a *Vastu*. The Vastu is enclosed in a low fence. In order to make maximum use of the sun's energy, the Vastu is measured on a true east-west, north-south axis and faces east. The ideal Vastu brings positive influences from the sun, moon, and planets. It defines the individual's connection to the universe, and creates a positive influence for every person who lives or works there.

The buildings on the site are designed to harmonize with natural law using three major principles: orientation, placement, and proportion.

Orientation

Buildings are oriented toward the sun, the main source of energy on earth. When the door of the building faces east, the morning sun falls on it during the first twelve minutes after sunrise. North is also considered a life-supporting direction to face, but northeast, south, southeast, west, southwest, and northwest all create negative effects on the inhabitants. These effects include anxiety, depression, illness, chronic disease, blocks to creativity, bad luck, financial loss, obstacles to progress and success, disharmony in relationships, breakdown of family life, and antisocial behavior.

Placement

Each room is also placed in alignment with the sun as it moves across the sky. The kitchen, for instance, where food is cooked, is placed in the southeast corner of the house, where the sun's rays fall during the preparation of the noon meal of the day. The living room is in the western half of the house, since people tend to relax there when the sun is setting. Rooms that are used for quiet study are in the northern end of the house. Thus every room is oriented to take advantage of the sun's energy to support the specific activity usually performed in that room. If the rooms are placed in the wrong place, it can cause an imbalance. A kitchen in the wrong place can cause digestive problems, for instance. A kitchen in the right place can help balance the doshas.

Proportion

Just as the design of the human body reflects perfect proportions, so the proportions of a building should harmonize. Lack of proportion in the height, width, or length of the rooms could cause an imbalance in the people living in them. You've probably had the experience of feeling cramped or restricted in a room that is too narrow, and you may also experience a sense of relief when you walk into a room that is balanced and harmonious in its proportions. The proportions of Maharishi Sthapatya Veda design create a deep and pervasive experience of relaxation, balance, and freedom in the brain, emotions, and body of the inhabitants of the home.

Even the furniture and appliances can create better health when placed in the right direction. Recent research has reported that brain cells fire differently according to different orientations of the brain. In other words, the firing patterns of neurons in the thalamus of the brain are altered by the direction you are facing, thus influencing the entire brain functioning and the whole physiology. When you are facing east, the brain is functioning differently than when you are facing north, south, or west.

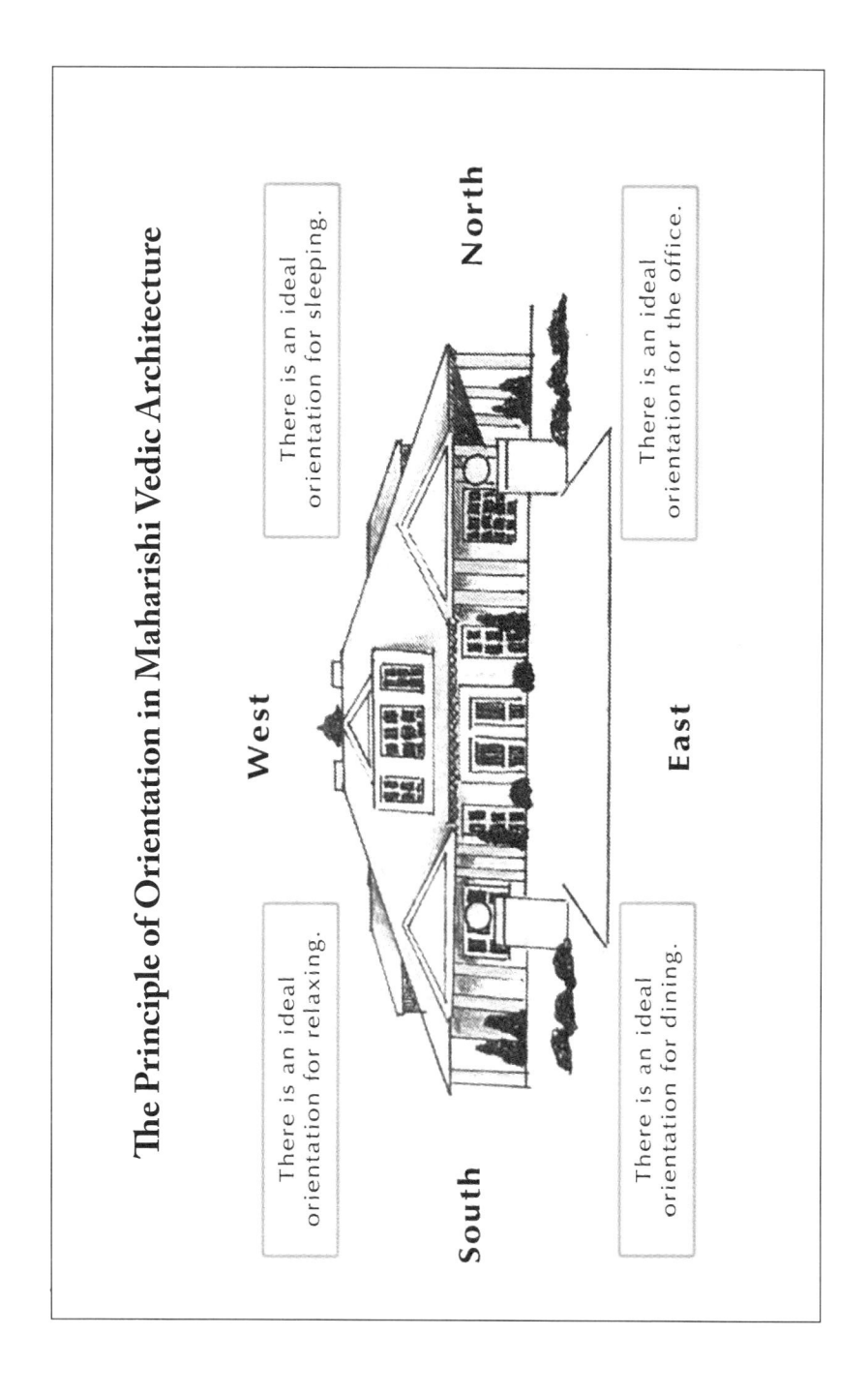

SUPER HEALTHY KIDS: A PARENT'S GUIDE TO MAHARISHI AYURVEDA

The Principle of Orientation in Maharishi Vedic Architecture

There is an ideal orientation for sleeping.

There is an ideal orientation for the office.

There is an ideal orientation for relaxing.

There is an ideal orientation for dining.

North

East

South

West

Research shows that brain waves become more coherent and orderly when a person faces east. You can capitalize on this principle from Maharishi Sthapatya Veda design by facing your child's desk east so that when he studies he feels most alert.

Reports from Families Who Have Used *Maharishi Sthapatya Veda Home* Designs

Families who have built homes based on the principles of Maharishi Sthapatya Veda design have noticed a wide range of results. They report more clear and creative thinking, better decision-making, greater health and happiness, increased alertness, more restful and refreshing sleep, more energy, greater peace of mind, and less fatigue and stress.

Sandra, mother of Matthew, twelve, and Anna, three, notices that their Sthapatya Veda home radiates a nourishing quality for the whole family. "The center area of silence, called the Brahmasthan, is nourishing the whole house. I feel like there's an underlying quality of wholeness that's protecting my son, Matthew. Whenever his friends are here there's a light, happy feeling, just because the house itself feels light and happy, and that permeates everything. The children can't help but feel it.

"I also notice that he wants to stay home with the family more since we've moved into our Sthapatya Veda home. He's still very social and loves his friends, and does well in school, yet he knows when he needs to be by himself, nourished by our home. He seems to be very balanced. The house moves in wholeness, I just feel like that."

Another mother said, "We don't live in a Sthapatya Veda home, but one night we stayed overnight in a Sthapatya Veda hotel. We noticed a difference in our daughter. Usually, no matter how tired she is, she likes to stay up late and avoid going to sleep. At the Sthapatya Veda hotel, it was the opposite. We were watching a family movie and she said, 'Mommy would you like to turn off the TV and go to bed?' In that environment she became more coherent, happy, and settled. She was more in tune with her body's needs. The change in her was dramatic."

PART 6
The *Maharishi Ayurveda* Approach to Common and Chronic Disease in Children

CHAPTER SIXTEEN
Prevention and Treatment of Common Childhood Illnesses

This chapter explains the underlying causes of common childhood illnesses from the Ayurvedic perspective. While these descriptions will give you an idea of possible treatments that might be recommended by a physician trained in Maharishi Ayurveda to create balance and prevent illness in your child, they are not intended to be prescriptions for you to follow at home, nor is this book in any way meant to substitute for proper medical care. Remember that in Maharishi Ayurveda treatment protocol, the underlying imbalance in the doshas must first be identified through pulse diagnosis and other diagnostic procedures before specific treatments can be recommended, and for that you will need to consult a physician trained in Maharishi Ayurveda. For acute disorders, it's important to consult your child's pediatrician immediately.

General Guidelines for Preventing Childhood Illness

Childhood is a time when Kapha dosha predominates, a time when the human body is building and developing. Almost all traditional childhood illnesses (such as colds, runny noses, sinus infections, and flu) are due to excess Kapha. As mentioned in Chapter Six, they can often be prevented by three dietary habits: no cold food, no heavy food, and no refined sugar. (Remember that the "no refined sugar" directive includes high fructose corn syrup, found in most processed foods and drinks.)

These three dietary habits help to reduce Kapha dosha, which is cold, heavy, sweet, and sticky—and is aggravated by cold, heavy, and sugary foods. Foods made with unrefined sugar, such as jaggary and rock sugar, will sate your child's sweet tooth without making him sick. These guidelines are especially important during Kapha season (March to June) and for children who have Kapha dosha predominating. These children should avoid cold dairy products such as cold milk and ice cream, chocolate, cheese, fermented foods, and sour foods such as vinegar. The child should still drink milk, but boil it first, and add spices such as cardamom and turmeric to make it more digestible, and serve it warm.

Vata dosha can also be a factor in illness, because Vata leads the other doshas. Also, it is more easily thrown out of balance by irregular routine, stress, pressure, and diet. That's why adequate rest is important on a daily basis, and why rest and quiet are so important to a child when he is sick. By resting, Vata dosha becomes balanced again, and then leads the other doshas back into balance.

Daily practice of the Transcendental Meditation technique is the most important component of prevention, because it settles the mind and brings deep rest to the body, triggering the body's inherent healing mechanisms.

When a Child Is Constantly Sick

If a child is experiencing a continual cycle of colds, antibiotic treatments, and more colds, it is not difficult to wean him or her from antibiotics and restore immunity. The physician trained in Maharishi Ayurveda will probably recommend a change in the diet to decrease digestive toxins (ama).

Besides providing your child with a balanced diet of fresh, home-cooked foods, essential daily habits for restoring immunity include following a regular daily routine and getting enough exercise. Daily Ayurvedic oil massage (abhyanga), followed by a warm bath to mobilize toxins and flush them from the body, is also effective (but once a child is congested, oil massage is not recommended). Other recommendations may include taking herbal food supplements to increase digestion, assimilate nutrients, and increase immunity.

For children with frequent colds and other Kapha-related problems, adding more fresh ginger or ground ginger to their food can help prevent colds and reduce other symptoms of ama. Sipping warm water from a thermos throughout the day is also helpful in dissolving impurities.

Sniffle Free® tablets and tea are Maharishi Ayurveda products that will help reduce the symptoms of a cold while correcting the underlying imbalance. Other helpful herbal formulas include Clear Breathe™, Clear Throat™, Flu Season Defense®, and Throat Ease®. They are especially useful when taken during the early stages of the cold. Unlike antibiotics, they have no harmful side effects; rather, they strengthen immunity.

In the rest of this chapter, you'll find a description of the causes, symptoms, and treatment approaches for a variety of common childhood illnesses from the perspective of Maharishi Ayurveda.

Common Childhood Illnesses and a Description of Treatments Using Maharishi Ayurveda

Aggressive Behavior, Temper Tantrums

Aggressive behavior such as temper tantrums may be normal during the "terrible twos" when children are trying to assert their independence and often respond to every suggestion with a resounding "No!" These tantrums can be kept at a minimum by keeping the child from getting overtired, overstimulated, or overly frustrated.

If the temper tantrums continue after age four, or if the child is acting aggressively toward other children, teachers, or parents, it may be a result of parents either being too strict or else not setting any limits at all. It could also be the result of a learning difficulty, behavioral disorder, or a vision or hearing problem. In any case, it is wise to consult your child's pediatrician.

Cause and Treatment of Aggression According to Maharishi Ayurveda: Aggression has its root in Pitta imbalances, so it is important to balance Pitta dosha.

Making sure the child drinks plenty of milk and includes ghee in the diet is usually recommended, as these sweet foods balance Pitta. Regular meals are important for all children, and if the child is hungry, healthy snacks are also important. Hunger can create irritability, frustration, and aggressive behavior. A regular daily routine, including regular practice of the Transcendental Meditation technique, daily abhyanga with a warm bath, early bedtime (well before 10:00 p.m., when the Pitta time of night sets in), Maharishi Ayurveda herbal supplements as recommended by a physician trained in Maharishi Ayurveda, and Maharishi Gandharva Veda music are other treatments that may be recommended. The aggressive child also needs large helpings of unconditional love and reinforcement from parents.

Chicken Pox, Measles, and other Children's Diseases

Chicken pox and measles are highly contagious diseases that are caused by viruses and are characterized by fever and skin eruptions. In our society, we take it for granted that children are often sick with these childhood diseases and need to use antibiotics to combat them. If your child has a fever and skin rash, consult your pediatrician immediately.

Cause and Treatment According to Maharishi Ayurveda: If the child's immune system is strong, if the parents have been following Ayurvedic guidelines from the start, then it's possible that the child will suffer less severe symptoms and may even avoid these childhood illnesses altogether. There are families whose children take Maharishi Amrit Kalash regularly, who follow the daily routine and dietary guidelines and almost never get sick—even when the other children around them are contagious.

Traditional Ayurvedic treatments include eating puffed rice and drinking *kanji*. (Kanji is rice broth made by cooking one part rice with eight parts water. As soon as the rice is cooked, pour off the water and serve it. Discard the rice.)

Zucchini, squashes, and other light foods are often recommended while the fever lasts. Hot spices are avoided.

Constipation

Constipation is characterized by hard stools, difficulty or pain during bowel movements, infrequent bowel movements, or incomplete bowel movements. It is considered a common ailment of childhood in Western medicine. Symptoms include gas, weak digestion, back pain, dizziness, nausea, tiredness in the lower part of the body, and a blocked feeling in the stomach. For acute abdominal pain, consult a physician immediately because it could be appendicitis.

Cause and Treatment According to Maharishi Ayurveda: According to Maharishi Ayurveda, bowel movements should take place once or twice a day and should be comfortable and easy. Constipation means that the child does not have at least one bowel movement a day. The healthiest time for bowel movements is upon arising in the morning and again late in the afternoon. According to Maharishi Ayurveda, most disorders start with constipation. Insomnia, headache, backache, dry skin, skin diseases, and menstrual cramps can be caused by or aggravated by constipation.

Constipation is caused by an imbalance in Vata dosha with related causes such as dehydration, eating too many cold foods and drinks, eating irregularly, lack of exercise, sitting in the same position for a long time, eating meat, eating the wrong diet for the child's body type, mental stress, fear, or anxiety.

Since constipation is a dry condition, treatment approaches often include recommendations to drink more water. Usually it's recommended to sip warm water throughout the day, as well as other warm fluids. The dietary regimen often includes eating more servings of fresh, juicy fruits and leafy green vegetables, drinking lassi regularly, including more ghee in the diet, and eating hot soups with ghee. It's usually recommended to avoid all Vata-aggravating foods, as well as dates, honey, root vegetables, roasted nuts with salt (and all nuts if digestive strength is low), yogurt (although lassi is actually helpful in relieving constipation), butter, salty foods, and dry foods such as cereals and chips.

Besides drinking enough water between meals, the child can drink Vata Tea to help balance Vata and provide sufficient hydration. A half-cup of warm milk with fresh ghee before bed, or a half-cup of soaked raisins, are remedies for constipation. Both act as mild laxatives. Drinking a cup of warm water on rising will also help stimulate the bowel.

For the daily routine, regular exercise is a must. Doing Yoga Asanas on a daily basis is also recommended, and in particular the seated pose (*vajra asana*), the twist (*vakra asana*), the shoulder stand (*sarvang asana*), the locust pose (*uttet ekapada asana*), and lying down while holding the knees to the chest and rolling from side to side (*pavan mukta*).

An evening oil massage and early bedtime can help reduce anxiety and Vata imbalance, and thus help with constipation. A mild laxative such as castor oil may help, but parents should receive the prescription from a physician trained in Maharishi Ayurveda.

Common Cold and Stuffy or Runny Nose

A cold is thought to be a viral infection of the upper respiratory tract. Sneezing, sore throat, earache, fever, stuffy or runny nose, and headache are symptoms of the cold. It's one of the most common childhood illnesses, thought to be caused by a child's immature immunity being unable to fight the nearly 200 types of cold viruses. If the fever or sore throat continues more than 48 hours, be sure to consult your pediatrician as it could be strep throat, which needs immediate attention.

Cause and Treatment of the Common Cold According to Maharishi Ayurveda: Most colds in childhood are caused by an imbalance in Kapha dosha along with ama.

For prevention, the recommendations for diet and daily routine presented in this book will strengthen immunity and prevent Kapha and Vata from going out of balance.

For treatment, Sniffle Free herbal tablets and Sniffle Free tea are often recommended to reduce mucus. Nasya (sniffing sesame oil) is sometimes recommended to prevent dryness and the spread of disease. Oils used for nasya include cured sesame oil and MP 16™, a special formula that helps increase Pitta, decrease Kapha, and kill bacteria, preventing it from spreading from the nose to the lungs. For children, MP 16 should be diluted with sesame oil.

If there is a fever with the cold, then the child can skip one meal and drink hot water or rice water instead. Easily digestible, warm, fresh, soupy foods—such as barley soup or juice made with tender, young radishes—are often recommended. A drink of 1/2 cup milk and 1/2 cup water, boiled with a slice of fresh ginger, is also a nourishing drink. Lassi diluted with seven parts water, one part freshly made yogurt, is sometimes recommended. Otherwise, eating yogurt or butter is not recommended. Meat, salty, sweet, and sour foods are also avoided.

Sipping hot water throughout the day can help reduce mucus (ama). Warm ginger tea is often recommended. It helps to reduce milk products (except for the diluted lassi and milk drinks mentioned above) during the duration of the cold. Cheeses and ice cream should be avoided while symptoms continue, as these are hard to digest and may create ama.

An herbal mix that children enjoy includes dry roasting a quantity of cumin, grinding it to a powder, and mixing it with an equal amount of ground rock sugar. Even very young children can eat a pinch throughout the day to reduce Kapha.

Cough and Bronchitis

Coughing can be associated with allergies, asthma, the common cold, bronchitis, or croup. If the cough sounds like a bark and occurs on inhalation, consult your child's pediatrician immediately because it may be croup, which can be life-threatening when severe.

Cause and Treatment of Dry Cough According to Maharishi Ayurveda:
Dry cough is caused by an imbalance in Vata dosha along with impurities in the lung area. It is characterized by itching in the throat, irritation, and blockage. It also can come with sore throat, hoarseness, headache, and irritation of the eyes.

Western medicine has a difficult time treating dry cough, because the underlying cause, Vata imbalance, is not understood. Dry foods, cold foods, too much of the bitter and astringent tastes, too much exercise, and irregular routine can cause this problem. Air pollution, smoking, secondary smoke, and other environmental toxins may be factors.

A Vata-reducing diet, herbal preparations, and a regular routine to balance Vata can be effective in treating this problem.

Cause and Treatment of Wet Cough According to Maharishi Ayurveda:
Excessive Kapha with impurities (ama) and mucus in the bronchial tubes is characteristic of this type of bronchitis. The same guidelines recommended for colds are often recommended. Wet cough may also be characterized by mild chest pain, heaviness in the chest area, and

mucus in the throat, and can be accompanied by nausea and vomiting. Eating Kapha-aggravating foods, such as foods that are heavy, cold, oily, and sweet can cause it. Too little exercise, sleeping too much during the day (this does not apply to infants and preschoolers, who need naps), and being too sedentary are other causes.

Recommendations often include eating lightly and if there is a fever, sipping water. If the child is very hungry, then drinking rice broth may be recommended. After skipping one meal, eating a light meal such as barley soup, pureed cooked vegetables, or other light food can help.

While symptoms continue children often are advised to avoid sweet, sour, and salty foods as these increase Kapha dosha, and to avoid dairy products except for light lassi (eight parts water to one part fresh yogurt) or ginger milk (half milk, half water, boiled with a slice of ginger). Drinking large amounts of hot water or fresh ginger tea may also help. Roasted cumin and powdered rock sugar is another common recommendation (see "Common Cold" section, above, for a description).

For a wet cough, the child should stay inside and rest, although it's important not to sleep during the day as this increases Kapha dosha. It's essential to avoid all abhyanga until the congestion is over, and avoid washing the hair.

Mixing a few drops of Clear Breathe with sesame oil and rubbing it on the chest, the back, and the sides of the chest can help. This is not recommended if the child is younger than one year. Making a steam tent and adding a few drops of Clear Breathe or eucalyptus oil to a pot of hot water and allowing the child to inhale the steam can help loosen mucus. Please note: This is not for young children. The child has to be old enough not to burn himself on the pan.

For children above one year (not infants), Clear Breathe can be used as an aroma oil, twice a day for ten or twenty minutes. Nasya is helpful if there is not too much mucus, using sesame oil or a mixture of MP 16 diluted with sesame oil. The child can gargle with warm water, salt, and turmeric, or salt and black pepper.

Other recommendations may include keeping the neck and chest warm and applying a hot water bottle to the neck to help increase the flow of toxins out of the body. Placing it over the heart should be avoided.

Diarrhea

Diarrhea is characterized by increased frequency, liquidity, and amount of bowel movements. It occurs commonly among children, especially in conjunction with common childhood illnesses. Usually it is short-term. If it lasts more than a day, consult your child's pediatrician immediately.

Cause and Treatment of Diarrhea According to Maharishi Ayurveda:
Diarrhea can be caused by an imbalance in any of the three doshas, but is usually caused by a Pitta imbalance along with ama. Eating dry, cold, spicy foods, or a diet rich in meat can cause diarrhea. Poor eating habits, such as overeating, eating at variable times, and mixing foods of opposite qualities (such as milk and salty foods) can also cause diarrhea. Anxiety, fear, and grief can bring it on, as well as trying to suppress the natural urges.

Symptoms include mild pain in the abdomen, weakness, bloating, indigestion, loose stool, and the alternation of loose stool with constipation.

Recommendations may include encouraging the child to eat only when he is really hungry. Avoiding cold foods and drinks and eating a light diet of soupy, liquid, easily digestible foods such as mung dhal soup, vegetable soups, zucchini, asparagus, and well-cooked grains is often recommended.

Giving the child a slice of ginger sprinkled with salt and a few drops of lemon juice before meals stimulates digestion and helps regulate elimination. An herbal mixture of equal parts cumin and fennel together, dry-fried, is sometimes recommended. Depending on the child's age, he could have 1/2 teaspoon or more before meals and one or two other times throughout the day.

Lassi is an ideal antidote to diarrhea, as it balances Pitta but also stimulates the digestion. A good recipe is to mix 1/4 cup freshly made yogurt with 1 and 3/4 cups water. Bring it to a boil, and add a teaspoon of turmeric and 1/2 teaspoon curry leaves. Let it cool before drinking. Rice water can also be added to it. Lassi blended with toasted cumin and salt is also helpful in regulating the digestion.

The child can also drink rice broth until the stool returns to normal, with cooled ginger tea (made from boiling fresh ginger in water) in between meals of rice broth.

Earaches

Earaches and ear infections can be caused by infections of the external, middle, and inner ear. Middle earaches are the most common in children six to twenty-four months old and children four to six years old, and can be caused by a viral or bacterial infection. They often are accompanied by colds, sore throat, allergies, tonsillitis, or adenoiditis. Earaches are caused by a buildup of pressure and fluid in the middle ear. An additional cause is eardrum inflammation or fluid drainage from a temporarily perforated eardrum. Usually they clear up spontaneously; if complications arise they are treated with antibiotics. A common external ear infection is called swimmer's ear. The more serious inner ear infections are less frequent and are often treated with antibiotics or surgery. Consult your child's pediatrician for treatment.

Cause and Treatment of Earaches According to Maharishi Ayurveda:
After diagnosis, the same guidelines as for colds are often recommended for the common middle ear infections. Nasya (sniffing oil to lubricate and clear the nasal passages) can help. Nasya using MP 16 diluted with sesame oil is often recommended. Protecting the ears from wind and draft is important, as these aggravate Vata and increase pain in the ears.

Squeezing warm garlic oil drops into the ear with an eyedropper is sometimes recommended with the supervision of a physician trained in Maharishi Ayurveda. One clove of garlic is chopped into fine pieces, and the garlic is cooked in three tablespoons of sesame oil until it becomes a dark brown or black color. After the oil is strained in cheesecloth and poured into a bottle, it is ready to use. Usually two drops in each ear (using an eyedropper) before bed, twice a week at most, is recommended. Applying cotton keeps the oil from dripping out.

Hot fomentation (hot water bottle) on the ear can help loosen congestion. Steam inhalation may also help, and if there is nasal or chest congestion along with the earache, eucalyptus drops can be added to the steam. The physician trained in Maharishi Ayurveda may recommend Maharishi Ayurveda herbal formulas.

Fear

Fear is caused by a Vata imbalance and a weakness in the dhatus. If symptoms continue, consult your child's pediatrician.

Cause and Treatment of Fear According to Maharishi Ayurveda: A light, nourishing diet will help build the dhatus: milk, ghee, soups, and blanched, crushed almonds. Almond Energy drink, Maharishi Amrit Kalash, Maharishi Ayurveda rasayanas, and Maharishi Ayurveda herbal food supplements may be recommended by a physician trained in Maharishi Ayurveda according to the child's needs as determined by pulse diagnosis.

Giving your child more love and affection and making a habit of praising positive behavior rather than constantly criticizing wrong behavior can be helpful. A regular daily routine with practice of the Transcendental Meditation technique, listening to Maharishi Gandharva Veda music, and an early bedtime is recommended.

Fever

Fever is an increase in body temperature at least one degree above the normal level of 98.6° F. Fever is dangerous under the following conditions: if a child under six months has a fever 100° F or higher; if a child from six months to three years has a fever of 102° F or higher; if any child has a fever of 103° F or higher lasting longer than four to six hours after measures to break the fever have begun; if a child has a fever above 105° F; or if a child of any age has a fever along with extreme drowsiness, lack of alertness, or labored breathing. In any of these situations, consult a physician immediately. Acute fever can be caused by bacterial infections such as earache and pneumonia; viral infections such as colds, flu, or chicken pox; allergic or toxic reactions; heat stroke; and dehydration.

If the child is over three years old and the fever is mild (and not one of the emergency situations mentioned above), your child's physician may recommend a "wait and see" attitude. Sponge baths, changing to cotton clothing, or removing some clothing can make a child more comfortable. In any case, go by your doctor's advice.

Cause and Treatment of Fever According to Maharishi Ayurveda: Fever occurs when the body has excessive toxins (ama) and the body increases Pitta (heat) to try to purify itself of the ama.

It is recommended to rest in bed when there is a fever, to help balance Vata and increase immunity. If the older child practices the Transcendental Meditation technique, he or she can meditate in bed and gain extra rest. Staying indoors and away from sun, rain, cold, and wind is also important. Washing the child's head during a fever is usually avoided; a sponge bath is recommended instead. Even though the child should rest, it's best if he can prop himself up in bed as he rests, as day sleep can cause congestion to develop.

Soup, broth, kanji (rice water—see description under "Chicken Pox"), and other warm, liquid foods are often recommended during a fever. If there is diarrhea or vomiting along with the fever, adding turmeric to the kanji while cooking may help. If the fever continues, adding some fresh ginger and cumin to the soup or kanji is usually recommended. Cooked plums or peaches seasoned with cinnamon, fennel, and cardamom powder are also recommended foods for fever.

Avoiding cold foods, leftover foods, butter, and meat is advised during fever. Salty, sweet, and sour foods are also avoided. When the fever is gone the child can resume his regular eating patterns.

A common Ayurvedic antidote for fever is sipping hot water throughout the day, as this dissolves impurities (ama) and stimulates digestion. Drinking herbal water may help reduce Kapha and bring the fever down. This is prepared by adding 1 teaspoon cumin, 2 pinches of black pepper, and 1 teaspoon coriander seeds in 3 cups of water and boiling for 3 minutes. If it is stored in a thermos, the child can sip from it throughout the day. Diluting milk with 1/2 part water and boiling it with a slice of fresh ginger is also a commonly recommended drink for a child with fever. Lassi, diluted with seven parts water and one part fresh yogurt, is also recommended. Children also like the cumin-rock sugar mixture (see description under "Common Cold"). This stimulates the digestion while reducing fever, and even very young children can take a pinch whenever they feel like it.

Abhyanga and nasya should be stopped during a fever or any kind of congestion in the chest. They can be started again when these symptoms disappear.

Consult a medical doctor immediately if any of the dangerous symptoms of fever are present (see above).

Gas, Bloating, Flatulence

This is not considered a serious medical condition in Western medicine, yet it can bring a child great discomfort and can also lead to more serious digestive problems.

The Cause and Treatment of Gas, Bloating, and Indigestion According to Maharishi Ayurveda: Painful bloating and bad-smelling flatulence are caused by the accumulation of ama. Recommendations may include avoiding eating sweets and sugar; taking a mixture of powdered ginger, lemon juice, and raw honey before lunch and supper; taking Herbal Di-Gest™ after meals to strengthen digestion (half a tablet is usually recommended for children). For infants, a fenugreek/fennel tea is helpful, as well as daily abhyanga.

Headaches

Tension or stress headaches are rare among children. Often, if children have problems with stress, they manifest it as stomachaches. If emotional stress is manifesting as a headache, it is usually a dull, steady ache that intensifies throughout the day and is quite constant. It can be accompanied by poor appetite, constipation, and insomnia. Pain relievers are the usual prescription for tension headaches. Be sure to consult your child's pediatrician for persistent or recurring headaches.

The Cause and Treatment of Tension Headaches According to Maharishi Ayurveda: Tension headaches are usually due to Vata imbalance, and can be aggravated by feeling too much pressure while studying. Usually it's recommended to balance Vata dosha first by putting the child to bed early, providing some periods of rest during the day, serving regular, warm meals, and offering warm milk and spices before bed. Expressions of love and nourishment and soothing influences in the environment may also help. In general, less stimulation is usually recommended. For these headaches it's often recommended that the child remain in a dimly lit room accompanied by a parent for comfort. Yoga Asanas also help increase blood flow to the brain and relax the nervous system. The practice of the Transcendental Meditation technique helps relieve mental stress and helps relieve tension headaches. Maharishi

Ayurveda herbal formulas and herbal oils can be applied as pastes to the forehead, temples, and neck.

If the headaches are intense and continue to occur frequently, then it is important to see a medical doctor, because there could be other causes.

Motion Sickness

A child with motion sickness experiences nausea, sweating, vomiting, or dizziness while riding in a car, train, airplane, or boat. It is caused by a disturbance in the body's balance fluids, which are located in the inner ear. Usually children outgrow motion sickness by adolescence.

The Cause and Treatment of Motion Sickness According to Maharishi Ayurveda: Traveling increases Vata dosha, which is composed of air and space. Travel sickness can also involve excessive Kapha. If traveling in a car, fresh air helps as well as frequent stops. It's usually recommended that the child refrain from reading or eating in the car, as these contribute to travel sickness. Fresh ginger with raw honey (or candied ginger available in health food stores) can help alleviate both Vata and Kapha, and may help prevent motion sickness. Vata Tea or ginger tea, if the child can drink it before traveling or when the car is stopped, can also settle the doshas and the stomach.

Small Scratches

For very small scratches, it is sometimes recommended to disinfect the area with a drop of Clear Breathe on a bandage. Consult your child's pediatrician to see if your child needs a tetanus shot.

Sore Throat

Sore throat is frequently a symptom of viral infections such as colds. It can also be caused by irritants such as dust or pollen, or engaging in too much talking, singing, or shouting.

Sore throat is a symptom that accompanies more than one-third of contagious childhood respiratory illnesses. If it is not associated with a cold, and is associated with a skin rash or pustules on the tonsils or throat, it may be strep throat. Consult your child's pediatrician immediately.

The Cause and Treatment of Sore Throat According to Maharishi Ayurveda: Sore throat is usually due to a Kapha-Pitta imbalance caused by toxins (ama) being released in the throat. It's important to keep the ears warm. The child may be advised to gargle with a solution of warm water, turmeric, and ginger; or warm water, ginger, and licorice; or a drop of Clear Breathe added to the gargle water; or salt and turmeric. Rubbing Clear Breathe diluted in sesame oil on the throat or ears may be recommended to release ama, but it's important to avoid getting it near the eyes. Clear Throat and Throat Ease are often recommended.

Stomachache

Tummy aches are a common childhood disorder, and may be caused by overeating, indigestion, constipation, emotional stress, viral or bacterial infection, overexertion, lactose intolerance, allergies, or straining a muscle in the abdomen. Sometimes it is accompanied by diarrhea or vomiting. If a stomachache is severe or lasts an entire day, seek medical attention immediately.

The Cause and Treatment of Stomachache According to Maharishi Ayurveda: If the child is nauseous, this is due to a Kapha imbalance with an acute eruption of ama. The digestion has been overloaded.

Unless the child is very, very hungry, it's usually recommended that he eat something light, such as kanji (rice broth—see description under "Chicken Pox") flavored with ginger and cumin. A tea made by boiling fresh ginger may be recommended to help stimulate the digestion and reduce Kapha. Warm water with two drops of Clear Breathe every half hour may also help reduce nausea. Chewing a tablet of Herbal Di-Gest may be recommended, because it contains a combination of herbs to stimulate digestion.

Tonsillitis and Adenoiditis

Tonsillitis is usually caused by a viral infection or strep bacteria and is characterized by painful swelling of the tonsils (the mass of lymph tissue at the back of the throat). Adenoiditis is also caused by a virus and is characterized by swelling of the adenoids, which are located in the upper throat. Both the adenoids and tonsils are part of the immune system, and help to filter bacteria and infectious agents in the mouth. Consult your child's pediatrician for treatment.

The Cause and Treatment of Tonsillitis and Adenoiditis According to Maharishi Ayurveda: Tonsillitis and adenoiditis are caused by a disturbance in Kapha dosha, but all three doshas could also be disturbed. Eating too many cold foods, drinking ice-cold drinks, living in a cold climate, and taking cold showers can also bring these conditions on.

It's usually recommended that the child avoid cold showers and any exposure to cold temperatures or wind. Make sure his head, ears, and throat are covered when exposed to the cold. Sesame oil nasya is helpful, or nasya with MP 16 diluted with sesame oil. Gargling with turmeric, salt, and warm water also helps.

The physician trained in Maharishi Ayurveda will recommend specific foods depending on the child's imbalances as determined by pulse diagnosis. Avoiding foods that cause ama, especially cold foods and drinks, and leftover, stale food may help. It's usually recommended to avoid breads and other foods with yeast. Spicier, Kapha-pacifying foods, such as black mustard seed, mung dhal, barley soup, bitter greens, and rock salt are usually advised, as well as using bitter oils such as olive oil or mustard oil in cooking.

It's often recommended for the child to sip warm water throughout the day. A powder of dry-roasted cumin seed and crushed rock sugar (see description under "Common Cold") may be given, and the child can eat a pinch frequently throughout the day, whenever he feels like it, to reduce Kapha dosha.

It's usually recommended to avoid washing the child's hair or getting his head wet until the symptoms subside. Avoid exposing the child to secondary smoke.

Vomiting

Vomiting is a common childhood ailment. It is usually caused when the body needs to purge itself of agents it cannot tolerate—such as viral infection, bacterial infection, poisons, or allergies—expelling them through the vomiting reflex. It may be accompanied by sweating, cold and moist skin, rapid heartbeat, mild fever, hiccups, aching, weakness,

PREVENTION AND TREATMENT OF COMMON CHILDHOOD ILLNESSES

dizziness, cough, or sore throat. Consult your child's pediatrician for treatment.

The Cause and Treatment of Vomiting According to Maharishi Ayurveda:
Vomiting happens when digestive toxins (ama) have become concentrated and the body wants to rid itself of them. After the child has vomited, rinse his mouth with a solution of warm water with a few drops of Clear Breathe dissolved in it. This will help remove the sour taste and make his mouth feel fresh again.

After vomiting, it may be recommended to drink 1/2 cup of warm water every half hour to dilute the impurities (ama) and to calm the stomach, and also to replace lost fluids.

If the child is hungry and asks for food, kanji (rice broth—see description under "Chicken Pox") flavored with cumin and ginger is often advised. A rice cracker or dry toast may also settle the stomach. Keeping the diet light with these foods for the rest of the day may be helpful, so that the digestive enzymes can grow strong again. Drinking more warm water with two drops of Clear Breathe once or twice more in the day can also help reduce the ama.

CHAPTER SEVENTEEN
Prevention and Treatment of Chronic Disease in Childhood

In this chapter you will find a general description of therapies that may be recommended by a physician trained in Maharishi Ayurveda to help restore balance and treat chronic disorders. Please note that this book is not meant to substitute for proper medical care, nor are the entries in this chapter meant to be a prescription to follow when your child is ill. For specific recommendations to treat your child's chronic condition, it is important to consult a physician trained in Maharishi Ayurveda. Only through a proper assessment of your child's specific needs, using techniques such as pulse diagnosis, can the proper diet, daily routine, herbal supplements, and other therapies be recommended for chronic illnesses. You will also want to continue consulting your child's primary physician or pediatrician to regularly monitor your child's condition.

Preventing Chronic Disease

Preventing disease in childhood is a profound investment in health. The expression "an ounce of prevention is worth a pound of cure" actually contains a lot of wisdom. In talking about children's health, there is no greater truism. Childhood is a golden time, when strong health habits can be established, laying the foundation for a long and healthy life.

There are several reasons for this. For one thing, the habits your child starts in childhood will have a profound influence on his health throughout life. An obvious example is smoking. Tobacco use alone is estimated to be responsible for nearly one in six preventable causes of death and about one in four cardiovascular deaths. The earlier a person starts, the more harmful the effects in later life, and the harder it is to quit. About 90 percent of adults who smoke started before they were eighteen years old. Increasing numbers of children today are starting in the preteen years, creating formidable developmental damage to their health.

Another example is cardiovascular disease. Up until recently, research has focused on the effects of healthy lifestyle habits for adults, such as changing their diet, exercising, and reducing blood pressure. Now many studies are showing that arteriosclerosis begins in childhood, and the great need is to prevent it then. Research shows that environmental factors such as cigarette smoking, use of oral contraceptives, alcohol consumption, aggression, and lack of exercise influence cholesterol levels in children and adolescents in an even more profound way than they do adults.

If you teach your child the healthy lifestyle, stress management, and dietary habits presented in this book, they will stay with him, preventing disease throughout his life. The health patterns your child will enjoy as an adult have their start right now.

There's another reason that prevention of chronic disease is more effective in childhood. It is much easier to treat such diseases when they are just beginning. Childhood is a window of opportunity, when tendencies for ill health can be corrected or reversed.

You can reverse these unhealthy statistics by teaching your child to eat healthy foods, exercise, and refrain from smoking—and thus save him or her from the majority of chronic diseases. In traditional Ayurvedic medicine, even hereditary diseases can be avoided, by strengthening the tissues with rasayanas while the baby is still in the womb.

While these rasayanas are not currently available in the United States due to FDA guidelines, the very least the expectant mother can do is to eat a balanced diet and avoid environmental toxins. As mentioned in Chapter Fourteen, there is increasing evidence that children exposed to environmental toxins while in the womb (including alcohol, cigarettes, lead poisoning, and pesticides) display higher incidence of allergies and asthma, as well as serious neurological and behavioral disorders.

Tools of Treatment

While prevention is the main emphasis of Maharishi Ayurveda, if your child already has developed a chronic condition, the therapies of Maharishi Ayurveda can help support and complement conventional medicine in treating chronic disease and its complicating and aggravating factors.

I have seen over and over that these Ayurvedic therapies, when administered under the care of a physician trained in Maharishi Ayurveda, can actually correct chronic conditions and restore health. Whereas conventional medicine is ideal for crisis management, Maharishi Ayurveda is far more sophisticated in preventing and treating chronic conditions.

Many parents have found that the Maharishi Ayurveda treatments have been helpful in treating chronic disorders that Western medicine has not been able to treat successfully. For one thing, standard medical treatment usually involves suppressing the symptoms with prescribed drugs that address the symptoms only. These treatments do not go to the root cause of the disease and correct the imbalance there.

In many ways, suppressing the symptoms of illness only makes the disease worse, because the toxins and imbalances that are causing the problem stay in the body.

In Maharishi Ayurveda, the therapies for chronic disease help eliminate toxins, ama, and free radicals in the body. They restore balance, allowing the body to cure itself with its own healing intelligence. Maharishi Ayurveda goes to the root cause of the disease and corrects imbalance where it originates in the habits, lifestyle, or diet of the child.

A Description of Causes and Treatments of Chronic Diseases According to Maharishi Ayurveda

Allergies (Pollen-Related) and Hay Fever

Allergies can affect children of all different ages, and are defined as a heightened sensitivity to elements in the environment. Hay fever and spring allergies are usually caused by inhaled pollens, while other allergies may be triggered by foods, dust, dust mites, mold, stinging insects, and poison oak, ivy, or sumac. While one in three children now has an allergic disorder, some children outgrow their allergies by the time they reach puberty. Testing can help determine which allergens your child is sensitive to so you can prevent exposure. Consult your physician for help.

Cause and Treatment of Pollen-Related Allergies and Hay Fever According to Maharishi Ayurveda: After assessing the child's imbalances and the cause of allergies with pulse diagnosis, the physician trained in Maharishi Ayurveda will often recommend specific Maharishi Ayurveda herbal supplements to improve immunity and reduce toxins (ama) in the nose and lungs. Usually the child starts taking these three months before allergy season begins. Aller-Defense™ and Sniffle Free are typical Maharishi Ayurveda herbal formulas that are recommended for allergies. Nasya (sniffing sesame oil to lubricate the sinuses) may help reduce mucus (ama) if begun a month before symptoms start and continued throughout hay fever season.

The month before symptoms start, an ama-reducing diet may be recommended (see diet under "Asthma"). Maharishi Amrit Kalash is often recommended to build immunity and detoxify the body.

Anxiety and Depression

Anxiety is characterized by a racing pulse, sweating, tremors, butterflies in the stomach, and dry mouth. In younger children, fears come and go as a normal course of growing up—fear of the dark, fear of strangers, fear of imaginary monsters, even fear of being flushed down the toilet! Usually children grow out of these fears by school age.

If there is a generalized, free-floating anxious feeling, this is usually due to a more serious cause, such as family tension or illness. If it becomes severe enough, it can manifest as panic attacks and can interfere with school and friendships.

Depression is characterized by a chronic condition of hopelessness, futility, sadness, anger, weight loss or gain, problems sleeping, poor concentration, and erratic behavior. Today depression affects younger children as well as adolescents. Depression can be the result of a chronic illness, a death, or a divorce. It can also be triggered by a problem at home or at school. For depression or anxiety, consult your family physician or pediatrician.

Cause and Treatment of Anxiety and Depression According to Maharishi Ayurveda: The causes of anxiety and depression are complex, because they arise as symptoms of underlying imbalances. All three doshas can be involved. It's important to treat the underlying condition first. For this, a physician trained in Maharishi Ayurveda should be consulted.

For the child's diet, fresh, sattvic foods are often recommended. Sattvic foods include rice, mung dhal, warm milk, ghee, saffron, and small quantities of soaked, crushed almonds. Fresh juicy fruits (such as grapes, pomegranate, mango, melon, sweet oranges) and fresh vegetables (such as pumpkin, zucchini, and okra) are often recommended for anxiety and depression.

Keeping a regular daily routine is also recommended. This includes going to the bathroom on awakening, doing a daily Ayurvedic oil massage (abhyanga), practicing the Transcendental Meditation technique, eating meals at a regular time, and going to bed early and at a regular time. These habits help balance Vata, which can then help balance the other doshas.

An early-morning walk in nature can be helpful in treating anxiety and depression. Exercising every day according to body type and avoiding day sleep can also help balance the system and especially help dissolve depression.

Specific Maharishi Ayurveda herbal food supplements, as recommended by the physician trained in Maharishi Ayurveda during a personal health assessment, are particularly effective in these disorders.

Asthma

Asthma, caused when the air passages leading to the lungs are blocked, is marked by coughing, wheezing, and difficulty breathing. Asthma may be triggered by inhaled allergens such as pollen, dust, and animal dander. Asthma is one of the major reasons for childhood hospitalization, and, like all allergies, has been sharply on the rise in the past thirty years. One in nine children in industrialized countries now has asthma. Consult your physician for treatment to ensure the safety of your child and to prevent severe attacks. Call 911 if your child has trouble breathing.

Cause and Treatment of Asthma According to Maharishi Ayurveda: Asthma is caused by a Kapha-ama or Kapha-Pitta-ama condition. Allergies such as asthma may be triggered by dust mites, molds, certain foods, or environmental toxins. A milk allergy may be the cause of asthma if there is digestive disturbance (ama) in the pulse. If there is a milk allergy, substitutes such as goat milk, soymilk, or rice milk might be used.

An ama-reducing diet is usually recommended. Avoiding sweets, avoiding heavy and ama-producing foods, and avoiding eating between meals unless there is real hunger also may help. Drinking plenty of warm water throughout the day and also ginger tea (water boiled with fresh ginger) can help flush out toxins. A recommended snack is milk diluted with water and boiled with turmeric and a slice of fresh ginger.

Other recommendations include eating meals in a settled atmosphere, scheduled at the same time every day. The evening meal should be lighter and is best served early in the evening so the food is thoroughly digested before bedtime. Often the physician trained in Maharishi Ayurveda will recommend several small meals (rather than three main meals) and a light diet. Ginger, cumin, saffron, cloves, cardamom, and fennel are recommended spices. Avoiding chocolate, cheese, sour foods, and cold, refrigerated foods is often advised. If the child is overweight, the physician will often recommend a diet to reduce weight. After assessing the strength and condition of the heart, exercise is often recommended.

Practice of the Transcendental Meditation technique increases resistance and immunity. Research shows that asthmatic conditions decrease with regular practice. Regular exercise (but not to the point of exhaustion) may be advised, although it's best if the child can avoid exposure to irritants and to rain, cold, and wind. The child should avoid day sleep. Pranayama (as described in Chapter Thirteen) is also helpful in strengthening and purifying the lungs. Regular bowel movements are encouraged. If possible, washing the child's head is avoided. Instead, using a warm, wet towel that has been squeezed dry is recommended to clean the hair and head. A physician trained in Maharishi Ayurveda should be consulted to see if daily Ayurvedic oil massage (abhyanga) is recommended.

Aller-Defense, Aller-Breathe®, and Protection Plus™ Respiratory are Maharishi Ayurveda herbal food supplements that may be recommended for preventing and treating asthma. They help build immunity; enhance long-term resistance to allergens such as dust, pollen, and chemicals; and help reduce toxins in the body. The physician may recommend additional Maharishi Ayurveda herbal supplements.

Steam inhalation with Clear Breathe may be recommended for children five years and over. For children one to five, it can be used as aroma oil. For children ten years and older, nasya with specific herbal oils such as MP 16 diluted with sesame oil, twice daily, may be recommended.

In general, a warm room temperature is considered best for children with asthma. Warm cloths and a hot water bottle on the back can help soothe asthmatic cough. Since Maharishi Amrit Kalash improves overall balance and immunity, it is often recommended for children with asthma.

Attention Deficit Hyperactivity Disorder (ADHD) and Hyperactivity

Attention Deficit Hyperactivity Disorder (ADHD) is a problem that affects five percent of today's children. Not all attention problems are characterized by hyperactivity, but it is the most common one. It is characterized by problems focusing, inability to sit still or pay attention, impulsiveness, excessive energy, learning problems, disruptive behavior, temper tantrums, and social problems. Usually, four out of five cases are boys, and diagnosis is not made until the child goes to school, since it is difficult to distinguish the ADHD child from other healthy-but-active children in the preschool years.

Since most children outgrow ADHD by adolescence, one cause may be the slow development of frontal areas of the brain, which are concerned with attention. It may also be hereditary, or may be linked with dietary deficits or food additives, although studies have not conclusively shown a link. Unfortunately, because there is no definitive test for ADHD, and diagnosis relies mainly on parental reports and physician's observations, many children today may be mistakenly diagnosed with ADHD and prescribed powerful drugs such as Ritalin just for being high-spirited or active.

Cause and Treatment of ADHD According to Maharishi Ayurveda: The most common forms of hyperactivity and ADHD are usually caused by a Vata disorder. (Other attention problems may be associated with different doshas, and are not discussed here.) A light but stabilizing and nourishing diet that pacifies Vata dosha is usually recommended.

Warm, cooked, fresh foods are considered ideal. Nourishing foods such as soaked almonds, walnuts, raisins, figs, or cashews are added to the diet, and refined sugar is avoided. Even rock sugar and jaggary are kept at a minimum. Carbonated drinks increase Vata and disrupt digestion, so it's recommended that they, too, are avoided.

A regular daily routine with regular meals served at the same time every day is often advised. For preschool children, healthy snacks are recommended in between meals. It's usually recommended that the evenings are settled, with little or no TV, and that the child goes to bed early and at the same time every night. In general, it's advised to keep computer games and TV at a minimum.

Even if the child is younger than ten, breathing exercises (pranayama) and Yoga Asanas for five minutes a day can be helpful. These help balance Vata dosha. Research published in *Current Issues in Education*, 2008, shows that regular practice of the Transcendental Meditation technique helps settle the mind and body, and is especially helpful in improving focus and concentration in children with ADHD.

It can help to keep the environment orderly, especially the child's room. White clothes may be more soothing to the child.

A physician trained in Maharishi Ayurveda may recommend herbal formulas to help balance the doshas and calm the nervous system.

Diabetes

Diabetes is caused by the lack of insulin, a hormone produced in beta cells and the pancreas. The onset of Type I Diabetes, formerly called Childhood Diabetes, is usually sudden and occurs between the ages of six and thirteen. Treatment includes insulin injections, the monitoring of the blood and urine, and dietary management. Recent research shows that with proper management, complications of diabetes such as kidney failure and visual impairment can be avoided. Exercise is an important part of diabetic treatment, and diabetics can live a full life and excel in nearly all sports.

Type II Diabetes, formerly called Adult Onset Diabetes, is now affecting children as young as ten years old, and has increased in the entire population to the point that experts are calling it an epidemic. A high-sugar, high-fat, high-junk-food diet, and lack of regular exercise are the most common reasons given for the rise in Type II Diabetes.

Consult your child's pediatrician immediately if you observe signs of Type I or Type II Diabetes in your child.

Cause and Treatment of Diabetes According to Maharishi Ayurveda: Diabetes is a metabolic Kapha disorder associated with weak agni and weak dhatu agnis. A Kapha- and Vata-pacifying diet and regimen is usually recommended by the physician trained in Maharishi Ayurveda (along with the prescribed dosage of insulin recommended by the medical doctor).

This includes sipping warm water throughout the day. Filling a copper vessel with water at night and letting the child drink the copper water in the morning can help create more heat in the system and improve digestion. A recommended way to enhance digestion is to chew 1/2 teaspoon of fenugreek seeds, soaked overnight and mixed with 1/2 teaspoon of honey. The recommended time to chew this mixture is in the morning before breakfast. Another helpful herbal compound includes 2 grams of turmeric and 2 grams of amalaki powder (made from the amla fruit, also known as Indian Gooseberry and considered to be a great rasayana and immunity booster) with 1/2 teaspoon of honey. The child takes this mixture at 7:00 or 8:00 a.m. At bedtime, a soothing drink to balance metabolism can be made of 1/2 gram of turmeric blended with 1 teaspoon aloe vera gel and 1/2 cup warm water.

Avoiding processed foods is usually recommended, since corn and high fructose corn syrup is found in 80 percent of processed foods and drinks today. Corn in its various forms is considered one of the deadliest foods for diabetics, and is thought by many researchers to be one of the main causes of the diabetes epidemic today.

Regular exercise is considered essential for the diabetic child, to help balance Kapha dosha and to increase digestion. Yoga Asanas are especially balancing to all three doshas, and in particular the twist pose (*vakra asana*), the fish pose (*matsyendra asana*), the seated pose (*vajra asana*), the crescent pose (*sashank asana*), and lying down while holding the knees to the chest and rolling from side to side (*pavan mukta asana*). Sun salutations (*Surya Namaskara*) are also recommended to stimulate digestion and balance the mind-body system.

Research published in the 2006 *Archives of Internal Medicine*, a journal of the American Medical Association, shows that the practice of the Transcendental Meditation technique can help during the initial stages, by lowering insulin resistance. The study showed that the TM technique can reduce the components of "metabolic syndrome," a cluster of symptoms including obesity, high blood pressure, elevated blood sugar and triglycerides, and low HDL (good) cholesterol. Due to poor diet, lack of exercise, and increased exposure to stress, 39,000 American children now have Type II Diabetes and could be helped by the Transcendental Meditation technique.

Phase I of a $1.6 million, two-year study is now under way on the effects of the Transcendental Meditation technique on diabetes among American Indians (80% of the Native American population suffers from diabetes). The study is funded, in part, by the U.S. Government's Indian Health Services. Preliminary research has shown a dramatic drop in diabetes among people who practice the Transcendental Meditation technique.

Dyslexia

Dyslexia is a learning problem associated with difficulty understanding and interpreting visual stimuli, making it difficult for the child to read. There are many types of dyslexia, and it must be diagnosed and treated by an expert. Dyslexia varies in severity and often is outgrown in time. A child may have a high IQ and have excellent learning skills in other areas, so it is important to seek professional help and not to label such children as "learning disabled."

Cause and Treatment of Dyslexia According to Maharishi Ayurveda: Dyslexia is due to a Vata imbalance. Treatment includes balancing Vata dosha, both with diet and daily routine. The practice of the Transcendental Meditation technique can be helpful in treating dyslexia, as is listening to or reading the Vedic sounds in Sanskrit. The Children's Rasayana (MA 674) is often recommended to help balance all three doshas and help support healthy brain functioning in children.

Heart Disease (Congenital)

Congenital heart disease refers to defects in the cardiovascular system caused by abnormal development in the womb. Such defects may be evident at birth or they may go undetected for years. The cause of congenital heart disease is unknown 90 percent of the time; it has also been linked with genetic mutations, heredity, excessive X-rays, maternal infections such as German measles, and fetal alcohol syndrome. Fatigue, shortness of breath, and failure to gain weight are some of the symptoms of congenital heart disease in children. Consult a medical doctor if you observe these symptoms in your child.

Cause and Treatment of Congenital Heart Disease According to Maharishi Ayurveda: Congenital heart disease in children is caused by a prenatal Kapha imbalance. A Kapha-pacifying diet and daily routine is usually recommended. Following diagnosis of the current state of imbalance, the physician trained in Maharishi Ayurveda will often recommend a diet that includes plenty of fresh fruits and vegetables, which are easily digestible, to reduce ama, and increase production of ojas.

Besides an ama-reducing diet, the child is often advised to avoid day sleep (after infancy and early childhood) and to exercise daily. Regular practice of the Transcendental Meditation technique has been found to be especially helpful in reducing stress and strengthening the heart, as reported in research journals of the American Heart Association.

Mild laxatives are sometimes recommended by a physician trained in Maharishi Ayurveda. Drinking copper water or gold water may be recommended to stimulate the digestion and provide needed trace minerals. Usually it's recommended to soak water overnight in a copper or gold cup and give the water to the child to drink in the morning. Or soak a pure gold coin in a cup of water overnight (see the section on "Diabetes" for description of copper water).

A physician trained in Maharishi Ayurveda may recommend herbal preparations that balance the doshas involved in regulating the health of the heart, improve the strength of the cardiac muscle, and regulate the nervous system. Maharishi Ayurveda herbal formulas can be effective in rejuvenating the cardiovascular system and can be used as both prevention and treatment. They have no harmful side effects, and are complementary to Western medical treatment.

Insomnia

Insomnia is characterized by difficulty falling asleep, restless sleep, broken sleep, or waking up too early. Almost every child (and adult) experiences temporary insomnia at some point, especially during a time of emotional or physical stress. Children may have trouble sleeping when facing an exam, a performance in a play, a move to a new home, or when traveling across several time zones.

Chronic insomnia can be associated with reduced performance at school, reduced mind-body coordination, hyperactivity, learning problems, and depression. Chronic insomnia can be caused by fear of the dark, an underlying disease, or chronic stress in the child's life. Sleep medication is used sparingly in treating children. If the cause is emotional, the physician may refer the child to a psychiatrist.

Cause and Treatment of Insomnia According to Maharishi Ayurveda:
Insomnia is often caused by Vata imbalance. It can also be caused by indigestion, mental stress, or pain (as from an accident or illness).

It's usually recommended to avoid feeding the child cold, dry, rough foods or any foods that create Vata imbalance. Avoiding large quantities of bitter, astringent, and pungent foods may also be advised. Dinner may consist of light, warm foods such as soup. Before bed, the child may be advised to drink a half cup of milk to help induce sleepiness.

For treating insomnia, it's recommended to structure a consistent daily routine for the child, with waking up and bedtime at the same time every day, as well as meals. Once children are school-age, they can rise by 6:00 a.m. Day sleep is not recommended, as it only promotes unhealthy sleep patterns and blocks the channels of circulation (srotas). Regular, early wake-up times can be very effective in treating insomnia.

Other recommendations include a quiet, unstimulating evening routine. After dinner the child is advised to avoid watching TV, getting involved in intense conversation, or engaging in stimulating activities such as computer games. Scheduling the homework session earlier in the evening, before dinner, is recommended. Light reading, light conversation, listening to music, and quiet games are considered best. Bedtime should be early. Even twelve-year-old children benefit from going to bed before 9:00, and younger children can go to bed much earlier.

Giving your child an Ayurvedic oil massage (abhyanga) at 5:00 p.m. can help relax him or her for sleep. Special oil for massaging the head, to help calm the mind, may be recommended by the physician trained in Maharishi Ayurveda. Avoid showing your child any frightening or violent movies that might make him afraid to fall asleep in the dark. Make bedtime a pleasant, relaxing time, something your child can look forward to. Slumber Time Therapeutic Aroma Oil can help create a soothing, restful influence at bedtime.

Obesity and Weight Gain

Due to lack of exercise and a diet rich in excessive junk foods and high-cholesterol fast foods, childhood obesity is on the rise in America. It is estimated that the amount of overweight children is now double what it was twenty years ago, with 15 to 25 percent of children in North America clinically overweight. Research shows that there is a strong link between excessive childhood weight gain and adult obesity—and with 50 percent of American adults overweight, this is an epidemic.

Obesity is linked with cardiovascular disease and other diseases such as asthma and diabetes. Adults who were overweight during adolescence are twice as likely to suffer from coronary heart disease than those who are normal weight.

This does not mean that you should be trying to make your preschooler diet. On the contrary, preschoolers need much more fat than adults for the developing brain, especially before age two. One unusual cause of weight gain in adults is gaining too little weight in early childhood. Somehow the deficit in calories causes the body to be more efficient in storing calories (i.e., in storing fat). This is why it is also important to prevent inadequate weight gain in early childhood. Called "failure to thrive," curiously enough, this form of malnutrition is found not only in poverty-stricken areas today, but also in about 15 percent of the general American population, among well-to-do families that are concerned about their children's cholesterol. Consult your child's pediatrician before starting him or her on any weight-loss diet.

Cause and Treatment of Obesity According to Maharishi Ayurveda: Obesity in children is generally due to a disorder in Kapha dosha. Therefore, it's best to start with a Kapha-pacifying diet and daily routine. For the diet, eating warmer, light, dry, bitter, astringent, and pungent foods can help balance Kapha dosha. Sweet, salty, and sour tastes will increase Kapha, as will oily, cold, or heavy foods. Adding spices to the food such as fresh ginger, cumin, black pepper, and turmeric aids metabolism of fat. Other common recommendations include teaching your child to avoid eating between meals and to avoid eating while watching TV, as these habits disturb digestion and cause ama. Make meals a relaxed, happy time without a lot of commotion. A light evening meal should be served early in the evening so there are at least two hours to digest it before bed.

It's recommended to avoid fried foods, heavy foods, packaged desserts, aged cheeses, butter, yogurt, ice cream, chocolate, chips, and meats because they are difficult to digest and contribute to obesity. A steady diet of packaged foods—and especially breads, crackers, chips, and sweets made with hydrogenated oils and high fructose corn syrup—can be a major contributor of weight gain and high cholesterol and triglyceride levels as well. The idea is to give your child healthy fats in early childhood and later. (See Chapter Seven for a discussion of healthy and unhealthy fats.) Just preparing home-cooked, whole foods can help your child immensely in maintaining a normal weight.

As for the daily routine, it's recommended to avoid day sleep. This will only cause the body's micro-channels (srotas) to fill with impurities, thus increasing Kapha imbalance. Starting the day with a drink made of warm water, lemon, and raw honey is a simple way to stimulate the digestion—and children love the taste. Sipping warm water throughout the day, or drinking warm water boiled with cumin and coriander, can also dissolve impurities (ama) and stimulate digestion.

Exercise is highly recommended for an overweight child. Depending on the child's body type and imbalances, it can be fairly vigorous, and it's recommended that the child engage in it every day. Specific Yoga Asanas for obesity are also especially helpful. These include the shoulder stand (*sarvang asana*), plough pose (*hala asana*), seated pose (*vajra asana*), twist pose (*vakra asana*), and the head-to-knee pose (*hasta pada asana*). Pranayama, a light breathing exercise that calms the mind, is also helpful in stimulating and purifying the digestive tract.

Skin Problems (Eczema and Minor Rashes)

Minor skin rashes can flare up throughout childhood, starting in infancy. They could be caused by the child's diet or from outside irritants, such as too much moisture (in the case of diaper rash). These types of skin rashes are more easily treated by application of an herbal talc and a change in diet.

Eczema is a chronic group of skin disorders that cause the skin to become irritated. The most severe type, atopic dermatitis, is thought to be a problem caused by weak immunity and seems to be hereditary, although the cause is unknown. It is characterized by hot, itchy skin made red, inflamed, and blistered by scratching. It can also cause dry, scaly skin. The condition is triggered by certain foods, sweating, acidic foods, emotional stress, and known allergens such as harsh soaps, irritants, and tobacco smoke. It tends to start when the child is from two to six months old, often gets better at age five, and often subsides by early adulthood. A medical doctor should be consulted for treatment. It is usually treated through medication, such as topical corticosteroids, antihistamines, and antibiotics. Older children may also be treated with ultraviolet light or sunlamps under the supervision of a doctor.

Cause and Treatment of Eczema and Skin Problems According to Maharishi Ayurveda: Skin diseases can be caused by all three doshas, although it is often a Pitta disturbance. Ama, indigestion, mental stress, and heredity also can be causes. Eating toxic foods, canned foods, preservatives, genetically modified foods, and food grown with chemical pesticides and fertilizers can cause skin problems, as well as wearing synthetic clothing or coming into contact with detergents or chemicals.

Often a Pitta-pacifying diet (avoiding foods that are sour, salty, and pungent) is recommended. Because Kapha is also a factor, avoidance of oily, sweet, cold, heavy foods is often recommended. Raw salads, seafood, and foods that are known to cause allergies (such as strawberries, peanuts, and eggplant) are usually avoided. Bitter and astringent tastes, such as pomegranate, are considered helpful, as they balance Pitta dosha. A diet of fresh, organic foods such as whole grains, fresh cooked vegetables, fresh fruits, and fresh lassi may be recommended, with olive oil for cooking.

Giving the child a daily Ayurvedic oil massage, using oil that is suitable for the child's skin type may also help. Although sesame oil is the most nourishing for all skin types, coconut oil is more cooling for Pitta types, and is often recommended for skin problems. The massage is usually followed with a shower or bath. Dressing the child in clean, dry clothing made from natural fibers, such as organic cotton, is recommended to allow the skin to breathe and avoid irritation.

Sufficient exposure to the sun in the early morning and late afternoon may also be recommended to improve skin tone. Using less soap to avoid skin irritation or using mild herbal soaps rather than the harsh commercial varieties may also help.

For the daily routine, it's usually recommended that the child eat three regular meals, go to bed early, rise early, avoid day sleep, and avoid blocking the natural urges. Regular Yoga Asanas—especially sun salutations—and breathing exercises (pranayama) can help increase the blood flow to the skin and eliminate impurities. Practicing the Transcendental Meditation technique helps reduce the emotional stress that contributes to breakouts.

Drinking warm milk with a few threads of saffron at bedtime may also be helpful in balancing Vata and Pitta dosha and treating skin disorders. One teaspoon to one tablespoon of aloe vera gel at bedtime is also helpful in balancing Pitta dosha.

Medicated ghee is often applied externally to heal the skin and balance the doshas. Applying a sandalwood powder such as talcum powder may be recommended, or applying a paste of sandalwood powder, turmeric, licorice, and ghee. The physician trained in Maharishi Ayurveda will advise whether the paste should be applied to open lesions.

Aller-Defense, Elim-Tox and Elim-Tox-O are other Maharishi Ayurveda herbal formulas that may be recommended for rashes and eczema.

PART 7
A Vision of Your Child's Future with Maharishi Ayurveda

CHAPTER EIGHTEEN
Your Cosmic Child

Putting his mouth near the newborn child's right ear, [the child's father] says thrice, "speech," "speech," "speech." Then mixing curds, honey, and clarified butter he feeds him out of a spoon of gold, which is placed within the mouth saying, "I place in you the earth, I place in you the sky, I place in you the heaven. I place in you everything—earth, sky, and heaven." Then he gives him a name saying, "You are Veda." So this becomes his secret name.
—Brihadaranyaka Upanishad 6. 4. 25–26

This excerpt is from the Brihadaranyaka Upanishad, the largest of the Upanishads (one of the forty aspects of the Veda and Vedic Literature). It illustrates a beautiful point: every child is cosmic; every child is the embodiment of the Veda, the total wisdom of life.

Surely it is not hard for a mother to think of her child as a wonder of God's creation. To a mother, her child expresses the beauty, the intelligence, and the cosmic potential of the vast universe.

The principles of Maharishi Ayurveda revolve around this very point: that every child is cosmic in nature, and every child can learn how to use his or her cosmic potential. It is actually easy for a child to realize his or her cosmic status, since every individual contains within himself or herself the intelligence of the Veda, the wisdom of the entire universe. Becoming cosmic is actually easy to accomplish because all that is required is to attune the individual mind with cosmic intelligence—to tap into the vast energy and orderliness of the cosmos.

This concept, that each child is an expression of the whole universe and is part of a grand continuum of nature, is both comforting and expanding. It explains how each person is connected to every other, how each of us has a common basis in pure consciousness, the intelligence of nature, the transcendental Self. The same cosmic intelligence that is operating the universe is operating your human body and everyone else's.

In the definition of health at the beginning of this book, you learned that health is more than the absence of disease. Health is living one's full potential. Maharishi Ayurveda makes use of all aspects of human life—mind, body, behavior, and environment—to nourish the growing child to live his full potential. This is a life truly worth living—a life in freedom and happiness, without mistakes or suffering, a state of enlightenment.

Total Knowledge inside Your Child

As mentioned earlier, the word "Veda" means "knowledge," which includes the knowledge of all the laws of nature that maintain and create the vast universe. Veda is the totality of silence, and the totality of the entire creation. Until just recently, the Veda and Vedic Literature were thought to exist solely as books of knowledge. Maharishi Mahesh Yogi has restored the true meaning of Veda as existing in consciousness, in human awareness.

It was the discovery of Professor Tony Nader, M.D., Ph.D., to find that the structures of the Vedic Literature are located in the structures of the human body. The various aspects of the Vedic Literature—of which there are forty—do not reside in books, but rather are structures of our own human brain and body. In other words, the same Vedic frequencies form the human body, the sounds of the Vedic Literature, and the entire universe. The Vedic sounds are the blueprint of creation, and one of their manifestations is the human body—its organs, systems, and cells.

To give you an idea of how this can be possible, the human DNA has more than one trillion bits of information, but only one billion or so form the physiology. Scientists don't know what the other billions are for, but one thing is certain: there is enough intelligence contained in the human DNA to structure the entire universe. Thus the universe is literally contained in every part of the human nervous system, like a hologram.

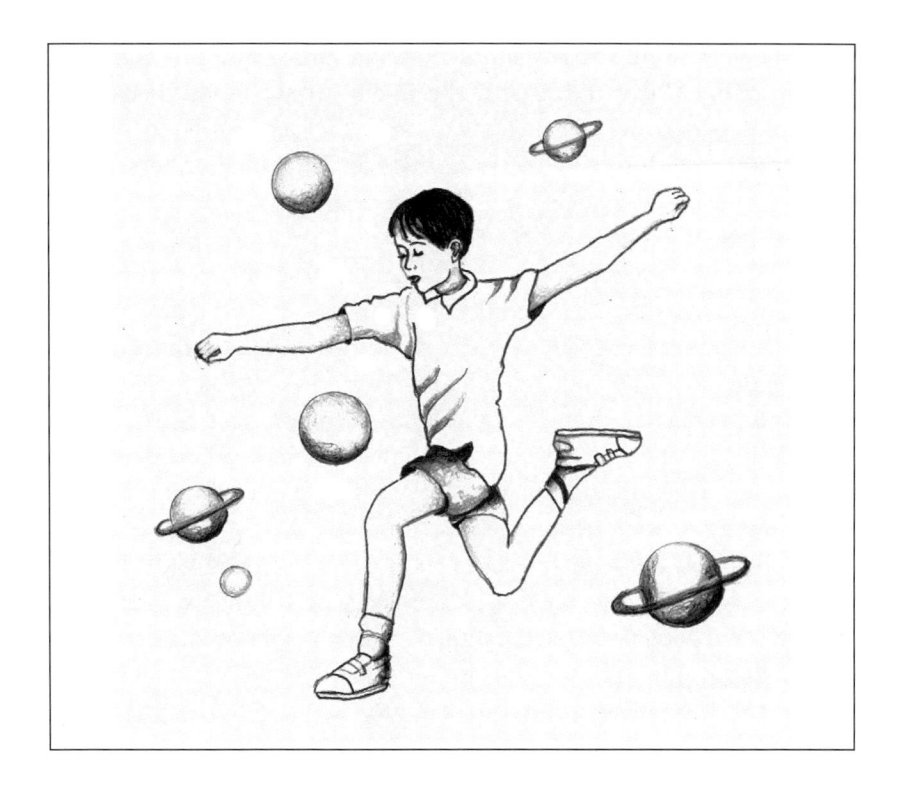

It is a common experience of people who practice the Transcendental Meditation technique that they begin to feel at home with everything in their surroundings. The reason for this experience is simple: the human physiology contains within it the intelligence that structures everything in the universe. That inner intelligence is nothing other than Atma, the Self. This is the true meaning of Veda.

Vedic sounds, the fundamental frequencies of the body in their subtlest forms, have a special value for children, who are in the process of forming the neuronal connections that structure their brains. To have a fully functioning brain, in order to use 100 percent of mental potential, it requires a special kind of holistic stimulus—a stimulus to awaken the total brain.

The Veda and Vedic Literature can provide just such a holistic stimulus. As Maharishi has explained, "When the Vedic texts are pronounced correctly in their proper sequence, it stimulates all elements of the brain physiology to be fully alert and to function holistically in a coherent, orderly manner. This means that the intelligence of each fiber of the brain physiology, each specific law of nature, is performing its natural activity along with the holistic performance of the total brain physiology. This means that during the Vedic recitation the total potential of Natural Law is enlivened in the brain."

Preliminary research shows that brain patterns during the reading of the Vedic texts, as measured by EEG, and stress levels measured by skin conductance levels (a measure of stress), are similar to those during practice of the Transcendental Meditation technique. Increased alpha activity and coherence reflect higher levels of brain functioning during the reading of the Vedic Literature. Subjects who read modern languages such as French, German, and Spanish did not exhibit increased brain coherence or reduction in stress.

For this reason, it's ideal to begin reading the Veda and Vedic Literature as early in life as is practical. By reading these lively expressions of natural law, which nourish evolutionary growth and support the whole brain and the entire physiology, children can grow up naturally in perfection, enlightenment, and fullness of life.

The Maharishi Vedic Vibration Program for Better Health

The Veda reverberates in sound. These primordial sounds can also have healing qualities, and can help prevent disease. Quantum physicists have discovered that the body is composed of vibrations, or waveforms. All matter has a vibratory or sound quality at its basis.

If the body is ultimately a complex waveform, made of many subtle vibrations, the possibility arises that certain vibratory frequencies might be used to restore normal functioning to treat chronic disorders. In Maharishi Ayurveda, it is said that superior forms of healing use sound rather than herbs, because sound can actually reset the imbalances at the fundamental level of the body.

Maharishi Vedic Vibration Technology[SM] (MVV[SM]) uses the ancient knowledge of Vedic sound to improve the life of individuals who are suffering from chronic disorders. This has been especially effective in situations where people with long-standing disorders have not been able to find relief.

Using the proper sound technology, the expert in Maharishi Vedic Vibration Technology enlivens the intelligence at the basis of the physiology to transform disorderly functioning into orderly functioning.

Research has shown that people have found immediate relief from arthritis and back pain, migraine headaches, shortness of breath due to asthma, abdominal discomfort and digestive problems, burning and itching related to skin disorders, insomnia, and anxiety. The average improvement reported by more than 2,000 participants in the study was 42.3 percent. This was for chronic disorders that had lasted an average of 13.8 years. In eighty-three instances, 100 percent relief was reported.

This technique has been especially helpful in the cases of children with ADHD, hearing problems, grief, and neurological damage.

One mother reports: "Due to a complication at birth, our son had some mild neurological damage which caused low muscle tone. It was extremely hard for him to learn how to sit up, how to crawl. He couldn't even walk until we got ankle braces.

"The low muscle tone also made speech very difficult for him. He found it hard to get his mouth and tongue to move, and to keep his breath going. He got to the point where he could speak two or three words at a time, and then his voice would fade out.

"Mentally, he was even a little advanced for his age. But because he couldn't express himself, it was very frustrating for him. We took him through the Maharishi Vedic Vibration Technology program, and now at age three he's talking in full sentences, two sentences at a time. He is so happy. He's not losing his voice. He's thrilled to be able to communicate. When he talks, he sometimes yells, he's just so excited. He's coming out with these big, long, complicated words—four or five syllable words—in the middle of a sentence. It's really a dramatic difference.

"His walking has also improved. The other day he came to some stairs and I was behind him. He used to wait for me to take his hand and we'd go up together, one step at a time. This time he saw the stairs and went up four or five steps all by himself, not holding on, one right after the other. He's made a giant leap forward. His coordination and balance are so much better. He's running around the yard more quickly.

For him, the difference is very dramatic, and he's much happier that he can do so many new things.

"He always made very steady progress, but the rate of development has sped up so much. It's a wonderful thing to see."

Maharishi Vedic Astrology^{SM} Program

Even when parents devote their lives to providing a healthy and happy environment for their children to grow up in, there is sometimes the lurking fear that something beyond their control could go wrong. Most parents would do anything in their power to protect their children from accidents, serious illnesses, and natural disasters.

Up until now, parents were at the mercy of fate. Now many fortunate parents are learning how to avert danger in their children's lives by using the science of prediction to find out the time periods when their children may be vulnerable to negative influences. Then they can take steps to protect their children.

Maharishi Vedic Astrology (also known as the Maharishi Jyotish[SM] program) is the knowledge of the influence of the sun, moon, planets, and stars on our lives. Maharishi Jyotish is one of the forty aspects of Maharishi Vedic Science[SM], and it is based on the principle that there is a one-to-one relationship between cosmic law, which governs the universe, and the holistic and specific laws of nature that govern the individual.

With the Maharishi Vedic Astrology program, a skilled *pandit* (Vedic expert) can predict the future trends of your child's life, based on the time of birth. The reason that these future trends can be mathematically calculated is that the universe unfolds in an orderly, predictable sequence. A *pandit* can take any point in the sequence and calculate the trends of the future or the past.

Having the birth chart analyzed can help you understand your child's strengths and weaknesses, and can help you prepare your child for the right profession. It also can offer comfort if your child is going through a rough period. The Maharishi Vedic Astrology program shows how long the negative period will last, and when it will end. It helps to know where the problem is coming from and how long it will continue.

Life by nature is cyclical. We all go through times that are easier and times that are more challenging. The value of knowing the good trends is that you can enhance them and take advantage of them. As for the negative trends, if an accident or illness is predicted, then there is another Vedic technology available to dissolve the negative influences and avert the danger.

Averting the Danger with *Maharishi Yagya* Performances

Parents naturally think ahead to protect the health and well-being of their children. Mothers purchase coats and mittens before the cold winter comes, so their children will be protected. If some storm is on the horizon, parents turn the boat into a safe port to protect their children from an accident at sea.

The practical value in knowing the future is to avoid ill health and accidents. If there is a possibility for disease or accidents predicted in the astrology chart, then you can avert the danger through a Vedic technology called the Maharishi Yagya® program.

Yagyas are Vedic performances carried out by trained pandits from India. Deeply grounded in Vedic wisdom and trained to perform the yagyas from the silent level of their own consciousness, the Vedic pandits employ the recitation of Vedic sounds to dissolve negative influences and to enhance positive trends in the person's life.

Although they may seem mysterious at first glance, the Vedic performances use the physics principle of action and reaction. As a stone thrown into a pond creates ripples that eventually reach the shore and rebound to their starting point, all of your thoughts, feelings, and actions generate influences in the environment that come back to you, either right away or sometime in the future.

If Maharishi Vedic Astrology calculates and predicts a negative influence coming to you due to past actions, you can take recourse to Maharishi Yagya performances to generate life-supporting influences to dissolve the negative influence before it happens. In this way you can avert danger before it arises. The purpose of the Vedic performances is to counteract negativity and enhance positive trends in your life and in the lives of your children.

Parents Who Use Maharishi Vedic Astrology and Maharishi *Yagya* Program

Karen and Rich have consulted Maharishi Vedic Astrology pandits for their three daughters, and have Maharishi Yagya performances done each year to improve positive trends and eliminate negative influences in their children's lives.

"When our daughter Kaeli was only one week old, a Maharishi Vedic Astrology pandit visited our home and did a life reading of her chart," says Karen. "One of the things they said was that in the first few years of her life she would have various respiratory problems. Sure enough, last year she developed a rattle that wouldn't go away, that lasted for months even with the doctor's care. We had a Maharishi Yagya performance done for her and that knocked it out within days."

Karen also says that having the prediction for the baby's entire life span was a moving experience. "It was powerful to put our attention on the manifestation of her life as embodied in her chart. We realized she is a wave of pure consciousness, and her chart is like a blueprint of what she is about to become. In the past one-and-a-half years we've seen some of these predicted tendencies begin to blossom in her life. It's wonderful to watch it happen."

Karen says that the family has used Maharishi Vedic Astrology for many purposes since learning about it. "We've used Maharishi Vedic Astrology to find out the correct time to start our business, enter into important business contracts, break ground for our new Maharishi Sthapatya Veda design home, and predict trends in the life of our children," she says.

"Each of our children receives a Maharishi Yagya every year on her birthday," says Karen. "The two older ones are old enough now to be aware of it and enjoy it. My oldest daughter, Sara, was five the first time she had a Maharishi Yagya performance. She is a quiet child, and was dominated by her younger sister, Jenny. Jenny, who is three years younger, has a strong personality and was acting like she was the older sister. After that first yagya performance, Sara started to step into a true big-sister role with Jenny, which she's maintained ever since. Now she's more the leader, the guide, the caretaker, and the nurturer in the relationship with her little sister."

Karen notices that Maharishi Yagya performances help her children achieve more success in school. "Sara had been struggling with her times tables just before one of the yagyas was performed. After the performance, she mastered them in one day. Both girls are doing extremely well in school, and I attribute part of that to the Maharishi Yagya program."

Karen says that she and her husband consult the Maharishi Vedic Astrology pandits whenever they hit a patch in their lives that needs sorting out.

"I've been practicing the Transcendental Meditation technique for more than thirty years, and in addition to everything else, I feel that Maharishi Yagya performances are an amazing enhancer of spiritual growth. And parents need this extra support to take care of themselves and their children."

Parents Can Influence Their Children

It's important to take the lead in influencing your child to eat a good diet and be on a healthy routine. Sometimes you may need to be firm or even a little strict. If you know and understand this knowledge of Maharishi Ayurveda, it is your responsibility to pass it on to your children.

One mother says, "You can't just think that your children will meditate or eat right all by themselves. You have to work with them, remind them gently."

She tells the following story of persuading her own daughter to meditate.

"In my case, it was inconceivable to me that our children wouldn't meditate. Yet when I told my daughter that her fourth birthday was coming and that she would be getting her Word of Wisdom, she didn't respond the way I expected.

"She said, 'Well, I'm going to have to think about that.'

"I didn't say much until the next day, when I sat down with her and said, 'Because this is so important to me, I just want to explain to you how I feel. I have given you a lot of choices—which videos you want to watch, what you want to wear. I let you choose those things.

"'But some things you don't have a choice about. I expect you to brush your teeth, so you won't get cavities. And we always go to bed on time. These things are very important because your ability to be happy is based on being very healthy. Meditating will help you to be healthier, happier, and to do well in school. That's why I'm not going to give you a choice about this.'

"She said, 'OK' and that was that. Now she is nineteen and not only meditates regularly, but she has blossomed into a confident, happy young adult who is active in community service and gets excellent grades. She attributes her success to the Transcendental Meditation technique and other programs offered by Maharishi Ayurveda. I really feel it's just a matter of how you talk to your children. The young child is like a tree. A parent provides a stake next to the tree so it grows strong and straight. As parents we must give them this guidance."

On the other hand, your child may not be ready to learn the Word of Wisdom technique by age four. As a parent you will need to balance your knowledge of your child with your knowledge of the vital role that the growth of consciousness plays in achieving perfect health. There will come a time when your child will feel ready to start, and that is the best time for instruction.

Consciousness-Based Education: A Vision of the Future

As stress in children and school violence are increasing, many educators are implementing the Transcendental Meditation technique in their schools. The children, staff, and faculty learn the technique and meditate together during a designated "TM/Quiet Time." In many inner city schools, the results of the TM/Quiet Time have been nothing short of miraculous. Grades have gone up while school violence has gone down.

The Fletcher Johnson Learning School in Washington, D.C.
Dr. George Rutherford, one of the most distinguished and beloved principals in the Washington, D.C., area, is credited as being the "Grandfather" of the TM/Quiet Time program in America. In 1993, Dr. Rutherford introduced the program at the Fletcher Johnson Learning School where he was principal, and later expanded it to include the

entire school—a first in U.S. education. He also serves as the National Codirector of the U.S. Committee for Stress-Free Schools.

Dr. Rutherford says, "All the students from 5th grade through 12th grade practice the TM/Quiet Time program. In the morning for those 15 minutes before class the whole school is quiet and the calm is carried throughout the day. The greatest benefit is relieving the stress. We know that some of the children would be more hyper without their meditation. Some of our children have ADHD. I always say a lot of children are special needs who don't have the papers on them. They have not been identified. With Quiet Time the academic achievement has gone up, and behavioral problems and absenteeism have gone down. I could never work in a school that doesn't have the TM/Quiet Time program."

The Nataki Talibah Schoolhouse in Detroit

Another school that has adopted Quiet Time℠ with similar results is the Nataki Talibah Schoolhouse in Detroit, a charter school founded in 1978 by principal Carmen N'Namdi. With the aid of nearly $200,000 in grants, she introduced the Transcendental Meditation program at Nataki in 1997.

"To see that 10- and 11-year-old boys know the meaning of 'quiet' is amazing. So many people don't," notes Ms. N'Namdi. "We want to help children manage their lives, and the Transcendental Meditation technique is a tool to get to the real self. Students are focusing better in class, and the whole school is more harmonious," says Ms. N'Namdi.

Today more than 100 students now meditate twice daily at the school, which has a long waiting list for new students. A research team led by Dr. Rita Benn, educational researcher and director of the education department at the Center for Complementary and Alternative Medicine at the University of Michigan, found in a randomized pilot control study that the meditating children showed "significantly more positive emotions and positive mood state and greater emotional adaptability than non-meditating peers."

Earlier research by Benn also showed that the meditating students experienced higher self-esteem, more positive well-being, improved management of stress and interpersonal skills, and less verbal aggression, anxiety and loneliness.

"If the Transcendental Meditation technique has the capacity to facilitate children feeling better about themselves, it has huge implications for other areas of their lives," says Dr. Benn. "It may prevent mental health difficulties—and it may reduce the likelihood of the need for medication."

Says Dr. Rutherford, "I would love to see that all students are able to learn in a stress-free environment. You can rest assured that in years to come the transformation in education will take place in schools with the TM/Quiet Time program. People are going to see that the Quiet Time program removes stress and everything else falls right in place. With Quiet Time, the potential of every student is unlimited."

The Chelsea School in Silver Spring, Maryland

A research study was also conducted at the Chelsea School in Silver Spring, Maryland, a school for students with language-based learning disabilities that was the site of a pioneering study on the use of the Transcendental Meditation technique in combating attention deficit-hyperactivity disorder (ADHD).

Researcher Sarina Grosswald, Ed.D., and colleagues used standard instruments to assess executive brain functions, and found that the children showed improved organization and planning, improved problem-solving, improved task execution, improved attention, and improved memory. The research was published in the December 2008 edition of *Current Issues in Education*.

Says Dr. Grosswald, "There have been exciting results with the Transcendental Meditation technique for children with ADHD and related disorders such as Asberger's and mood disorders. The teachers report that the children are less stressed and more open to learning than they were before learning TM. There are also fewer episodes of anger, fewer fights, and fewer tantrums. The children themselves say they are able to focus better, and able to work more independently on tasks like doing their homework. Unlike drugs, the Transcendental Meditation technique doesn't just treat the symptoms, it influences the cause of the disorder. Which means it doesn't just create a temporary effect, but can improve the condition permanently."

A *Consciousness-Based* Curriculum at Maharishi School of the Age of Enlightenment

In several schools throughout the U.S. and abroad, the entire curriculum is Consciousness-Based, meaning that every student, teacher, and staff member practices the Transcendental Meditation technique and other Maharishi Vedic℠ technologies to develop consciousness. Developing the consciousness of the student is the core of the curriculum.

The first Consciousness-Based school, Maharishi School of the Age of Enlightenment (MSAE), was established in 1979 in Fairfield, Iowa. Several hundred students from kindergarten to twelfth grade take the traditional subjects, including literature, mathematics, science, social studies, and sports. Along with their academic studies, they also learn principles of Maharishi Ayurveda such as self-pulse diagnosis. They also study Sanskrit, the Maharishi Jyotish program, and Maharishi Gandharva Veda music. The heart of the curriculum is the twice-daily practice of the Transcendental Meditation technique.

Four hundred students from kindergarten to twelfth grade attend Maharishi school of Age of Enlightenment in Fairfield, Iowa. The students take the traditional subjects, including literature, mathematics, science, social studies, and sports. Along with their academic studies, they also learn principles of Maharishi Ayurveda such as self-pulse diagnosis. They also study Sanskrit, the Maharishi Jyotish program, and Maharishi Gandharva Veda music. The heart of the curriculum is the twice-daily practice of the transcendental Meditation technique.

When you walk into the school, you immediately sense something different. The children are not only vibrantly healthy, but they display a love of learning that makes each class lively and joyful. Visitors comment on the level of positive interactions between students and teachers—and between students and their peers.

"As a reading consultant, I have visited many public and private schools, and I have never felt such a calm and silent atmosphere in a school full of bright, lively, alert children as was evident at Maharishi School of the Age of Enlightenment," noted Julia Herbert, an educator from Washington, D.C.

Another visitor, Dr. Manfred Bayer from the Education Department of the University of Duisburg in Germany, said that "the Fairfield model proves the practicality of its approach: I was most impressed by the creative and open-minded atmosphere which I found within this institution. Any kind of aggression among students and between teachers and students was completely missing. Any school system which strengthens the mutual understanding of different ethnic groups while maintaining their cultural integrity deserves all support."

Through the practice of the Transcendental Meditation technique and other Vedic technologies, the students have developed a sense of Self, of self-esteem, and this translates into behaviors that are more positive than those of students who are struggling to maintain emotional balance. Teachers find that at this school, students are highly receptive to learning and create a harmonious feeling that can only be described as blissful. The students' achievements have been recognized in state and national competitions in science, art, history, athletics, speech, and drama. Here are just a few of their achievements.

Maharishi School of the Age of Enlightenment Highlights of Achievements[*]

In the past decade, students at Maharishi School have won more than 100 state titles in science, speech, drama, writing, poetry, spelling, art, photography, history, mathematics, chess, tennis, golf, track, and Destination ImagiNation, a national and international creative problem-solving competition.
- Grades 10–12 score in the top 1% nationally, and in Iowa, on standardized tests (ITED)
- 95% of graduates accepted at four-year colleges
- Over ten times the nation's average for National Merit Scholar Finalists over the past five years

State Record: Sixty state championships in creative problem-solving competitions Destination ImagiNation and Odyssey of the Mind

---

[*] Excerpted with permission from the book *A Record of Excellence: The Remarkable Success of Maharishi School of the Age of Enlightenment* by Ashley Deans, Ph.D., Maharishi University of Management Press: Fairfield, Iowa, 2005.

- **World Record**: Four-time winners of the Global Finals of Destination ImagiNation and Odyssey of the Mind, and more top-ten finishes than any other school in the world
- **First Place**: American High School Math Exam, Iowa Division, four years in a row
- **First Place**: Five first-place finishes, Iowa State History Fair, Senior Division
- **First Place**: Twelve first-place finishes in the senior division of the Eastern Iowa or Hawkeye state science fairs
- **Grand Champions**: Eight grand champion awards in the past decade in the junior division of the Eastern Iowa Science and Engineering Fair
- **First Place**: Twice winner of the state spelling bee
- **State Record**: Most Critics' Choice State Banner Awards for speech in the past decade
- **National Champion**: Bravo Cable Channel High School Theater Competition
- **State Record**: Congressional Art Competition, "An Artistic Discovery," grand prize three years in a row
- **First Place**: Iowa Poetry Association's high school contest
- **First Place**: Iowa "Young Writer of the Year" award
- **State Champion**: Iowa Junior Chess Championship
- **First Place**: Iowa Educational Media Association (Photography)
- **Grand Prize**: International Photo Imaging Education Association competition
- **State Champions**: 16 boys' state tennis championships, tying for the most in Iowa history
- **State Champion**: Girls' state singles tennis
- **State Record**: Boys' track 800 meters
- **State Champions**: Golf team and individual

Writes Ashley Deans, the executive director of Maharishi School, "The equanimity and evenness that our students display, both in victory and defeat, is a sign of the growth of personal enlightenment and invincibility, where the ups and downs of everyday life do not overshadow the ever-present inner stability of the Self. This ability to exhibit skill in action without being thrown off balance by stressful situations has profound implications for health."

A senior girl who is planning to attend college next year describes how she feels after her education at Maharishi School of the Age of Enlightenment: "I know I am really strong inside and always will have that strength. I feel connected with myself and with the world. Meditating gave me that, and no matter where I go, I'll always feel that way."

This kind of achievement, joy of learning, and vibrant health is possible for every child. Every child can learn to express his or her cosmic potential. This is the goal of Maharishi Ayurveda.

The Future Is Bright

When students have a way to prevent stress from building, this kind of achievement, joy of learning, and vibrant health is possible for every child. Every child can learn to express his or her cosmic potential. This is the goal of Maharishi Ayurveda.

As you have seen, the principles and treatment modalities of Maharishi Ayurveda are simple and easy to implement. In many cases, it is simply a matter of creating new habits. And because Maharishi Ayurveda is designed to prevent illness, your efforts to establish ideal habits now will help your children enjoy health and happiness for a lifetime.

It may seem like a small thing to make the changes in diet and lifestyle recommended in this book. Yet the dividends are enormous. There is nothing more important than contributing to a better life for our world's children. I wish you great success in creating true health for your family, and through them a healthier, more peaceful world.

Glossary
Quick Reference Guide
Appendix
Notes
Index

Glossary

Abhyanga—Ayurvedic oil massage

Agni—digestive fire; also the element of fire generally (see dhatu agni and jatharagni)

Akasha—the element of space

Ama—the sticky, bad-smelling, toxic remains of undigested food that obstructs the channels in the body

Asana (also *Yoga Asana*)—a neuromuscular integration exercise; a pose that stretch the body and prepares the body for smoother experience in meditation

Asthi Dhatu—one of the seven tissues (dhatus), asthi is bone tissue

Ayurveda—"knowledge of life span"; a major category of Vedic Literature dealing with medicine and health

Bala—strength or immunity

Bulgur—parched cracked wheat

Chapati—unleavened bread

Charaka Samhita—one of the forty aspects of the Vedic Literature; the best known of the six aspects that deal explicitly with medicine and health

Churna—a spice mixture used to flavor food and balance the doshas

Dhal—a soup made with split, husked, and dried legumes, traditional in Indian cuisine

Dhatu—any of the seven tissues that make up the body

Dhatu Agni—digestive or metabolic fire associated with each of the seven bodily tissues

Dinacharaya—Ayurvedic daily routine

Dosha—any of the three fundamental operators underlying all aspects of the mind-body system (see Vata, Pitta, and Kapha)

Dravyaguna—"qualities of matter"; sophisticated science of preparing Ayurvedic herbal compounds

Gandharva Veda—music of the ancient Vedic civilization; the eternal rhythms and melodies of nature

Ghee—clarified butter

Jaggary—an unrefined sweetener made from crushing the juice from sugar cane; available in Indian grocery stores

Jala—the element of water

Jatharagni—the primary digestive fire functioning in the digestive juices in the large and small intestines and the stomach, which are responsible for converting food into the nutrient plasma that nourishes all the cells and tissues throughout the body

Jyotish—aspect of Vedic Literature concerned with Vedic astrology

Kapha—one of the three mind-body operators (doshas); governs physical structure, including bones, muscles, the lymphatic system, and fluid balance; primarily situated in the chest; primary qualities: heavy, oily, slow, cold, steady, solid, dull, soft, sweet, and smooth

Kapha Kala—childhood stage of life (birth-30)

Lassi—a drink made from fresh yogurt and water and flavored with rose water or spices

Maharishi Vedic Science—the complete science of consciousness as it is found in every field of life, revived in its completeness by Maharishi Mahesh Yogi

Maharishi Ayurveda health care program—Ayurvedic science of health and system of medicine revived in its completeness by Maharishi Mahesh Yogi

Maharishi Jyotish program—science of prediction—Vedic astrology—revived in its completeness by Maharishi Mahesh Yogi

Maharishi Sthapatya Veda design—aspect of Maharishi Vedic Science that includes the health effects of the orientation, design, proportion, and positioning of buildings; the most ancient and supreme system of country, town, village, and home planning in harmony with natural law

Maharishi Yagya performances—aspect of Maharishi Vedic Science whose aim is to avert the danger that has not yet come through Vedic performances by expert Vedic pandits

Majja Dhatu—one of the seven dhatus, majja includes bone marrow and the tissues of the nervous system

Mala—any of the several types of normal waste produced during formation of the dhatus, including urine, feces, sweat, phlegm, bile, and various other excreta

Mamsa Dhatu—one of the seven dhatus, mamsa is muscle tissue

Meda Dhatu—one of the seven dhatus, meda is fat tissue

Mono-doshic—characterized by the predominance of one dosha

Nadi Vigyan—Ayurvedic system of diagnosing the underlying state of balance and imbalance by taking the radial pulse (at the wrist)

Ojas—the most refined and nourishing product of digestion; the finest material form of consciousness

Pandit—an expert thoroughly trained to use Vedic technologies of sound and action to restore the functioning of natural law through, for example, the precise performances of yagyas

Pitta—one of the three mind-body operators (doshas); governs heat, metabolism, and energy production; primarily situated in the area around the navel; primary qualities: hot, sharp, light, acidic, slightly oily, liquid, and flowing

Prakriti—nature

Prana—life force

Pranayama—neurorespiratory technique involving simple, rhythmic breathing exercises to balance, relax, and revitalize the mind-body connection

Prithivi—the element earth

Quinoa—an ancient grain that contains many minerals and is a complete protein

Raga—musical composition

Rajas—one of the three mental qualities (gunas); governs the action principle, serves as the spur to action, but in an imbalanced state can give rise to agitation, anger, impulsiveness, and excess (see also sattva, tamas)

Rakta Agni—one of the seven dhatu agnis; the dhatu agnis transform one tissue into the other in the process of digestion

Rakta Dhatu—one of the seven dhatus, rakta equates with blood

Rasa—essence or taste

Rasa Agni—one of the seven dhatu agnis, the dhatu agnis transform one tissue into the other in the process of digestion

Rasa Dhatu—one of the seven dhatus, rasa is associated with chyle, or plasma, and is the first product of digestion

Rishi—wise person, enlightened teacher

Samadosha—a mind-body type characterized by a balance of all three doshas—Vata, Pitta, and Kapha

Sama Veda—aspect of the Vedic Literature

Samhita—wholeness of Rishi, Devata, and Chhandas; also used in titles of many aspects of the Vedic Literature

Sattva—one of the three mental qualities (gunas); described as pure, illuminating, beneficial (see also rajas, tamas)

Shirodhara—a Maharishi Rejuvenation treatment in which a stream of warm oil is poured back and forth in a special pattern on the forehead to settle and relax the nervous system

Shukra—the subtlest of the seven dhatus; reproductive tissues

Srotas—channels and microchannels within the body, such as veins, arteries, and capillaries

Tamas—one of the three mental qualities (gunas), generally associated with effects generated by its imbalance or excess, which produce slowness, lethargy, inertia; but when in balance, help to stabilize growth (see also sattva, rajas)

Tejas—the element of fire

Upma—a cream of wheat dish made with spices and vegetables

Vaidya—health expert from India extensively trained in traditional Ayurvedic principles and practices

Vastu—the correct relationship between a building site and the environment

Vata—one of the three mind-body operators (doshas); governs movement of all kinds, mental, physical, emotional; primarily situated in the area around the colon; primary qualities are dry, rough, moving, clear, and course.

Vayu—the element of air

Veda—"knowledge"; total knowledge and structure of Natural Law expressed in unmanifest frequencies of sound that precede and produce the physical manifestation of the universe

Vikriti—a state of imbalance in the dosha characterized by an excess of one or more doshas

Yagya—Vedic performance which aims to transform the planetary influences on one's life so as to correct imbalances before they arise

Yoga Asana—see asana

Quick Reference Guide
to *Maharishi Ayurveda* Products for Children

Many herbal formulas and products manufactured by Maharishi Ayurveda Products International are suitable and effective for children if used under the guidance of an expert trained in Maharishi Ayurveda. There are no known side effects for these holistic, natural, gentle herbal formulas.

To order Maharishi Ayurveda products or for more information: Please go to www.mapi.com or call 800-255-8332. To receive a 10% discount, use this code when ordering: HP2060309.

For personal recommendations and dosages: Schedule an appointment with a Maharishi Ayurveda health expert (Vaidya) or health professional, see contact information below.;

Or contact Kumuda Reddy, M.D.: email: kreddy72@yahoo.com; phone: call toll free at 866-REDDY, MD or 301-474-2184; address: 5009 Paducah Road, College Park, MD 20740; website:www.allhealthyfamily.com.

Recommended Guidelines
- For children aged 0–3, it's best to seek advice from an expert trained in Maharishi Ayurveda before giving your child any herbal formulas.
- Children aged 3–5 years can take 1/4 tablet twice daily.
- Children aged 5–10 years can take 1/2 tablet twice daily.
- Children 10 years and older can take 1 full tablet twice a day.
- To make the herbs more digestible, crush the tablets and stir them into applesauce, raw honey, maple syrup, or yogurt.

Please note: The contents of this book are not in any way meant to substitute for a medical professional's diagnosis and treatment. Consult an expert trained in Maharishi Ayurveda to receive a proper diagnosis and treatment assessment for your child. For acute cases, call your pediatrician or primary care physician immediately.

Maharishi Ayurveda Product	Benefits
Aci-Balance®	Supports natural resistance of the GI tract to acquired food allergies
Aller-Breathe®	Enhances respiratory resistance to environmental allergens
Aller-Defense™	Supports the body's response to allergens
Almond Energy™	A wholesome energy drink combining the nourishing effect of almonds with Ayurvedic herbs and sugar
Ayurdent	A natural toothpaste that cleanses the mouth and strengthens and nourishes the teeth and gums
Calming (Vata) Spice Mix	Calming herbal spice mix containing cumin, ginger, and fenugreek, along with other spices
Calming Vata Therapeutic Aroma Oil	Calming aroma oil to relax the mind and body, or for greater balance during cool, dry weather
Children's Rasayana MA 674	Increases intelligence in children, as shown by research (this liquid form of Intelligence Plus™ herbal supplement is available only through the recommendation of a Maharishi Ayurveda expert or health professional)

QUICK REFERENCE GUIDE

Citronella Aromatherapy Cleansing Bar	Stimulates, refreshes, and revitalizes oily skin
Clear Breathe™	Opens the channels of the upper respiratory tract
Clear Throat™	Soothes the occasional cough
Cooling (Pitta) Spice Mix	Cooling herbal spice mix containing coriander, fennel, and cumin, along with other spices
Cooling Pitta Therapeutic Aroma Oil	Cooling aroma oil for balancing the emotions and during hot weather
Digest Tone®	Supports the digestive system and elimination
Elim-Tox®	Helps detoxify the blood, colon, and whole body
Elim-Tox®-O	Helps detoxify the body (recommended for those with a tendency toward acne, heartburn, and excess stomach acid)
Flu Season Defense®	Supports the body's natural defenses
Genitrac®	Supports genitourinary function
Herbal Di-Gest™	Supports improved digestion and balanced appetite
Intelligence Plus™	Increases intelligence in children, as shown by research

Jasmine Aromatherapy Cleansing Bar	Cleanses and nurtures the skin
Kapha® Tea	A delicious, stimulating blend of ginger and other spices
Lemongrass Aromatherapy Cleansing Bar	Calms and soothes dry skin
Liver Balance™	Balances, nurtures, and supports healthy liver function
Maharishi Amrit Kalash®	Full-spectrum antioxidant for overall health and immunity
Mind Plus®	Supports mental functioning under stress
Moisturizing Herbal Massage Oil	Formulated to balance, lubricate, and purify dry skin
Organic Ghee	Organic clarified butter for cooking
Organic Sesame Oil	Used in massage to enhance immunity and experience of well-being
Pitta® Tea	A delicious, cooling blend of cardamom and other spices
Protection Plus™ Respiratory	Supports a healthy respiratory system
Raja's Cup®	A powerful antioxidant coffee substitute
Rose Aromatherapy Cleansing Bar	Cleanses and cools the skin

QUICK REFERENCE GUIDE

Rose Petal Preserve™	Creates a cooling effect on mind, body, and emotions
Rose Water	Cooling, refreshing spray, good for sunburn, also a food flavoring
Sandalwood Aromatherapy Cleansing Bar	Cools and pacifies sensitive skin
Slumber Time® Tea	A delicious, herbal blend for a deeper, more rejuvenating quality of sleep
Slumber Time™ Therapeutic Aroma Oil	Relaxing aroma oil to assist deeper sleep
Sniffle Free®	Improves natural resistance against colds
Sniffle Free™ Tea	A delicious herbal blend to aid the body's resistance against cold weather and to restore balance to the respiratory system
Soothing Herbal Massage Oil	Formulated to balance, lubricate, and purify sensitive skin
Stimulating Herbal Massage Oil	Formulated to balance, lubricate, and purify oily skin
Stimulating (Kapha) Spice Mix	Stimulating herbal spice mix containing ginger, pepper, and coriander along with other spices
Stimulating Kapha Therapeutic Aroma Oil	Stimulating aroma oil to get the body moving or for damp, cool spring days

Throat Ease®	Soothes and clears the throat
Vata® Tea	A delicious, calming blend of licorice and other spices

About MAPI's Safety Record

Since its inception, MAPI has been known for its safe and stringent testing of Ayurvedic products. By the time an herbal product reaches a consumer in America, it has undergone a series of ISO-certified laboratory tests, which are conducted at every phase of production to screen out residual pesticides, biological contamination, and heavy metals such as lead, cadmium, and mercury.

MAPI's manufacturing plant in India was the first to receive certification from the world's top safety and quality regulators, the International Organization for Standardization (ISO) 9000 and the Hazard Analysis and Critical Control Points (HACCP) Certification. Even today, their laboratory remains the only Ayurvedic facility in India to hold certification from the ISO for Good Laboratory Practice, which ensures that their internal testing is valid.

The production facilities use modern, state-of-the-art equipment and strict cleanliness standards to produce traditional Ayurvedic herbal formulas in a germ-free, sterilized environment.

To Contact a *Maharishi Ayurveda* Health Expert (Vaidya) Available by Telephone or On Tour in Your Area

Maharishi Ayurveda Health Assessment Program
Phone: 800-379-6353
Email: wellness@mapi.com
Website: www.vaidyaconsultation.com

Deepen your understanding of your child's health-care needs by scheduling a session with an experienced Maharishi Ayurveda expert from India (Vaidya). A Vaidya has many years of training in the traditional and holistic knowledge of Ayurveda.

The assessment will take 20 to 30 minutes and will include both evaluation of needs and recommendations for a home care program.

Using Maharishi Ayurveda pulse diagnosis (Nadi Vigyan) and other time-tested methods of evaluation, the expert will detect imbalances that need to be addressed to prevent them from becoming full-blown health problems.

Based on the evaluation of needs, the Vaidya will offer recommendations for deeply balancing and rejuvenating treatments that include:

- Specific foods to favor, reduce, or avoid in order to bring your child's physiology back into balance
- Lifestyle education, including daily and seasonal routines for optimal health
- Herbal food supplements and essential oils prepared according to classical Ayurvedic texts
- Rejuvenation treatments
- Meditation techniques for reducing stress and developing consciousness
- Yoga postures and breathing exercises for restoring mental, physical, and emotional health

To Contact a *Maharishi Ayurveda* Health Professional In Your Area

Maharishi Ayur-Veda Health Professional Program
Phone: 877-767-7555
Email: healthpro@mapi.com

Many health professionals (i.e., doctors, osteopaths, chiropractors, naturopaths, and other licensed health professionals who are using Maharishi Ayurveda programs and products in their practice) have become experts in Maharishi Ayurveda by taking extensive training. The health professional trained in Maharishi Ayurveda will use Maharishi Ayurveda pulse diagnosis (Nadi Vigyan) to detect imbalances in your child's pulse, and based on that assessment, he or she will prescribe a complete home care program (see above).

Appendix

Contact Information for Maharishi Ayurveda and Related Programs

HOW TO LOCATE AN AYURVEDIC HEALTH EXPERT IN YOUR AREA

To contact Kumuda Reddy, M.D.
5009 Paducah Road, College Park, MD 20740
www.allhealthyfamily.com
866-REDDYMD
301-474-2184

Maharishi Ayurveda Health Assessment Program
Locate a Maharishi Ayurveda expert from India (Vaidya) available by telephone or on tour in your area
800-379-6353
wellness@mapi.com
www.vaidyaconsultation.com

Maharishi Ayurveda Health Professional Program
Health assessment by a medical doctor, osteopathic physician or naturopathic physician who has been trained in Maharishi Ayurveda
877-767-7555
healthpro@mapi.com

WHERE TO ORDER *MAHARISHI AYURVEDA* PRODUCTS AND HERBAL FORMULAS

Maharishi Ayurveda Products International (MAPI)
800-255-8332 or 719-260-5500
1680 Highway 1
Fairfield, IA 52556-8947
www.mapi.com

CENTERS OFFERING REJUVENATION AND TREATMENT PROGRAMS IN MAHARISHI AYURVEDA

The Raj Maharishi Ayurveda Health Center and Spa
800-248-9050 or 641-472-9580
Fairfield, Iowa
www.theraj.com

Maharishi Ayurveda Health Center Lancaster
877-890-8600 or 978-365-4549
Lancaster, Massachusetts
www.lancasterhealth.com/learn/

Maharishi Peace Palace Houston, TX
281-362-2100
www.woodlandspeacepalace.org

MAHARISHI VEDIC VIBRATION TECHNOLOGY

Maharishi Vedic Vibration Technology
800-431-9680
www.vedicvibration.com
applications@vedicvibration.com

TO LOCATE A TEACHER OF THE *TRANSCENDENTAL MEDITATION* TECHNIQUE IN YOUR AREA

Call toll-free 888-LEARN-TM (888-532-7686)

www.tm.org

FOR INFORMATION AND RESEARCH ON THE *TRANSCENDENTAL MEDITATION* TECHNIQUE

Information and research on the Transcendental Meditation technique
www.tm.org
The Transcendental Meditation technique and health benefits
www.doctorsontm.org

APPENDIX

The Transcendental Meditation technique and educational benefits
www.tmeducation.org
www.adhd-tm.org

Information for implementing and funding programs for teaching the Transcendental Meditation technique in schools
www.davidlynchfoundation.org
www.cbeprograms.org (US)
www.consciousnessbasededucation.org.uk (UK)

MAHARISHI SCHOOLS AND UNIVERSITIES

Maharishi School of the Age of Enlightenment (for Children K–12)
In the United States:
804 Robert Keith Wallace Drive
Fairfield, IA 52556
866-472-6723
Fax: 641-472-1211
www.maharishischooliowa.org

Maharishi School of the Age of Enlightenment (for Children K–12)
In the United Kingdom:
Cobbs Brow Lane, Lathom
Ormskirk, Lancashire, L40 6JJ
UK
+44 (0)1695 729912
Fax: +44 (0)1695 729030
www.maharishischool.com

Maharishi University of Management
1000 North 4th St.
Fairfield, IA 52557
800-369-6480 or 641-472-1110
www.mum.edu

HEALTH EDUCATION COURSES IN *MAHARISHI AYURVEDA*

Health Education Short Courses:
1. Human Physiology: Expression of Veda and the Vedic Literature
2. Good Health through Prevention
3. The *Maharishi Yoga*[SM] Program
4. Self-Pulse Reading Course for Prevention
5. Diet, Digestion, and Nutrition
6. Maharishi Vedic Astrology Overview
7. Maharishi Vedic Architecture[SM] Services

These courses, the Transcendental Meditation technique, and other programs are available at the following Maharishi Peace Palaces:
- Maharishi Peace Palace, Bethesda, MD
301-770-5690
www.bethesdapeacepalace.org
- Maharishi Peace Palace, Lexington, Kentucky
859-269-3803
www.lexingtonpeacepalace.org
- Maharishi Peace Palace, Houston, TX
281-362-2100
www.woodlandspeacepalace.org
- Maharishi Peace Palace, Encinitas, CA
619-518-8266

Full descriptions of these courses can be found at www.maharishi.org.

For Training Courses in Maharishi Ayurveda for Physicians and other Health Professionals:
Maharishi Ayurveda Association of America
maaa@globalcountry.net
877-540-6222

APPENDIX

For Degree Programs in Maharishi Integrative Medicine:
Maharishi University of Management
Bachelor's degree and pre-med program
800-369-6480 or 641-472-1110
admissions@mum.edu
www.mum.edu/premed

THE *MAHARISHI VEDIC ASTROLOGY* AND *MAHARISHI YAGYA* PROGRAMS IN THE UNITED STATES AND CANADA

Maharishi Vedic Astrology and Maharishi Yagya programs
www.maharishiyagya.org
www.globalgoodfortune.com

For more information, choose the Time Zone you live in:

Time Zone 9 Eastern States (CT, DC, DE, FL, GA, KY, MA, ME, MD, NJ, NC, NH, NY, OH, PA, RI, SC, VA, VT, WV)
530-877-8332
530-327-7736 (fax)
MaharishiYagyaTZ9@Maharishi.net

Time Zone 10 Central States (AL, AZ, AR, CO, ID, IL, IN, IA, KS, LA, MI, MN, MS, MO, MT, NE, NM, ND, OK, SD, TN, TX, UT, WI, WY)
503-639-0464
503-639-3860 (fax)
MaharishiYagyaTZ10@Maharishi.net

Time Zone 11 Western States (AK, CA, HI, NV, OR, WA)
530-877-8332
530-327-7736 (fax)
MaharishiYagyaTZ11@Maharishi.net

(Outside the U.S.A. and Canada, please contact the Maharishi Yagya program's international office in Switzerland at +4141-825-1525 phone, +4141-825-1526 fax, Jyotish-yagya@maharishi.net email.)

MAHARISHI VEDIC ARCHITECTURE, MAHARISHI VASTU[SM,] AND THE *MAHARISHI STHAPATYA VEDA* PROGRAM

Fortune-Creating[SM] **Homes and Communities**
www.fortunecreatingbuildings.com
641-472-7570

Notes

Title Page

"Maharishi Vedic Vibration Technology: Instant Relief Program for Chronic Disorders—A Non-Medical Approach for Enlivening the Body's Inner Intelligence," *Maharishi Ayurveda Foundation*, 1999.

Chapter 2. Nature Knows Best

"The World Health Report 2000 Health Systems: Improving Performance." *The World Health Organization*, 2000.

Craig, K.D. and Weiss, S.M. (Eds.) *Health Enhancement, Disease Prevention, and Early Intervention: Biobehavioral Perspectives.* Springer Publishing Company, New York, 1990, p. 95.

"Healthy People 2000: National Health Promotion and Disease Prevention Objectives." *U.S. Department of Health and Human Services*, Washington, D.C., DHHS, 2000.

Sagan, L.A. *The Health of Nations.* Basic Books, Inc., New York, 1987, p. 78.

Ball, T.M., Castro-Rodriguez, J.A., Griffith, K.A., Holberg, C.J., Tylerez, F.D., Wright, A.L. "Siblings, Day-Care Attendance, and the Risk of Asthma and Wheezing during Childhood." *The New England Journal of Medicine*, 2000, vol. 343:538–43, no. 8.

"Plagued by Cures: The Downside of Curing Disease." *The Economist*, Nov. 22, 1997, vol. 344, no. 8044, pp. 95–98.

Szilagyi, P.G. and Schor, E.L. "The Health of Children." *Health Services Research*, October 1998, volume 33, issue 4, part 2, pp. 1001–1039.

Perrin, J.M., Bloom, S.R., Gortmaker, S.L., "The Increase of Childhood Chronic Conditions in the United States." *Journal of the American Medical Association* (JAMA), 2007, 297, pp. 2755–2759.

Newachek, P., Budetti, P., and McManus, P. "Trends in Childhood Disability." *American Journal of Public Health* 74, 1984, pp. 232–236.

Brent, D.A. "Depression and Suicide in Children and Adolescents." *Pediatrics in Review* 14 (10) 1993, pp. 380–388.

McCormick, M.C., Workman-Daniels, K., and Brooks-Gunn. "The Behavioral and Emotional Well-Being of School-Age Children with Different Birth Weights." *Pediatrics 97.* 1996, (1), pp. 18–25.

Craig, K.D. and Weiss, S.M. (Eds.) *Health Enhancement, Disease Prevention, and Early Intervention: Biobehavioral Perspectives.* Springer Publishing Company, New York, 1990, p. 95.

Halfon, N., Inkelas, M., and Wood, D. "Nonfinancial Barriers to Care for Children and Youth." *Annual Review of Public Health*, 1995, 16, pp. 447–472.

Anderson, G. "In Search of Value: An International Comparison of Cost, Access, and Outcomes." *Health Affairs*, vol. 16, no. 6, pp. 163–171.

Cooper, M. "Screaming for Relief." *Time*. November 22, 1999, pp. 38–42.

President's Committee on Mental Retardation, "Preventing the New Morbidity: A Guide for State Planning for the Prevention of Mental Retardation and Related Disabilities Associated with Socioeconomic Conditions." *U.S. Department of Health and Human Services*. Washington, D.C., 1988.

Szilagyi, P.G. and Schor, E.L. "The Health of Children." *Health Services Research*, October 1998, volume 33, issue 4, part 2, pp. 1001–1039.

"WHO Issues New Healthy Life Expectancy Rankings: Japan Number One in New Healthy Life System." Press Release WHO, June 4, 2000, Washington, D.C. and Geneva, Switzerland.

Forrest, C.B., Simpson, L., Clancy, C. "Child Health Services Research: Challenges and Opportunities." *JAMA*, June 11, 1997, vol. 277, no. 22, pp. 1787–1793.

Finland, M. "Emergence of Antibiotic Resistance in Hospitals 1935–1975." *Review of Infectious Diseases 1*, 1979, pp. 29–51.

Ticciati, L. and Ticciati, R. *Genetically Engineered Foods*. Keats Publishing, Inc., New Canaan, CT, 1998, p. 6.

Eickhoff, T. "Antibiotics and Nosocomial Infections." In *Hospital Infections*, ed. J. Bennett and P. Brachman, Little Brown, Boston, 1986, pp. 171–192.

Hauser, W. and Remington, J. "Effect of Antibiotics on the Immune Response." *American Journal of Medicine* 72, 1982, pp. 711–716.

Moore, P. "Children Are Not Small Adults." *The Lancet*, vol. 352, no. 9128, pp. 630–632.

Leape, L.L. "Error in Medicine." *JAMA*, 1994, 272:1851–1857.

Lazarou, J., Pomeranz, B., and Corey, P. "Incidence of Adverse Drug Reactions in Hospitalized Patients, a Meta-Analysis of Prospective Studies." *JAMA*, 1998, 279:1200–5.

Cole, R. "Too much Tylenol Can Harm Children." *The Detroit News*, October 19, 1997.

Houk, V.N. and Thacker, S.B. "Program to Prevent Primary and Secondary Disabilities in the United States." *Public Health Rep.* 1989, 104:2207–2212.

Power C. and Peckman C. "Childhood Morbidity and Adulthood Ill Health." *Journal of Epidermal Community Health*, 1990, 44:69–74.

Hayward, M.D. et al. "Does Childhood Health Affect Chronic Morbidity in Later Life?" Paper presented at the annual conference of the American Sociological Association, August 13, 2000.

Forrest, C.B. et al. "Child Health Services Research: Challenges and Opportunities." *JAMA*, June 11, 1997, vol. 277, no. 22, pp. 1787–1793.

Borenstein, S. "Cost for Treatment of Chronic Disease Soars." Knight Ridder Newspapers, Dec. 4, 2000, Reported at the 15th National Conference on Chronic Disease Prevention and Control.

Chapter 3. Treating Individual Differences

Charaka Samhita, Sharirasthana, 5:1–2.

Chapter 4. Why Kids Get Sick and How to Prevent It

Charaka Samhita, Sutrasthana, 27:342.

Chapter 5. How to Eliminate Stress and Restore Immunity

Galinsky, E. *Ask the Children: What America's Children Really Think about Working Parents*. William, et al., Morrow & Co., Inc., New York, 1999.

Grosswald, S. J., Stixrud, W. R., Travis, F., and Bateh, M.A. "Use of the Transcendental Meditation technique to reduce symptoms of Attention Deficit Hyperactivity Disorder (ADHD) by reducing stress and anxiety: An exploratory study." *Current Issues in Education* [On-line], 10(2), Dec. 2008.

Chapter 7. Foods That Build Immunity and Foods That Destroy It

Chandra, R.K. "Interactions between Early Nutrition and the Immune System." *The Childhood Environment and Adult Disease: 156*, Ciba Foundation Symposium Series, 1991, pp. 77–89.

Howard, L. et al. *Journal of Agricultural and Food Chemistry*, 2000, 48:1315–1321.

Nath, S.B. and Murthy, R.M.K. "Cholesterol in Indian Ghee." *The Lancet*, 1988, vol. 2, p. 39.

Sharma, H.M. "Butter Oil (Ghee)—Myths and Facts." *Indian Journal of Clinical Practice*, July 1990, vol. 1, no. 2.

Reddy, B.S. and Wynder, E.L. "Large-bowel Carcinogenesis: Fecal Constituents of Populations with Diverse Incidence Rates of Colon Cancer." *Journal of the National Cancer Institute*, 1973, 50:1437–42.

Nair, P.P. et al. "Diet, Nutrition Intake, and Metabolism in Populations at High and Low Risk for Colon Cancer." *American Journal of Clinical Nutrition*, 1984, 40:931–36.

Cancer Control Objectives for the Nation: 1985–2000. NCI Monographs, no. 2, 1986, National Cancer Institute, Bethesda, MD.

Thorogood, M. et al. "Risk of Death from Cancer and Ischaemic Heart Disease in Meat and Non-meat Eaters." *British Medical Journal*, 1994, 308:1667–71.

Dwyer, J.T. et al. "Nutritional Status of Vegetarian Children." *American Journal of Clinical Nutrition*, 1982, 35:204–16.

van Staveren, W.A. et al. "Food Consumption and Height/Weight Status of Dutch Preschool Children on Alternative Diets." *Journal of American Dietetic Association*, 1985, 85:1579–84.

Tayter, M. and Stanek, K.L. "Anthropometric and Dietary Assessment of Omnivore and Lacto-Ovo Vegetarian Children." *Journal of American Dietetic Association*, 1989, 89:1661–63.

Dwyer et al. "Size, Obesity, and Leanness in Vegetarian Preschool Children." Journal of American Dietetic Association, 1980, 77:434–37; J. Ruys and J.B. Hickie, "Serum Cholesterol and Triglyceride Levels in Australian Adolescent Vegetarians," *British Medical Journal*, 1976, 2:87.

Erasmus, U. *Fats That Heal, Fats That Kill*. Alive Books, Buraby, BC, Canada, 1993, p. 404.

Gaynor, M.L., Hickey, J., Fryer, W., Hickey, G. *Dr. Gaynor's Cancer Prevention Program*. Kensington Publishers Corp., 1999.

Sabate, J. et al. "Anthropometric Parameters of Schoolchildren with Different Life-Styles." *American Journal of Diseases in Children*, 1990, 144:1159–63.

Sabate, J. et al. "Attained Height of Lacto-Ovo Vegetarian Children and Adolescents." *European Journal of Clinical Nutrition*, 1991, 45:51–58.

Lozoff, B., Jimenez, B., and Wolf, S.W. "Long-term Developmental Outcome of Infants with Iron Deficiency." *New England Journal of Medicine*, 1991, vol. 325, pp. 687–94.

Olivier, S. "Cereal Killers?" *Child*, Jan-Feb 2000, p. 19.

Smith, K. "New Survey Finds Room for Improvement in Children's Lunch Box Lunches." *Quaker Foresight*, Sept–Oct 1993, vol. 6:5.

Pica, R. "Physical Fitness in Early Childhood: What's Developmentally Appropriate?" *Early Childhood News*, May-June 1998.

Erasmus, U. *Fats That Heal, Fats That Kill*. Alive Books, Buraby, BC, Canada, 1993, p. 103.

Chapter 8. Foods for Different Ages

Kant, A., Schatzk, A., Granbard, B., Schairer, C. "A Prospective Study of Diet, Quality and Mortality in Women." *JAMA* 2000, 283:2109-2115.

Mayor, E.J., Hamman, R.F., Gay, E.C. et al. "Reduced Risk of IDDM among Breast-fed Children." *Diabetes*, 1998, vol. 37, pp. 1625-32.

Birch, L.L. and Marlin, D.W. "I Don't Like It; I Never Tried It: Effects of Exposure to Food on Two-year-old Children's Food Preferences." *Appetite*, 1982, 4:323-31.

Charaka Samhita, Sutrasthana 7:36.

Borra, S.T., Schwartz, N.E., Spain, C.G., and Natchipolsky, M.M. "Food, Physical Activity, and Fun: Inspiring America's Children to More Healthful Lifestyles." *Journal of the American Dietetic Association*, July 1995, vol. 95, no. 7, p. 816 (3).

Chapter 9. Ten Healthy Eating Habits for Powerful Digestion

Losey, J.E. et al. "Transgenic Pollen Harms Monarch Larvae." *Nature*, 1999, 399, 214.

Rolls, B. et al. "Serving Portion Size Influences 5-year-old but Not 3-year-old Children's Food Intakes." *Journal of the American Dietetic Association*, 2000, vol. 100, no. 3.

Chapter 10. Boosting Immunity and Creating Balance with Maharishi Ayurveda Herbal Food Supplements and Rasayanas

Southon, S. "Increased Fruit and Vegetable Consumption within the EU: Potential Health Benefits." *Institute of Food Research*, Norwich, UK, 2000, Elsevier Science Ltd.

Sharma, H.M., Hanna, A.N., Kauffman, E.M., and Newman, H.A.I. "Inhibition of Human Low-Density Lipoprotein Oxidation In Vitro by Maharishi Ayurveda Herbal Mixtures." *Pharmacology, Biochemistry and Behavior*, 1992, vol. 43, pp. 1175–1182.

Niwa, Y. and Hansen, M. *Protection for Life*. Thorsons, Wellingborough, UK, 1989, p. 9.

Glaser, J.L. Robinson, D.K., Wallace, R.K. "Effect of Maharishi Amrit Kalash on Allergies, Described in Maharishi Ayurveda: An Introduction to Recent Research." *Modern Science and Vedic Science*, 2(1):89–108.

Dileepan, K.N., Varghese, S.T., Page, J.C., Stechschulte, D.J. "Enhanced Lymphoproliferative Response, Macrophage Mediated Tumor Cell Killing and Nitric Oxide Production after Ingestion of an Ayurvedic Drug." *Biochemical Archives*, 1993, 9:365–374.

Sharma, H.M., Hanissian, S., Rattan, A.K., Stern, S.L., Tejwani, G.A."Effect of Maharishi Amrit Kalash on Brain Opioid Receptors and Neuropeptides." *Journal of Research and Education in Indian Medicine 1991*, 10(1):108.

Hauser, T., Walton, K.G., Glaser, J., Wallace, R.K. "Naturally Occurring Ligand Inhibits Binding of (3H)-Imipramine to High Affinity Receptors." Society for Neuroscience, 18th Annual Meeting, Toronto, Canada, November 14, 1988, p. 244 (abstract 99. 19).

Nidich, S.I., Morehead, P., Nidich, R.J., Sands, D., and Sharma, H.M. "The Effect of the Maharishi Student Rasayana Food Supplement on Nonverbal Intelligence." *Personality and Individual Differences*, Vol. 15, No. 5, pp. 599–602, 1993.

Sharma, H.M., Hanna, A.N., Kauffman, E.M., Newman, H.A.I. "Effect of Herbal Mixture Student Rasayana on Lipoxygenase Activity and Lipid Peroxidation." *Free Radical Biology and Medicine*, Vol. 18, No. 4, pp. 687–697, 1995.

Chapter 11. Sleep and the Bedtime Routine

Leach, P. "Sleep Talk." *Child*, March 2000, pp. 74–76.

Golbin, A.Z. *The World of Children's Sleep: Parent's Guide to Understanding Children and their Sleep Problems*. Michaelis Medical Publishing Corp., Salt Lake City, 1995, pp. 56–59.

Ferber, R. *Solve Your Children's Sleep Problems*. Simon and Schuster, 1986, p. 44.

Golbin, A.Z. *The World of Children's Sleep: Parent's Guide to Understanding Children and their Sleep Problems*. Michaelis Medical Publishing Corp., Salt Lake City, 1995, pp. 115–117.

Golbin, A.Z. *The World of Children's Sleep: Parent's Guide to Understanding Children and their Sleep Problems*. Michaelis Medical Publishing Corp., Salt Lake City, 1995, pp. 91–92.

Figliulo, S. "A New Look at Sleep Schedules from Babies to Teens." June 2006, www.Health Gate.com.

Chapter 12. Ayurvedic Massage and the Wake-Up Routine

Field, T.M. et al. "Tactile/Kinesthetic Stimulation Effects on Preterm Neonates." *Pediatrics*, May 1986, vol. 77, no. 5, pp. 654-658.

Charaka Samhita, Sutrashanam 7. 3–4

U.S. Department of Health and Human Services, *Healthy People 2000: National Health Promotion and Disease Prevention Objectives*. 1990, Washington, D.C.: DHHS.

Chapter 13. Improving Health with Ayurvedic Exercise

Charaka Samhita, Sutrasthana 7.32.

Sushruta Samhita, Chikitsa Sthanam, 24:25.

Pica, R. "Physical Fitness in Early Childhood: What's Developmentally Appropriate?" *Early Childhood News*, May-June 1998.

Taras, H.L. "Physical activity of young children in relation to physical and mental health., in C.M. Hendricks (ed.) *Young children on the grow: Health, activity, and education in the preschool setting*. ERIC Clearinghouse, Washington, D.C., 1992. pp. 33–42.

Borra, S.T., Schwartz, N.E., Spain, C.G., and Natchipolsky, M.M. "Food, Physical Activity, and Fun: Inspiring America's Children to More Healthful Lifestyles." *Journal of the American Dietetic Association*, July 1995, vol. 95, no. 7, p. 816 (3).

Harris, L. "Parents Say: No More Excuses." *NASPE* News, 1996, 49, 3.

Pica, R. "Physical Fitness in Early Childhood: What's Developmentally Appropriate?" *Early Childhood News*, May/June 1998.

Sothern, M.S., Loftin, M., Suskind, R.M., Udall, J.N., Blecker, U. "The Health Benefits of Physical Activity in Children and Adolescents: Implications for Chronic Disease Prevention (Review)." *European Journal of Pediatrics*, 1999, 158 (4):271–4.

Chapter 14. Emotions, Behavior, and a Nourishing Family Environment

Biondi, M., Zannino, L.G. "Psychological Stress, Neuroimmunomodulation, and Susceptibility to Infectious Diseases in Animals and Man: A Review." *Psychotherapy Psychosomatics*, 1997, 66:1, 3–26.

Fon, B.H. "Psychosocial Factors and the Immune System in Human Cancer." in Ader, R. (ed.), *Psychoneuroimmunology*, New York, Academic Press, 1981.

Weiner, H. "Social and Psychobiological Factors in Autoimmune Disease," in Ader, R., et al. (eds.), *Psychoneuroimmunology*, ed 2, San Diego, Academic Press, 1991.

Stein, M. "A Biopsychosocial Approach to Immune Function and Medical Disorder." *Pediatric Clinics of North America*, 1981, 4:203–221.

Sandberg, S. et al. "The Role of Acute and Chronic Stress in Asthma Attacks in Children." *The Lancet*, Vol. 356, No. 9234, pp. 982–988.

Charaka Samhita, Chikitsasthanam, 1:30–35.

Luecken, L.J. et al. "Stress in Employed Women: Impact of Marital Status and Children at Home on Neurohormone Output and Home Strain." *Journal of Psychosomatic Medicine*, 59:352.

Jevning, R., Wilson, A.F., and Davidson, J.M. "Adrenocortical Activity during Meditation." *Hormones and Behavior*, 1978, 10(1):54–60.

Reddy, K., Egenes, T., and Egenes, L. *All Love Flows to the Self*. Samhita Productions, Schenectady, NY, 1999.

Maharishi Mahesh Yogi. *Science of Being and Art of Living*. Meridian/Penguin Books, 1994, New York, pp. 227–228.

Eliot, L.P. *What's Going On In There? How the Brain and Mind Develop in the First Five Years of Life*. Bantam, 1999, New York, pp. 27–29.

Sharma, H.M. et al. "Effect of Different Sounds on Growth of Human Cancer Cell Lines in Vitro." *Alternative Therapies in Clinical Practice*. 1996, vol. 3, no. 4, pp. 25–32.

"Viewing Preferences, Symptoms of Psychological Trauma, and Violent Behaviors among Children Who Watch Television." *Journal of the American Academy of Child & Adolescent Psychiatry*, 1998. 37:1041–1048.

Cantor, J. *Mommy I'm Scared: How TV and Movies Frighten Children and What We Can Do to Protect Them*. Harvest Books/Harcourt Brace, 1998, p. 205.

Robinson, T.N. "Reducing Children's Television Viewing to Prevent Obesity." *JAMA*, 1999; 282:1561–1567.

Chapter 15. Ten Ways to Protect Your Child from Environmental Risk Factors

Herron, R.E. and Fagan, J.B. "Lipophill-Mediated Reduction of Toxicants in Humans: An Evalution of an Ayurvedic Detoxification Procedure." *Alternative Therapies in Health and Medicine*. 2002; 8(5): pp. 40-51.

National Research Council. *Pesticides in the Diets of Infants and Children*. Washington, D.C.: National Academy Press, 1993, pp. 64–65.

National Research Council. *Pesticides in the Diets of Infants and Children*. Washington, D.C.: National Academy Press, 1993, p. 7.

Schmidt, C.W. "Are We Poisoning Our Children?" *Child*, April 2000, pp. 30–35.

Environmental Working Group, press release, Jan. 2000, www.ewg.org.

Carpenter, D.O. "Plychlorinated Biphenyls and Human Health," *International Journal of Occupational Medicine and Environmental Health*, 1998, 11(4), 291-303.

Stellman, S.D., Djordjevic, M.V., Muscat, J.E., Gong, L., Bernstein, D., Citron, M.L., White, A., Kemeny, M., Busch, E., and Nafziger, A.N. "Relative Abundance of Arganochlorine Pesticides and Plychlorinated Biphenyls in Adipose Tissue and Serum of Women in Long Island, NY." *Cancer Epidemiology, Biomarkers, and Prevention*, 1998, 7(6), 489-496.

Sturgeon, S.R., Brock, J.W., Potischman, N., Needham, L.L., Rothman, N., Brinton, L.A., and Hoover, R.N. "Serum Concentrations of Organochlorinecompounds and Endometrial Cancer Risk." *Cancer Causes and Control*, 1988, 9 (4), 417-424.

Hunter, D.J., Hankinson, S.E., Laden, F., Coditz, G.A., Manson, J.E., Willet, W.C., Speizer, F.E., and Woff, M.S. "Plasma Organochlorine Levels and the Risk of Breast Cancer." *New England Journal of Medicine*, 1997, 337 (18), 1253-1258.

U.S. General Accounting Office. *Pesticides: Adulterated Imported Foods Are Reaching U.S. Grocery Shelves*, 1992. Washington, D.C.: U.S. General Accounting Office.

Wargo, J., *Our Children's Toxic Legacy: How Science and Law Fail to Protect Us from Pesticides*, (2nd ed.). Yale University Press, New Haven, Conn., 1998.

Carpenter, D.O. "Polychlorinated Biphenyls and Human Health." *International Journal of Occupational Medicine and Environmental Health*, 1998, 11 (4), 291-303.

Baldi, I., Mohammed-Brahim, B., Brochard, P., Dartiques, J.F., and Salamon, P. "Delayed Health Effects of Pesticides: Review of Current Epidemiological Knowledge." *Revue Epidemiologie et de Sant Publique*, 1998, 46 (2), 134–142.

Longnecker, M.P., Rogan, W.J., and Lucier, G. "The Human Health Effects of DDT (dichlorodiphenyl-trichloroethane) and PCBs (polychlorinated biphenyls) and an Overview of Organochlorines in Public Health." *Annual Review of Public Health*, 1997, 18, 211–244.

National Research Council. *Pesticides in the Diets of Infants and Children*. Washington, D.C.: National Academy Press, 1993, pp. 49–110.

Zetterstrom, R. "Child Health and Environmental Pollution in the Aral Sea Region in Kazakhstan." *Acta Paediatrics Supplement*, 1999, 88 (429), 49–54.

NOTES

Davis, D.L. and Muir, C. "Estimating Avoidable Causes of Cancer," *Environmental Health Perspectives*, 1999, 103 (Supplement 8), 301–306.

Davis, D.L., Axelrod, D., Osborne, M.P., and Teland, N.T. "Environmental Influences on Breast Cancer Risk." *Science and Medicine*, May-June 1997, 56–59.

DeWaily, E., Dodin, S., Verreault, R., Ayotte, P., Sauve, L., Morin, J., and Brisson, J. "High Organochlorine Body Burden in Women with Estrogen Receptor-positive Breast Cancer." *Journal of the National Cancer Institute*, 1994, 86, 232–234.

Wolfson, R. "Biotech News." *Alive: Canadian Journal of Health and Nutrition*, July 2000.

Townsend, M. "Why Soya Is a Hidden Destroyer." *Daily Express*, March 12, 1999.

Food and Drug Administration 57, *Federal Register* 22987.

"EPA Approves Bt Corn and Cotton with Conditions." *The Gene Exchange*, December, 1995.

Losey, K.E. et al. "Transgenic Pollen Harms Monarch Larvae." *Nature*, May 20, 1999, vol. 399, no. 6733, p. 214.

Moss, M.E. et al. "Association of Dental Caries and Blood Lead Levels." *JAMA*, 6/23-30/99.

Taube, J.S. et al. "Processing the Head Direction Cell Signal: A Review and Commentary." *Brain Research Bulletin 40(5-6)*, 1996, pp. 477–484.

Chapter 16. Prevention and Treatment of Common Childhood Illnesses

Office on Smoking and Health. *Reducing the Health Consequences of Smoking: 25 Years of Progress: A Report of the Surgeon General*. US Dept. of Health and Human Services, 1989, Washington, D.C., DHHS publication CDC 89-8411.

Breslau, N. and Peterson, E.L. "Smoking Cessation in Young Adults: Age at Initiation of Cigarette Smoking and Other Suspected Influences." *American Journal of Public Health*, 1996, 86:214–220.

Public Health Service. *Preventing Tobacco Use Among Young People: A report of the Surgeon General*. U.S. Dept. of Health and Human Services, 1994, Atlanta, GA.

Feinstein, J.A. and Quivers, E.S. "Pediatric Preventive Cardiology: Healthy Habits Now, Healthy Hearts Later." *Current Opinion Cardiology*, January 1997, 12:1, 70–77.

Frank, G.C. et al. "Dietary Intake as a Determinant of Cardiovascular Risk Factor Variables," in Berenson, G.S., (ed.), *Causation of Cardiovascular Risk Factors in Children: Perspectives on Cardiovascular Risk in Early Life*, Raven Press, New York, 1986, p. 290.

Respiration 32 (1975): 74-80; *Respiratory Therapy: The Journal of Inhalation Technology* 3 (1973):79–80; *Clinical Research 49* (1973):278.

Castillo-Richmond, A. and Schneider, R.H. et al., "Effects of Sress Reduction on Carotid Atheroschlerosis in Hypertensive African Americans." *Stroke*. 2000, 31:568–573.

Tamborlane, W. V., ed. *The Yale Guide to Children's Nutrition*. Yale University Press, 1997, p. 133.

Lewis, D.S., Bertrand, H.A., McMahan, C.A., McGill, H.C., Carey, K.D., and Masoro, E.J. "Preweaning Food Intake Influences the Adiposity of Young Adult Baboons." *Journal of Clinical Investigation*, 1986, vol. 78:899–905.

Chapter 17. Prevention and Treatment of Chronic Disease in Childhood

Maharishi Mahesh Yogi. *Vedic Knowledge for Everyone*. Vlodrop, The Netherlands: Maharishi Vedic University Press, 1994, p. 300.

Paul-Labrador, M. et al. "Effects of randomized controlled trial of Transcendental Meditation on components of the metabolic syndrome in subjects with coronary heart disease." *Archives of Internal Medicine* 166:1218–1224, 2006.

Travis, F. and Egenes, T. "Physiological Patterns during Practice of the Transcendental Meditation Technique Compared with Patterns while Reading Sanskrit and a Modern Language." *International Journal of Neuroscience*, 2001, vol. 109:71–80.

"Twelve Stories of Renewed Health." *Relief*, vol. 1:17.

INDEX

A

Abhyanga
  See Ayurvedic Oil Massage
Achara Rasayana
  See Behavioral rasayanas
ADHD
  See Attention Deficit Hyperactivity Disorder
Aggressive behavior, 222–223, 228
  cause and treatment, 247
  Pitta dosha and, 247-248
  temper tantrums, 65, 73, 80, 99, 161, 247, 269
Agni, 70-73, 75, 92, 96, 98, 116, 137, 144, 188, 247, 269, 271
  dhatu agni, 72–73, 271, 299–300
  jatharagni, 70, 72, 300
  mamsa agni, 71
  qualities of, 73
  rakta agni, 302
  rasa agni, 71, 303
  See also Digestion
Akasha (space)
  See Ayurvedic elements
Aller-Defense, 268, 278
Allergies, 21–22, 27, 32–33, 56, 98, 109, 207, 232, 235, 251, 254, 259–260, 264, 307
  cause and treatment, 232, 265-267
  See also Genetically modified foods, Milk
Almond Energy, 205, 255
Ama, 73–74, 101, 104–106, 116, 123, 125, 134, 137, 141, 145, 174, 181, 184–185, 234, 246, 251, 253, 255–256, 259–261, 265–268, 273, 276–277
  ama-reducing diet, 266, 268, 273
  defined, 98, 299
  free radicals and, 159
  ojas and, 75, 119
  See also Digestion
Antibiotics
  antibiotic-resistant genes, 233
  colds and, 27, 35
  over-prescribed, 20, 247
  side effects, 20, 35
  use of, 32, 75, 153, 248, 254

weakened immunity, 27, 35–36, 68, 98, 153, 232
  See also Immunity
Antidepressants, 23
Antihistamines, 27, 68
Antioxidants, 106, 117, 120, 125, 155
  herbal formulas, 159–160
  research, 157
  vitamin A and, 110
  See also Maharishi Amrit Kalash, Free radicals
Anxiety, 39, 55, 73, 81, 83, 86, 103, 161, 220, 239, 249–250, 253, 285, 291, 321
  cause and treatment, 266–267
Aroma therapy, 26, 220
Arteriosclerosis, 73, 110, 124, 126, 158, 160, 264
Asanas
  See Yoga Asanas
Asberger's, 292
Asthma, 21, 22, 27, 29, 32–33, 38–39, 56, 167, 204, 207, 235, 251, 264, 275, 285
  cause and treatment, 267–269
  See also Allergies
Astringent taste
  See Ayurvedic tastes
Atma, 44, 283
  See also Self
Attention Deficit Hyperactivity Disorder (ADHD), 33, 62, 80–81, 220, 269–270, 285, 291–292
Autism, 33, 228
Autonomic nervous system, 207
Ayurveda, 24, 299
  See also Maharishi Ayurveda
Ayurvedic daily routine
  bathing and exercise, 184
  bedtime routine, 165, 168–175
  case histories, 42, 54, 68, 165
  cycles of doshas, 166–167
  daily routine chart, 178
  digestion and, 179, 184-185
  early bedtime, 168
  exercise and, 178, 184–186, 193–197, 205
  homework/active time of day, 185

329

immunity and, 69–70, 76
meditation and, 209, 246, 248, 255
morning routine, 179–185
meals, 195
as prevention/treatment, 19, 25, 29, 58, 65, 162, 250, 263, 267, 270, 272–274, 276, 278
rising time, 170
See also Ayurvedic seasonal routine, 177
Ayurvedic dental hygiene, 179, 183
Ayurvedic elements,
air (vayu), 52, 93, 251, 329
doshas and, 51–53
earth (prithivi), 92, 302
fire (tejas), 52, 93, 304
space (akasha), 299
water (apu), 51–53, 92–93, 300
Ayurvedic oil massage (abhyanga), 22, 58–59, 64, 91, 165, 173, 175, 177–181, 184, 189, 238, 246, 248, 252, 257, 267–268, 274, 277
defined, 299
how to, 181–183
infant massage, 179–180
Ayurvedic seasonal routine
foods, 96, 189
Kapha season, 189
overview, 187–188
Pitta season, 188
prevent imbalances, 189–191
seasonal checkups, 26
Vata season, 188
See also Ayurvedic daily routine
Ayurvedic tastes, 92–97, 99–100
astringent, 58, 92, 94, 97, 99, 136, 189, 190, 251, 274–275, 277
for balance, 99–100, 220
bitter, 58, 92–94, 97, 99, 136, 189, 190, 251-252, 260, 274–275
food and, 95, 109, 102, 115, 135–136, 155
pungent, 58, 92–95, 97, 99, 136, 189–190, 277
salty, 58, 92–94, 96–97, 100, 109, 136, 174, 188, 190, 249, 252, 253, 275, 277
sour, 53, 56, 58, 92–97, 100–102, 109, 112, 134, 136, 143, 174, 188, 190, 246, 251–252, 256, 261, 268, 275, 277
sweet, 23, 53, 57–58, 74, 80, 92–97, 99–100, 109, 115, 132, 134, 136, 161, 172, 188–190, 205, 208, 215, 231, 245, 247, 251–252, 256, 267, 275–277, 300
See also Balance/Imbalance, Diet

B

Bala
See Immunity
Balance/Imbalance
Ayurvedic seasonal routine, 99-100, 220
Ayurvedic tastes for, 99–100, 220
diagnosing cause, 25–26, 28, 58–60, 62–65
herbal food supplements, 59, 149–150, 154
how food creates, 52-53, 57-59, 70, 80, 92-96, 129, 134
immunity and, 69–70
Kapha, 56–57
Pitta, 55–56, 60–61, 93–94, 123, 134, 172, 174, 220, 172, 237, 247–248, 253, 255, 259, 267
restoring, 263–267, 269–277
in senses, 220–221
total health and, 44
Vata, 54–55, 57–59, 63–65, 73–74, 80, 93, 99–100, 106, 113, 134, 137, 144, 146–147, 170, 172, 220–221, 246
Behavior
behavioral approach to health, 15, 22, 25, 28, 38, 44, 46, 282
digestion and, 142–146
discipline, 217–218
doshas and, 54–56
food and, 92
positive social interactions, 207
problems, 31, 33–34, 73, 86, 220, 223, 230, 239, 247–248, 264, 266, 269, 291
seasons and, 188–191
storytelling model, 212–215

INDEX

Transcendental Meditation technique and, 81, 83, 86, 209–211, 291, 294
See also Aggressive behavior, Behavioral rasayanas, Attention Deficit Hyperactivity Disorder
Behavioral rasayanas, 208–209, 222
Bitter taste
See Ayurvedic tastes
Benn, Dr. Rita, 291–292
Body type (prakriti), 25, 28, 60, 119, 151, 199–200, 249, 267, 276, 303
Brahman, 212–217
Brain, 42, 69, 71, 75, 103, 105, 108, 110, 116–117, 129, 160–161, 171, 201-203, 218–219, 223, 227–228, 239, 241, 257, 269, 275, 282– 284, 292
Breastfeeding, 20, 116–117, 130
Brihadaranyaka Upanishad, 281
Bronchitis *See* Cough/Bronchitis

C

Cancer, 37, 219
  diet and, 110, 119–120, 129, 142
  free radicals and, 158
  emotions and, 207
  genetically modified food and, 232
  skin cancer, 236–237
  toxins and, 227–230
Cardiovascular disease, 37, 117, 120, 264, 275
  cause and treatment, 272–273
Car sickness
  See Motion sickness
Centers for Disease Control and Prevention, 34
Chapati, 114, 132, 134, 239, 299
Charaka Samhita, 70, 137, 299
Cheeses, 70, 92, 97–99, 119, 125, 132, 138, 142, 232, 251, 276
Chelsea School, Silver Spring, Maryland, 292
Chicken pox, 70, 255
  cause and treatment, 248, 256, 259, 261
Child abuse, 33
Childhood illnesses, 29, 33, 37, 69–70
  cause and treatment, 116, 137, 248–261
  cycle of sickness, 30, 68, 162, 246
  guidelines for preventing, 245–247
Children's health
  advances in twentieth century, 31
  national indicators, 34
  new paradigm, 38
  window of opportunity for treatment, 264
Cholesterol, 110–111, 116–118, 120, 123–125, 135, 159–160, 264, 275–276
  HDL (good cholesterol), 200, 272
  LDL (bad cholesterol), 155, 157, 200
  See also Fats
Chronic disease
  chronic ailments, 21, 27, 29, 31, 32–33, 37, 68, 149–150, 162, 207, 227, 239
  cause and treament, 265–278
  curing without drugs, 38, 162
  increase in problems, 33
  preventing, 61, 129, 200, 243, 263–264
  tools of treatment, 256
  See also specific chronic diseases
Circadian rhythms, 166–167
  See also Natural rhythms
Circulation, 60, 74, 179, 201–202, 274
Clear Breathe, 247, 252, 258–259, 261, 269
Clear Throat, 247, 259
Clothing, 184, 236–237, 255
  colors, 220
  organic, 235, 277–278
Colds
  antibiotics and, 27, 35
  cause and treatment, 151, 250–251
  case histories, 21, 39, 41, 56, 68
  diet and, 96, 98–99, 116, 137
  digestion and, 73, 188
  food supplements and, 149
  Kapha dosha and, 69–70, 110, 189–190, 245–247
  prevention, 26, 29, 184, 204, 207, 250
  related disorders, 254–255, 258
  See also Cough, Sore throat

Cold sores, 94
Computers, 145
 games, 165, 175, 189, 194–195, 270, 274
 health risks, 221–223
Concentration, 41, 82–83, 86, 199, 202–203, 266, 270
 inability to focus, 220
Congestion, 29, 56–57, 68, 96, 130, 135, 220, 252, 254, 256
 See also Colds; Cough/Bronchitis
Consciousness, 15, 24, 38, 44–46, 48–49, 65, 74, 81, 103, 105, 146, 201–203, 212, 238, 282, 287–288, 290, 293
 pure consciousness, 81, 212, 238, 282, 288
Consciousness-Based, 293
 education, 290
 model of health, 52
Constipation, 21–23, 55, 73–74, 80, 100, 146, 187, 234, 248–250, 257, 259
Cortisol, 211–212
Cough/bronchitis, 68, 96, 98, 116, 153, 204, 261
 cause and treatment, 251–252
 dry cough, 251
 wet cough, 252
 See also Colds
Current Issues in Education, 81, 270, 292, 321

D

Daily routine
 See Ayurvedic Daily Routine
Dairy, 109, 121, 131, 133, 154, 232, 234, 246, 252
 See also specific dairy products
DDT, 229
Deans, Ashley, 294–295
Dental hygiene
 See Ayurvedic dental hygiene
Depression, 33, 73, 86, 160, 220, 239, 266–267, 274
 See also Emotions
Desserts, 97, 115, 124, 132–133, 137, 142

Dhal, 97, 114, 121, 130, 132, 134, 139, 253, 260, 267, 299
Dhatus, 71–74, 105, 123, 154–155, 161, 254–255, 300, 303
 asthi, 71, 299
 majja, 301
 mamsa, 301
 meda, 301
 rasa, 205, 208, 303
 rakta, 303
 seven dhatus chart, 72
 shukra, 71, 303
Diabetes, 27, 33, 37, 120, 132, 158
 cause and treatment, 270–273
 obesity and, 275
Diarrhea, 20, 23, 98, 132
 cause and treatment, 253
 fever and, 256
 stomachache and, 259
Diet
 cancer and, 110, 119–120, 129, 142
 case histories, 39, 42,100–102
 cravings for chocolate and candy, 136
 children choose what to eat, 135
 colds and, 110, 119–120, 129, 142
 flu and, 96, 98, 116, 137, 245
 immunity and, 103–105, 108–118
 Kapha-pacifying, 99, 101, 113, 271, 273, 275
 Pitta-pacifying, 99, 113, 277
 prevention and, 129
 Vata-pacifying, 59, 99–100, 173, 271
 See also Food, Sattvic foods, Vegetarian diet
Digestion
 appetite, 20–21, 27, 29, 38, 55–56, 73, 80, 101, 106, 133, 144, 257
 Ayurvedic daily routine and, 179, 184–185
 behavior and, 142–146
 colds and, 73, 188
 digestive spices, 100, 102, 115, 136, 271, 276
 digestive toxins (ama), 75, 98-99, 116, 125, 134, 137, 141-142, 144-145, 155, 159, 246, 261, 263
 energy and, 74, 98 100-101, 103
 exercise and, 193

INDEX

fatigue and, 74, 98, 105, 174
free radicals and, 74, 145, 155, 159
herbal supplements and, 157, 161, 205, 246
immunity/digestive strength, 56–57, 68–74, 112, 131, 133, 135, 141–147, 151, 155, 165, 246, 270
Kapha dosha and, 73-74
ojas and, 74–75
Pitta dosha and, 52, 60, 169
problems, 23–25, 67, 74, 100, 137, 145–147, 179, 232, 248, 253, 257, 259
seasons and, 96–98
See also Agni, Ama, Food, Toxins
Digest Tone, 101
Dinacharaya, 300
See also Ayurvedic daily routine
Discipline
See Behavior
Disease
See Chronic disease, Childhood illness
Diverticulitis, 73
DNA, 42, 46, 72, 75, 111, 155, 158–159, 231, 282
Doshas
behavior and, 54-56
in daily, seasonal life cycles, 53–54, 58–59, 187
diagnosing, 59–60
energy and, 56, 167
fatigue and, 55, 89, 177, 197
in food, 57, 59
like increases like, 93
mono-doshic, tri-doshic, 57
primary location of, 60
qualities, 53–57, 69–70, 94–95, 99, 108–109, 112–115
sleep and, 55, 58, 64, 69-70, 100, 134, 186-189, 252
subdoshas, 60, 80, 100–101,165
See also Vata, Pitta, Kapha
Dravyaguna, 152, 300
Dyslexia, cause and treatment, 272

E

Earaches

cause and treatment, 254
infections, 20–21, 29, 98, 116, 150
Eating habits, 65, 126, 136, 141–147, 253, 264, 267, 276
how to change, 137
Eczema, 56, 91, 94, 104, 278
cause and treatment, 276–278
See also Skin
Elements
See Ayurvedic elements
Elimination, 23, 38, 55, 73–75, 101–102, 110, 183, 248, 253
See also Constipation
Elim-Tox, 278
Elim-Tox-O, 102, 278
Emotions, 15, 24, 28, 38, 86, 103, 179, 207
behavior and, 207–209, 218–220, 222
cancer and, 207
food and, 91–92, 98, 127
food supplements and, 149, 157, 160–161
loving relationships, 207
mind and, 44, 48, 61, 220
rasayanas and, 160, 255
role in creating health, 48, 75, 207
Endocrine system, 207, 229
Energy, 24, 44, 51, 174, 189, 241, 269, 302
digestion and, 74, 98, 100–101, 103
doshas and, 56, 167
exercise and, 196, 198
food and, 105, 108, 115, 145
food supplements, 153
Enlightenment, 30, 282, 284, 295
Environment
eating, 142, 145
exercise and, 197
fresh air, 175, 196, 236
family, 58, 87–88, 207–208, 218, 221–223, 257
health and, 15, 24, 282
immunity and, 32, 48, 76, 191
Transcendental Meditation technique and, 83, 292
risk factors, 227–234, 251, 264, 267
sensory, 218–220
See also Toxins

Environmental Working Group, 228, 326
EPA, 229, 233, 327
Exercise
  Ayurvedic daily routine and, 178, 184–186, 193–196, 205
  Ayurvedic guidelines for, 199–201
  body type and, 58, 70, 197–199
  breathe through your nose, 201
  breathing exercises (pranayama), 178, 204, 270, 278, 302, 312
  energy and, 196, 198
  environment and, 197
  fatigue and, 193, 199-200, 202, 204
  free play, 196–197
  Kapha and, 70, 189–191, 193, 197-200
  lack of, 191, 246, 252, 264, 272, 275
  nutrition and, 204–205
  as prevention and treatment, 29, 101, 109, 174–175, 268, 271–273, 275–276
  sports, 58, 189–190, 196–201, 205, 223, 270, 293
  See also Yoga Asanas and Salute to the Sun

F

Facial tic, 21–22
Families and Work Institute, 79
Fatigue, 86, 170, 175, 186, 191, 234, 241
  case histories and, 21–23, 29, 38, 165
  daily routine and, 178–179, 181
  digestion and, 74, 98, 105, 174
  doshas and, 55, 177, 89, 197
  exercise and, 193, 199–202, 204
  parents and, 79, 165–166
Fats, 130–131, 238
  healthy fats, 110, 116–117, 131, 276
  unhealthy fats, 123–125, 159
  See also Dairy and Oils
Fear, 81, 189, 207, 214, 222–223, 237, 249, 253, 266, 274, 286
  cause and treatment, 254–255
Fever, 35, 68
  cause and treatment, 60–61, 255–256
  diarrhea and, 256
  other diseases and, 248, 250, 252, 260
Fletcher Johnson Learning School in Washington, D.C., 290
Flu, 26, 28–29, 35, 39, 41, 255
  diet and, 96, 98, 116, 137, 245
  immunity and, 68–70, 76
  seasons and, 188–190
Food
  appealing, 138–140, 220
  Ayurvedic seasonal routine, 96, 189
  behavior and, 92
  in case histories, 22–23, 39, 80, 100–102
  chewing, 145
  in childhood (Kapha Kala), 96–98, 115–116, 126, 245
  childrens choice of, 135–137
  cravings, 129, 136–137
  creates balance/imbalance, 52–53, 57–59, 70, 80, 92–96, 129, 134
  digestion and, 71–75, 141–142, 145–147, 155, 186, 268
  doshas and, 57, 59
  emotions and, 91-92, 98, 127
  empty calories, 116, 122, 138
  energy and, 105, 108, 115, 145
  food pyramid, 126
  free radicals and, 118, 135
  fresh foods, 105–108
  genetically modified, 230–234
  immunity boosting, 105–118
  junk, packaged, frozen, canned or leftover, 105, 123, 125, 256, 270
  mind and, 91, 105, 108, 146, 149
  nutrition in, 105, 121–122, 146, 155
  as prevention and treatment, 19–20, 26, 65, 91, 103–104, 131, 149, 252, 259–261, 270–271, 275–277
  seasons and, 96–99
  toxins in, 227–230
  See also Ayurvedic tastes, Meals, Organic foods, Processed foods, Sattvic foods, *specific foods*
Free radicals, 200
  cancer and, 37, 219
  digestion and, 74, 145,155, 159
  foods and, 118, 135
  how to stop, 157–161, 204, 237, 265
  See also Antioxidants, Maharishi Amrit Kalash

INDEX

French fries, 98, 104, 122, 124–125, 136
  recipe, 138
Fruit, 80, 106, 132–134, 205, 249, 271, 267, 273, 277
  pesticides and, 228–230
  sweet tastes and, 92-93

G

Gandharva Veda *See* Maharishi Gandharva Veda music
Gargling, 252, 259–260 *See also* Ayurvedic dental hygiene
Gas, Bloating, Flatulence, 23–24, 67, 74, 100, 137, 146–147, 179, 248, 253
  cause and treatment, 257
  See also Digestion, Indigestion
Genetically modified foods (GMOs), 118, 230, 277
  defined, 231
  health risks for children, 232–234
Ghee, 110–112, 131, 160, 300
Ginger, 102
  as treatment, 174, 246, 205–253, 256–259, 261, 275
  dairy and, 109, 112–113, 130, 133–134, 250, 252
  in recipes, 114, 134, 138–139
  in salad, 106, 133
  in spice mix, 101, 115, 136, 174, 268
  tea, 101, 250–253, 258–259, 268
Grosswald, Sarina, Ed.D., 292
Grief, 253, 285
Gunas, 108
  See also Sattva

H

Headaches,
  common cold, 249-250
  cause and treatment, 257–258
  migraine, 59, 220, 285
  symptomatic, 27, 137, 151, 220, 234-235
  tension, 257-258
Health care
  modern, 31-34, 38, 46
  natural, 15, 19

See also Maharishi Ayurveda
Hearing, 219–220, 247, 285
Heart, 42–43
  congenital heart disease, 272-273
  strengthening, 74, 120, 129, 135, 142, 160, 172, 268
  risk factors, 37, 124, 126, 158, 195, 275
Herbal Di-Gest, 257, 259
Herbal oil massage
  See Ayurvedic oil massage (abhyanga)
Herbal food supplements
  See Maharishi Ayurveda Herbal Food Supplements
Herbert, Julia, 293
Hereditary diseases, 37, 269, 273, 277
High fructose corn syrup, 231, 245, 271, 276
Household cleaners/detergents, 235
  See also Toxins

I

Ice cream
  craving, 137
  foods to avoid, 97, 99, 115, 132, 137, 246, 251, 276
  Kapha-increasing, 70
Imbalance
  See Balance/Imbalance
Immunity, 64, 73, 75-76. 141, 152, 299
  case histories, 20, 59
  defined, 70, 74
  environment and, 32, 48, 76, 191
  flu and, 68-70, 76
  food and, 105-118
  hygiene hypothesis, 32-33, 35
  lower, 27, 33, 35, 68, 72, 119, 229, 250, 277
  Maharishi Amrit Kalash boosting, 157, 237
  ojas and, 74-75, 105-106, 149, 167
  rasayanas and, 155-157
  strengthening, 26–27, 29, 38, 68-76, 103, 105, 107–109, 115, 120, 125, 127, 130, 141-142, 149, 153, 160, 162, 179–181, 188, 193, 200, 246–247, 250, 255, 266, 268-271
  See also Antibiotics

335

Indigestion, 73–74, 99–100, 109–110, 274, 276–277
　case histories, 24, 100–102
　cause and treatment, 135, 137, 142, 147, 253, 257, 259
　See also Agni, Ama, Digestion
Infant mortality rates, 34
Infections, 29, 69, 75, 116, 150, 184, 207, 245, 254–255, 258, 273
　case histories, 20–21, 41, 67
Infectious disease, 31–33, 68–69, 75, 207
Insomnia
　case histories, 23, 59-60
　cause and treatment, 249, 274, 285
　defined, 273
　occurrence of, 23, 25, 55, 169, 173, 189, 249, 257
　See also Sleep
Intelligence, 22
　healing, 42-46, 265
　inner, 27-28, 48–49, 64, 146, 153, 162
　nature's, 49, 51-53, 81, 88, 103, 136, 154, 281–285
Intelligence Plus, 160–161
Irritability, 56, 94, 170, 190, 247
Irritable bowel syndrome (IBS), 23–24, 73

J

Jaggary, 98, 115–116, 131–133, 246, 270
Jala (water)
　See Ayurvedic elements, Water
Johns Hopkins University, 37
Journal of American Medical Association (JAMA), 36
Jyotish
　See Maharishi Vedic Astrology program

K

Kanji, 248, 256, 259, 261
Kapha dosha
　balance/imbalance, 56–60
　daily routine/seasonal cycles, 53–54, 97, 133, 178, 181, 184-186, 189–190
　defined, 52–53, 300

digestion and, 73-74
disorders, 250–252, 256, 258–260, 267, 271, 273, 275–277
exercise and, 70, 189-191, 193, 197–200
foods that increase/decrease, 93–95, 99–102, 109–110, 112–113, 117, 123.
Kapha Kala (childhood), 69–70, 96, 98-99, 106, 231, 245–246,
learning styles, 62
sleep and, 167–169, 174-175
See also Doshas
Kapha Tea, 101, 133, 175
Ketchup, 97, 99–102, 104, 136
Kidder, Tracy, 223

L

Lassi, 97, 131, 133–134, 142, 205
　defined, 301
　for illness, 249–253, 256, 277
　recipe, 112–113
　See also Dairy
Lead, 236
Learning, 161
　ability, 27
　disorders, 33–34, 170, 236, 247, 269, 274
　styles, 62
　See also Dyslexia, ADHD
Lethargy, 57, 73–74, 100, 303
Linoleic acid, 111
Liquids, 58, 143, 145, 153, 188

M

Maharishi
　See Maharishi Mahesh Yogi
Maharishi Amrit Kalash
　boosting immunity, 157, 237
　diseases and, 248, 266, 269
　fear and, 255
　See also Free radicals, Antioxidants
Maharishi Ayurveda
　benefits, 19–30, 35, 37–39, 42–44, 46, 48–49, 59–64, 68–70
　defined, 1–4, 9–11, 15, 19–30, 37–39, 42–46, 48–49, 59–64, 68–70

fundamental principles, 19–30, 37–39, 42–46, 48–49, 51–53, 57, 59–64, 68–70, 73, 75, 80–82, 91
health care program, 301
Maharishi Ayurveda herbal food supplements
 defining qualities, 151
 digestion and, 157, 161, 205, 246
 emotions and, 149, 157, 160-161
 energy and, 153
 products, 2, 9, 247
 formulas, 23, 26, 102, 104, 150–154, 254, 258, 266, 270, 273, 278
 whole herb, 149, 151–152, 160
Maharishi Ayurveda health expert (Vaidya), 25, 100, 150, 180
Maharishi Ayurveda pulse diagnosis (nadi vigyan), 25, 63
 defined, 59-60, 301
 self-pulse diagnosis, 59–62, 100, 150, 165, 245, 255, 260, 263, 266, 293
 16-lesson course, 62, 64
Maharishi Gandharva Veda music, 186, 220, 248, 255, 293
Maharishi Jyotish Program
 See Maharishi Vedic Astrology Program
Maharishi Mahesh Yogi, 15, 24, 82, 217, 238, 282, 301
Maharishi School of the Age of Enlightenment, 198–199
 achievements, 293–294, 296
Maharishi Sthapatya Veda design, 238–241, 288, 301
Maharishi Vedic Approach to Health, 24
 See also Maharishi Ayurveda
Maharishi Vedic Astrology Program, 286, 289, 293, 301
Maharishi Vedic Medicine, 24
 See also Maharishi Ayurveda
Maharishi Vedic Science, 286, 301
Maharishi Vedic Vibration Technology (MVVT), 284–285
Maharishi Yagya performances, 287–289, 301
Mala, 301
Meals, 108, 138, 143, 145
 between meals, 234, 249, 268, 270, 276

first year, 130, 131
hot/warm, 58, 105, 104, 127, 129, 142, 189, 257
one to three years, 131–132
schedule, 23, 58–59, 67, 130-131, 170, 174, 185, 247, 267, 270, 274, 278
three to twelve years, 133–135
See also Diet, Food, Recipes
Measles, 70, 248, 273
 cause and treatment, 248
Medications
 prescription drugs, 21, 29, 39, 104
 side effects, 20-21, 26-27, 35-36, 38-39, 151-152, 154, 167
Meditation
 See Transcendental Meditation technique
Mendel, Gregor, 231
Menstrual cramps, 249
Mental problems, 26, 73
Mental retardation, 34, 236
Metabolic syndrome, 272
Metabolism, 52, 69, 75, 116, 131, 271, 276, 302
Migraine headaches
 See Headaches
Milk, 109, 110-113, 131, 135, 232, 234, 247, 250, 267
 allergies, 109, 267–268
 at bedtime, 172, 174, 189–190, 249, 257
 goat's, 130
 increase Kapha, 99, 231, 246
 soy, 231
 sweet taste, 92–93, 96
 warm, 59, 132–134, 172–174, 249, 257, 267, 278
 See also Dairy
Mind, 15, 30, 38, 74, 215–216, 241, 271, 274, 276, 281–282
 agni and, 98, 103
 balance/imbalance, 61, 64
 consciousness and, 44
 emotions and, 44, 48, 61, 220
 food and, 91, 105, 108, 146, 149
 rasayanas and, 157, 160
 sleep/daily routine and, 165, 169, 173, 179

Transcendental Meditation technique and, 81-84, 86, 88, 184, 204, 209, 214, 246, 270
yoga asanas and, 201-202
Mind-body
coordination, 37, 44-46, 86, 180, 198, 201, 204, 274
operators, 52, 54-55, 57, 197, 300, 302-303
See also Doshas
Minerals, 122, 125, 149, 151, 155, 273, 302
Mono-doshic, 57
See also Doshas
Mood disorders, 170, 292
See also Emotions
Mothers, 62, 161, 217
cooking, 99-109
expectant, 34, 264
as teachers, 217
working, 79, 211
See also Parents
Motion sickness,
cause and treatment, 258
eating in car, 147
MSG (monosodium glutamate), 123
Mucus, 70, 96, 110, 130–131, 134, 137, 143, 250–252, 266
See also Colds, Cough
Music therapy, 26
See also Gandharva Veda Music
MVVT
See Maharishi Vedic Vibration Technology

N

Nader, Tony, M.D., Ph.D., 282
Nadi vigyan
See Maharishi Ayurveda Pulse Diagnosis
Nataki Talibah Schoolhouse, Detroit, 291
Nidich, Sanford, 161
N'Namdi, Carmen, 291
Nasya, 184, 250, 252, 254, 256, 260, 266, 269
See also Ayurvedic Daily Routine
Nature

healing power, 38
individual's nature, 51–53
laws of nature, 46, 48–49,191, 208, 238, 282, 284, 286
natural desires, 144
nature's intelligence, 28, 42–45, 48–49, 88, 136
violation of natural law, 48
Natural rhythms, 166–167, 191, 197
daily cycle, 52–54, 169–170, 185–189, 267
disruption, 27, 170
seasonal, 96–97, 102, 188
See also Circadian rhythms
Neglect, 33, 223
NREM (non rapid-eye-movement sleep), 168–169
Nutrition
exercise and, 204-205
role of, 105
for young athletes, 204–205
See also Diet, Food

O

Obesity, 57, 73, 120, 124, 132, 135, 144, 194, 223, 272
epidemic of, 33
cause and treatment, 275–276
Oils
canola, 118, 231
flaxseed, 118
genetically modified, 230–232
hemp-seed, 117–118
hydrogenated, 124, 125, 276
olive, 117–118
organic, 118
safflower, 117–118
sesame, 117–118, 181, 183-184, 250, 254, 259,-260, 266, 269, 277
sunflower, 117–118, 121-122
See also Ghee, Fats
Oil massage
See Ayurvedic Oil Massage
Ojas
defined, 74, 302
immunity and, 74–75, 105–106, 149, 167
ojas-producing foods, 108–110

ojas-decreasing foods, 119, 141
rasayanas, 154, 156, 208
 See also Digestion, Immunity
Organic foods, 109, 111-114, 118, 123, 127, 129-13-, 138, 140, 153, 181, 227-232, 234-235, 238, 277-278
Overeating, 58, 144, 253, 259

P

Pandits, 287–289, 301
Panir, 113
 See also Dairy
Parents
 bonding, 171, 179–180
 fatigue and, 79, 165-166
 nurturing responsibility, 15, 19, 37, 51, 98, 105, 108, 142, 177, 237, 217–218, 222, 247–248, 286–287, 289–290
 role model, 48, 91, 126, 195, 208, 217–218, 222, 286–287, 289–290
 working, 79
 how the Transcendental Meditation technique benefits, 81, 83, 87–88, 211
 See also Mothers
Peace, 30, 186, 210–211, 214–215, 241, 296
Peer pressure, 191
Penicillin, 32
 See also Antibiotics
Pennsylvania State University's Population Research Institute, 37
Peptic ulcers, 73
Pesticides and chemical fertilizers, 227–230
 See also Toxins
Picky eater, 23, 55, 144–145
Pitta dosha
 aggressive behavior, 247–248
 balance/imbalance, 55–56, 60–61, 93–94, 123, 134, 172, 174, 220, 237, 247–248, 253, 255, 259, 267
 daily/seasonal cycles, 53–54, 99, 167, 169, 185, 188–189
 decreasing, 94–95
 defined, 52-53, 302
 digestion and, 52, 60, 169
 increasing, 94–95
 learning styles, 62
 physical activity, 177, 198, 200
 skin problems, 277–278
 See also Doshas
Pitta Tea, 133
Polio, 32
Polyps, 73
Poverty, 34, 275
Prakriti, 51, 57, 99, 102, 145, 220, 302
 See also body type
Prana, 105–106, 119, 123, 204, 302
Pranayama, 204, 268, 270, 276, 278, 302
Pregnancy, 20, 67
Prenatal care, 34, 67
Prescription drugs
 See Medications
Preservatives, 105, 108, 123, 159, 204
Prevention, 28, 37, 245, 263–264
 herbal formulas, 273
 role of diet, 129
 strengthening immunity, 69, 250
Prithivi (earth)
 See Ayurvedic elements
Processed foods, 70, 105–106, 118, 123, 125, 232, 245, 271
 See also Food
Protection Plus Respiratory, 268
Protein, 103, 110, 113–115, 118, 120–122, 126, 129, 132, 135, 158, 268, 302
Psychological imbalances, 220
 See also Emotions, Mind
Pulse diagnosis
 See Maharishi Ayurveda pulse diagnosis
Pungent taste
 See Ayurvedic tastes
Pure consciousness
 See Consciousness

Q

Quantum field theory, 46
Quiet environment, 58, 142, 145
Quiet Time
 See Transcendental Meditation technique
Quinoa, 115, 132–134, 302

R

Raga, 186, 302
Rajas, 108, 302
Raja's Cup, 204
Rasa, 71, 155, 303
  See also Ayurvedic tastes
Rasayanas
  children's rasayana (MA 674), 161
  defined, 155–157
  food supplements, 149
  immunity boosting, 155-157
  mind and emotions, 157, 160, 255
  See also Behavioral rasayanas
Rashes, 56, 94, 149, 190, 235, 276–278
  See also Skin
Recipes
  ayurvedic pizza, 139
  baked french fries, 138
  ghee, 111
  lassi, 113
  panir, 113
  mung dhal soup, 114
  veggie burgers, 140
  yogurt, 112
REM (rapid-eye-movement) sleep, 168
Research Studies
  Decreased Health-Care Expenditures, 41
  Decreased Hospitalization and Doctor Visits, 87
  Healthier Family Life, 87
  Increased Resistance to Disease, 156
  Mean Creativity Scores, 86
  Mean IQ Scores, 85
  Most Effective Antioxidant, 156
  Percentage of Prosocial Responses, 210
  Physiological and Psychological Improvement, 40
  Reduced Anxiety, 84
Respiratory infections, 67, 69, 258
Rock music, 219
Rose Petal Preserve, 113, 172, 174, 190
Routine, 25–26, 62–65, 191
  consistency, 170–171, 248–249
  irregular, 79, 170, 246
  See also Ayurvedic daily routine, Ayurvedic seasonal routine
Rutherford, George 290–292

S

Salty taste
  See Ayurvedic tastes
Salute to the Sun (Surya Namaskara), 201–204, 271
Samadosha, 303
  See also Doshas
Sanskrit, 15, 238, 272, 293
Sattva, 156, 303
Sattvic foods
  defined, 108
  formula for sattvic diet, 126
  ghee, 110–112
  honey, 116
  jaggary, 115
  lassi, 112–113
  milk, 108, 115, 127, 267
  mung dhal soup, 114
  panir, 113–114
  rice/whole grains, 115
  yogurt, 112
Satyakama, 213–217
School lunches, 108, 124
Scratches, 258
Seasons, 188-191
  See also Ayurvedic Seasonal Routine
Sesame seeds, 109-110, 118, 121, 135
  See also Oils
Self, 44, 49, 62, 213–216, 282–283
  self-awareness, 22
  self-esteem, 41, 193, 291, 294–295
Self-pulse diagnosis
  See Maharishi Ayurveda pulse diagnosis
Senses, 103, 146, 165, 169, 173, 203-204, 208, 216
  at home, 218-220
Sharma, Hari, 161
Shukra
  See Dhatus
Skin, 235
  cause and treatment of eczema, 276–278
  dry skin, 104, 249
  Pitta dosha and, 277-278
  rashes, 56, 94
  scraches, 258
Sleep

340

INDEX

bedtime routine, 24, 79, 165–172, 175, 274–275
case histories, 20–23, 55, 59, 67
day sleep, 191, 256, 267, 273–274, 276, 278
doshas and, 55, 58, 64, 69-70, 100, 134, 167-169, 174-175, 186–189, 252
mind and, 165, 169, 173, 179
sleep aids, 171–173, 179–181, 201, 205, 208–209, 241, 274, 275
sleep patterns, 157, 168, 274
sleep problems, 80–81, 142, 170–171, 173–174, 178, 220, 222–223, 226, 274
Vata dosha and, 172-175
See also Insomnia
Slumber Time Tea, 165
Slumber Time therapeutic aroma oil, 173, 275
Smallpox, 32
Smoking, 58, 251, 263–264
Sniffle Free herbal tablets, 250, 266
Social and emotional development, 223
See also Emotions
Sodas, 23, 57, 104, 109
Sore throat, 98, 250–251, 254, 261
cause and treatment, 258–259
See also Colds
Sour
See Ayurvedic tastes
Spices, 64, 100–101, 109–111, 115, 132, 136, 138–139, 174, 246, 248, 257, 268, 275, 301
Calming (Vata) Spice Mix, 115, 136
Cooling (Pitta) Spice Mix, 115, 136
spice mix, 114, 299
Stimulating (Kapha) Spice Mix, 101, 115, 136, 175
See also Ginger
Sports
See Exercise
Srotas, 116, 135, 170, 189, 274, 276, 303
Stanford Center for Research in Disease Prevention, 223
Steam inhalation, 254, 269
Sthapatya Veda
See Maharishi Sthapatya Veda
Stomachache, 25, 145, 150

cause and treatment, 257, 259
Storytelling, 212
Stress, 58–59, 79, 149, 158, 178, 219–220, 246, 249, 259, 284, 290–292
case histories, 22–24, 67, 80, 104
emotional/psychological stress, 80, 86, 207, 274, 277–278
stress problems, 33, 257, 259, 272
stress management, 26, 29, 79, 81, 167, 173, 177, 179–180, 186, 200–202, 241, 264, 296
Transcendental Meditation technique and, 81–84, 87, 209–211
Stuffy nose
See Colds
Subdoshas
See Doshas
Sugar, 92–93, 96, 98, 103, 115–116, 124, 131–133, 136, 215, 223, 232, 245–246, 251–252, 256–257, 260, 270, 300
Sunflower seeds, 118, 121–122
See also Oils
Sunlight, 188, 220, 236
Sun salutes
See Salute to the Sun
Sweet
See Ayurvedic tastes

T

Tastes
See Ayurvedic tastes
Temper tantrums
See Aggressive behavior
Tejas (fire)
See Auyurvedic elements
Television
health risks, 220-223
watching, 145, 171, 173, 175, 189, 193–195, 205, 241, 270, 274, 276
Tension, 59, 80, 180, 257, 266
See also Stress
The Science of Being and Art of Living (Maharishi Mahesh Yogi), 217
Tiredness; 73, 101, 249
Tissues, 69–72, 74–75, 106, 108, 111,

341

154, 158, 184, 194, 196, 205, 236, 259, 264, 300–301, 303
Tonsillitis/adenoiditis, cause and treatment, 259–260
Touch, 64, 180, 198, 220
Toxins, 158, 174, 179, 181, 227, 255, 259, 265
  cancer and, 227-230
  clearing away, 100–102, 104, 136, 153–154, 189, 193, 201, 203, 234, 252, 266, 268
  digestion, 75, 98–99, 116, 125, 134, 137, 141–142, 144–145, 155, 159, 246, 261, 263
  food, 227-230
  environmental, 159, 227, 229–230, 236–238, 251, 264, 267
  See also Ama, Genetically modified foods
Transcendental Meditation (TM) technique, 88, 179, 204, 209, 220, 246, 248, 255, 267, 284
  behavior and, 81, 83, 86, 209–211, 291, 294
  benefits, 81, 83, 87-88, 211–212, 257, 268, 270, 272-273, 278, 283, 292
  case histories, 81, 87, 211, 289-91
  children's meditation/Word of Wisdom, 84–86, 184, 199, 202–203, 293–294, 184
  defined, 82–83
  environment and, 83, 292
  mind and, 81-84, 86, 88, 184, 204, 209, 214, 246, 270
  stress and, 81-84, 87, 209–211
TV
  See Television

U

Underweight, 20, 55, 67
Unified field, 45-47
Upanishads, 212–213, 281
Upma, 132, 304

V

Vaccines, 32–33

Vaidya
  See Maharishi Ayurveda health expert
Vastu, 238, 304
  See also Maharishi Sthapatya Veda design
Vata
  balanced/imbalanced, 54-55, 57–59, 63–65, 73–74, 80, 93, 99–100, 106, 113, 134, 137, 144, 146–147, 170, 172, 220–221, 246
  daily/seasonal cycles, 54, 97, 167, 177, 179, 185–190
  defined, 52–53, 304
  disorders, 249–251, 254–255, 257–258, 267, 269–272, 274, 278
  exercise and, 197–198, 200–201
  increasing/decreasing, 94–95, 102, 130–132
  learning styles, 62
  qualities/location, 55, 60
  sleep and, 172–175
  See also Doshas
Vata Tea, 64, 133, 258
Vayu (air)
  See Ayurvedic elements
Veda
  defined, 24, 46, 304
  Veda and human physiology, 53, 281-284
  Vedic literature, 70, 212, 219, 281–284, 299–300, 303,
  Vedic sounds, 219, 272, 283-285, 287
  Sama Veda, 219, 303
Vedic architecture
  See Maharishi Sthapatya Veda design
Vegetables, 23, 93, 109, 118-19, 229-230, 131, 135
  Green leafy, 92–93, 97, 109, 121, 249
Vegetarian diet
  benefits 119–123,
  protein, iron, and other nutrients, 119–123, 126
Vikriti, 99, 304
  See also Balance/Imbalance
Vision impairment, 34, 270
Vitamins
  from food, 154-155, 158

synthetic, 75, 154, 160
Vitamin A, 110, 159
Vitamin B, 121-122
Vitamin C, 155, 158-159
Vitamin D, 110, 196, 236
Vitamin E, 110, 158
Vomiting, cause and treatment, 260–261

W

Water
  copper, 234
  pure, 93, 100-101, 234, 249
  herbal, 101, 256
  lemon, 276
  warm/hot, 101, 106, 133, 143, 247, 249–252, 256, 259, 261, 268, 271, 273, 276
  See also Ayurvedic elements
Word of wisdom
  See Transcendental Meditation technique

Y

Yagya, 287–289, 301, 304
Yoga Asanas
  benefits, 201-204
  defined, 184, 203, 299
  exercise, 198-199
  treatment of disease and, 249, 257, 271, 276, 278
  See also Salute to the Sun

Additional Titles Available from MUM Press

The following books and other titles are available from
Maharishi University of Management Press
800-831-6523
Press Distribution DB 1155
Fairfield, Iowa 52557
E-mail: mumpress@mum.edu
Web site: www.mumpress.com/

Books by Maharishi Mahesh Yogi

Life Supported by Natural Law. Washington, D.C.: Age of Enlightenment Press, 1986.

Maharishi Forum of Natural Law and National Law for Doctors. India: Age of Enlightenment Publications, 1995.

Maharishi Mahesh Yogi on the Bhagavad-Gita: A New Translation and Commentary, Chapters 1-6. New York: Penguin Books, 1973.

Maharishi Vedic University: Introduction. India: Age of Enlightenment Publications, 1995.

The Science of Being and Art of Living. New York: Penguin Books, 1995.

Books on Maharishi Ayurveda Scientific Research

Scientific Research on Maharishi's Transcendental Meditation and TM-Sidhi Program: Collected Papers, Volumes 1–6, available through Maharishi University of Management Press, Press Distribution, DB 1155, Fairfield, Iowa 52557.

Scientific Research on the Maharishi Transcendental Meditation and TM-Sidhi Programs: A Brief Summary of 500 Studies. Fairfield, Iowa: Maharishi University of Management Press, 1996.

Books by Other Authors

Deans, Ashley, Ph.D. *A Record of Excellence: The Remarkable Success of Maharishi School of the Age of Enlightenment*. Fairfield, IA: Maharishi University of Management Press, 2005.

Denniston, Denise. *The TM Book: How to Enjoy the Rest of Your Life*. Fairfield, Iowa: Fairfield Press, 1986.

Pearson, Craig, Ph.D. *The Complete Book of Yogic Flying*. Fairfield, Iowa: Maharishi University of Management Press, 2008.

Nader, Tony, M.D., Ph.D. *Human Physiology: Expression of Veda and the Vedic Literature*. Vlodrop, The Netherlands: Maharishi Vedic University Press, 2001.

Reddy, Kumuda, M.D.; Egenes, Linda; and Mullins, Margaret, MSN, FNP. *For a Blissful Baby: Happy and Healthy Pregnancy through Maharishi Vedic Medicine*. Schenectady, New York: Samhita Productions, 1999.

Reddy, Kumuda, M.D.; Egenes, Thomas; and Egenes, Linda. *All Love Flows to the Self: Eternal Stories from the Upanishads*. Schenectady, New York: Samhita Productions, 2000.

Roth, Robert. *Maharishi Mahesh Yogi's Transcendental Meditation*. New York: Donald I. Fine, 1994.

Schneider, Robert, M.D., *Total Heart Health: How to Prevent and Reverse Heart Disease with the Maharishi Vedic Approach to Health*. Laguna Beach, CA: Basic Health Publications, 2006.

Wallace, R. Keith. *The Neurophysiology of Enlightenment*. Fairfield, Iowa: Maharishi International University Press, 1986.

Wallace, R. Keith. *The Physiology of Consciousness*. Fairfield, Iowa: Maharishi International University Press, 1993.

Additional Books by Kumuda Reddy, M.D.

For a Blissful Baby: Healthy and Happy Pregnancy with Maharishi Vedic Medicine by Kumuda Reddy, M.D., Linda Egenes, and Margaret Mullins, MSN, FNP

Forever Healthy: Introduction to Maharishi Ayurveda Health Care by Kumuda Reddy, M.D., and Stan Kendz

All Love Flows to the Self: Eternal Stories from the Upanishads by Kumuda Reddy, M.D., Thomas Egenes, and Linda Egenes

Conquering Chronic Disease through Maharishi Vedic Medicine by Kumuda Reddy, M.D., and Janardhan Reddy, M.D., with Linda Egenes

Golden Transition: Menopause Made Easy through Maharishi Vedic Medicine by Kumuda Reddy, M.D., and Janardhan Reddy, M.D., with Sandra Willbanks

Ayurvedic Cooking Made Easy: 100+ Recipes for a Healthy You by Kumuda Reddy, M.D., Janardhan Reddy, M.D., and Bonita Pederson

The Timeless Wisdom Series of children's stories by Kumuda Reddy, M.D., and John Emory Pruitt: *The Indigo Jackal, The Lion and the Hare, The Monkey and the Crocodile, The Female Mouse, The Hares and the Elephants*

Timeless Wisdom Stories, Vol. I: Magical and Enchanting (audio collection), and *Timeless Wisdom Stories, Vol. II: Playful and Awe-Some Timeless Stories* (audio collection)

To order, visit www.AllHealthyFamily.com or your favorite online bookstore.

About the Authors

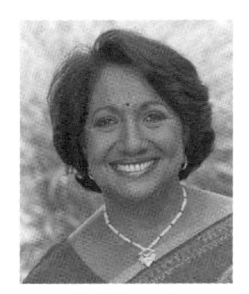

Kumuda Reddy, M.D., practiced Western medicine in the United States for over 25 years. After receiving her training in Maharishi Ayurveda, she has devoted herself to bringing the time-tested knowledge of Maharishi Ayurveda to the modern world. She has found that this natural, holistic system complements Western care and can solve many of the health problems we face today.

Dr. Reddy completed her residency and fellowship at Mt. Sinai Hospital, New York. For many years she was a faculty member at Albany Medical College. She has practiced Maharishi Ayurveda around the world since the mid-eighties.

Dr. Reddy has coauthored six books on Maharishi Ayurveda and Maharishi Vedic Medicine and a series of children's stories called the *Timeless Wisdom Series*, based on traditional Indian stories that she first heard as a child.

Dr. Reddy and her husband, Dr. Janardhan Reddy, are devoted to their extended family and three grown children, Sundeep, Hima, and Suma. Currently the Reddys are dividing their time between India and the U.S. They continue working toward their vision to help create a disease-free society generation after generation through Maharishi Ayurveda.

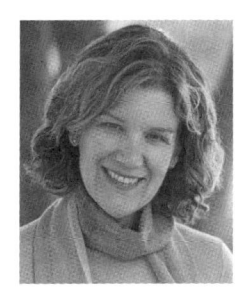

Linda Egenes is the author of over four hundred articles and two other books on Maharishi Ayurveda. She is an adjunct associate professor of writing at Maharishi University of Management in Fairfield, Iowa, where she lives with her husband, Tom.